Recent Advances in Withdrawn
Paediatrics
24

Recent Advances in Paediatrics 23
Edited by T.J. David

ISSN 1-85315-652-3

ISSN 0–309–0140

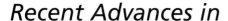

Recent Advances in

Paediatrics
24

Edited by

Timothy J. David MB ChB MD PhD FRCP FRCPCH DCH

Professor of Child Health and Paediatrics,
University of Manchester;
Honorary Consultant Paediatrician,
Booth Hall Children's Hospital, Manchester, UK

© 2007 Royal Society of Medicine Press Ltd
Published by the Royal Society of Medicine Press Ltd
1 Wimpole Street, London W1G 0AE, UK
Tel: +44 (0)20 7290 2921
Fax: +44 (0)20 7290 2929
Email: publishing@rsm.ac.uk
Website: www.rsmpress.co.uk

British Library Cataloguing in Publication Data
A catalogue record for this book is available from the British Library
ISBN 978–1–85315–725–7
ISSN 0–309–0140

Distribution in Europe and Rest of World:

Marston Book Services Ltd
PO Box 269, Abingdon
Oxon OX14 4YN, UK
Tel: +44 (0)1235 465500
Fax: +44 (0)1235 465555
Email: direct.order@marston.co.uk

Distribution in the USA and Canada:

Royal Society of Medicine Press Ltd
c/o BookMasters Inc
30 Amberwood Parkway
Ashland, OH 44805, USA
Tel: +1 800 247 6553/+1 800 266 5564
Fax: +1 419 281 6883
Email: order@bookmasters.com

Distribution in Australia and New Zealand:

Elsevier Australia
30-52 Smidmore Street
Marrikville NSW 2204, Australia
Tel: +61 2 9517 8999
Fax: +61 2 9517 2249
Email: service@elsevier.com.au

Editorial services and typesetting by GM & BA Haddock, Ford, Midlothian, UK
Printed in Great Britain by Bell & Bain, Glasgow, UK

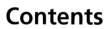

Contents

Contents

Preface

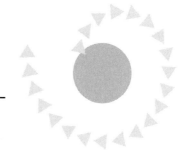

The aim of *Recent Advances in Paediatrics* is to provide a review of important topics and help doctors keep abreast of developments in the subject. The book is intended for the practising clinician, those in specialty training, and doctors preparing for specialty examinations. The book is sold very widely in Britain, Europe, North America and Asia, and the contents and authorship are selected with this very broad readership in mind. There are 16 chapters which cover a variety of general paediatric, neonatal and community paediatric areas. As usual, the selection of topics has veered towards those of general rather than special interest.

I am indebted to the authors for their hard work, prompt delivery of manuscripts and patience in dealing with my queries and requests. I would also like to thank Gill and Bruce Haddock of the RSM Press for all their help. Working on a book such as this makes huge inroads into one's spare time, and my special thanks go to my wife and sons for all their support.

2007

Professor Timothy J. David
University of Manchester
Booth Hall Children's Hospital
Manchester M9 7AA, UK
E-mail: t.david@manchester.ac.uk

Harper N. Price Andrea L. Zaenglein

1

Acne

Acne vulgaris is an extremely common inflammatory skin condition affecting more than 80% of individuals during their lifetime. Not surprisingly, most of those with acne are adolescents. While often thought of as trivial or just a part of growing up, the psychological impact of having acne can be profound and lead to anxiety, depression, anger, frustration and poor self-image.[1] The economic impact of acne is also great, accounting for more than 2 million office visits each year for those between the ages of 15 and 19 years. Given the vast numbers of people with acne, this is only a small portion of those who could benefit from treatment.[2] Surprisingly, only a minor fraction of those affected seek the attention of a medical doctor and an even smaller percentage see a dermatologist.[3] Therefore, it is important that primary care physicians recognise the impact of acne on teenagers and discuss treatment strategies with them.

In most cases, acne is easy to diagnose clinically and is immediately identifiable when the patient enters the room. Recognition of the different lesion types and assessment of severity, however, is a practiced art, vital to designing the most efficacious treatment strategy for the patient. Knowledge of how the variety of acne medications work and their side effects is critical to good patient care, while educating patients on strategies to increase tolerability will result in increased compliance (the primary foe to effective treatment.) Also, it is important to recognise atypical presentations of acne, neonatal and infantile acne, as well as acne with systemic associations.

Harper N. Price MD
Resident in Dermatology
Department of Dermatology, Penn State/Milton S. Hershey Medical Center, Hershey, Pennsylvania, USA

Andrea L. Zaenglein MD (for correspondence)
Associate Professor of Dermatology and Pediatrics
Department of Dermatology HU14, Penn State/Milton S. Hershey Medical Center, 500 University Drive, Hershey, PA 17033, USA
E-mail: azaenglein@psu.edu

AETIOLOGY AND PATHOPHYSIOLOGY

The key to developing an effective therapeutic regimen for any acne patient is to understand the pathogenesis behind the condition. Acne is a disorder of the pilosebaceous unit, which is made up of a hair follicle, a hair shaft and a sebaceous gland. The pathogenesis of acne is multifactorial and currently defined by four major steps (Fig. 1):[4]

1. Increased sebum production from the sebaceous gland.
2. Abnormal desquamation of keratinocytes within the follicle.
3. A collaborative role by the resident bacterium *Propionibacterium acnes.*
4. Inflammation.

Not surprisingly, hormones, specifically the androgens, are central to the pathophysiology of acne. The onset of puberty begins at approximately 7–10 years of age and is heralded by the up-regulation of sebum production.[4] This corresponds directly to a rise in dihydroepiandrostenedione sulphate (DHEA-S) produced by the adrenal gland, the initial hormone in the androgen pathway (Fig. 2). DHEA-S is converted first to androstenedione, then testosterone (via 17β-hydroxysteroid dehydrogenase). Testosterone can be converted to the more potent androgen, dihydroxytestosterone by the enzyme 5-α-reductase in the sebaceous follicle. These converting enzymes are all found and active in the follicular unit.[5] Once androgens are produced locally in the follicular environment, genes are upregulated to stimulate cell growth and differentiation of sebaceous glands, resulting in both sebaceous gland enlargement and an increase in sebum production. Clinically, the rising levels of DHEA-S have been shown to correlate directly with comedone formation in preteenage girls.[6]

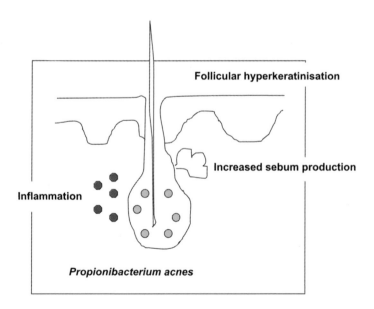

Follicular hyperkeratinisation

Increased sebum production

Inflammation

Propionibacterium acnes

Fig. 1 Pathogenesis of acne.

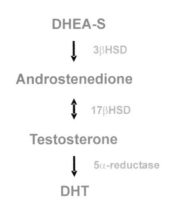

Fig. 2 The androgen pathway.

The amount of sebum produced differs between individuals and is affected by many variables including hormones (androgens, melanocortins) and growth factors (epidermal growth factor and insulin-like growth factor 1). Sebum consists of triglycerides, wax esters and squalene. Micro-organisms within the follicle then hydrolyse the triglycerides into free fatty acids. These substances are inherently comedogenic, stimulate inflammation, and encourage bacterial clumping. Oily sebum is also an excellent growth media for *P. acnes*, one of the other prominent conspirators to the development of acne.

Concurrent with the sebum increase, the cells that line the follicular opening become dysregulated and begin to accumulate within the outlet. As a result, the cells and sebum build up, plugging the opening. This leads to the formation of the non-inflammatory microcomedone, a microscopic precursor to the visible blackhead.[7] The stimulus for the keratinocyte proliferation is not completely understood yet, but androgen stimulation, decreased linoleic acid levels, and interleukin-1α (IL-1α) activity have all been suggested to contribute.[8–10] An increase in the number of androgen receptors in the outer root sheath of follicle, as well as the sebaceous gland, suggest a supporting role for androgens in follicular hyperkeratinisation. Linoleic acid is an essential fatty acid present in the skin and has been found in decreased levels in patients with acne. The dilution of this essential fatty acid by an increased volume of sebum may contribute to abnormal turnover of keratinocytes as well. IL-1α levels have been studied in an *in vitro* acne model and the addition of this cytokine to human pilosebaceous unit caused hypercornification of the infundibulum akin to that seen in comedones.[11] Further experiments support that *P. acnes* may stimulate viable keratinocytes to up-regulate production of specific cytokines, including IL-1α, and the presence of this cytokine has been demonstrated in open comedones of acne patients.[12,13]

P. acnes is a resident Gram-positive, facultative anaerobe universally found within the hair follicle. While acne was initially thought to be a direct infection caused by *P. acnes*, research has recently found that the organism has much more to do with causing inflammation. This organism has been found in larger concentrations in younger patients with acne than those without, but correlation between colonisation and severity of acne has not been found.[14]

The inflammatory response stimulated by *P. acnes* is thought to be the main contributing factor to its pathogenesis. The cell wall of the bacterium contains a carbohydrate that stimulates antibody production which results in complement activation.[15] Additionally, through the interaction with Toll-like receptor 2, found on the cell wall of neutrophils and monocytes, *P. acnes* induces the up-regulation of inflammatory cytokines.[16,17] Another recent finding is that the composition and timing of an individual's inflammatory response is an important factor in determining if scarring will result.[18] Inflammation occurs very early in the pathogenesis of acne even before the detection of a microcomedone.[45]

CLASSIFICATION OF ACNE LESIONS

One particularly useful tool for clinicians is to develop a consistent classification and grading scale when evaluating acne patients, which will then guide therapy and prognosis. First, identify the primary lesion types present, then assign a degree of severity based on extent and distribution. While no uniform grading system exists, an example is given in Table 1. The primary lesions of acne include open and closed comedones ('black heads' and 'white heads', respectively; Fig. 3). Inflammatory lesions include papules, pustules, and nodules ('acne cysts'). Secondary lesions which may evolve from the primary lesion or external trauma are important to note as well, especially at follow-up since these changes should not be counted when doing lesion assessments.

Table 1 Acne severity and grading system

VERY MILD ACNE (almost clear) – see Figure 5
• Few papules and pustules or comedones
• Often seen in early adolescence (ages 8–10 years)

MILD ACNE – see Figure 6
• Some non-inflammatory lesions (comedones)
• Few papules and pustules
• No nodules
• Often in the 't-zone' or seborrhoeic areas of the forehead, cheeks, chin and nose

MODERATE ACNE – see Figures 7 & 8
• Papules, pustules
• Many comedones are also usually present
• 1–2 nodules may be seen
• Extra-facial areas may also be involved

SEVERE ACNE – see Figure 9
• Papules, pustules and many comedones and importantly, larger and deeper nodules may be present but are few
• Extra-facial involvement can be extensive and moderate

VERY SEVERE ACNE – see Figure 10
• Large pustular and nodular lesions admixed with comedones and smaller papules
• Extra-facial involvement can be extensive and severe
• Risk of scarring is high

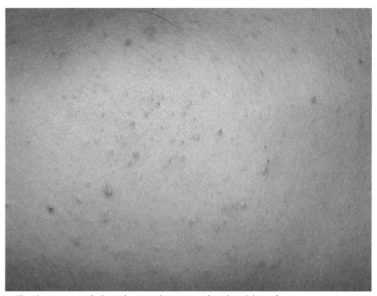

Fig. 3 Classic open and closed comedones on the shoulder of a teenager.

Secondary changes typically seen are erythema, hyperpigmentation and hypopigmentation. While mild discolouration will generally resolve in a few months after treatment, pigmentary changes can last several months to years, especially in darker skin types (Fig. 4). While not a primary acne lesion, these hyperpigmented changes can be very distressing to patients and appropriate counselling and re-assurance can help. Scarring is often an unfortunate and permanent side effect of acne. Various types of scarring include pitted, boxcar,

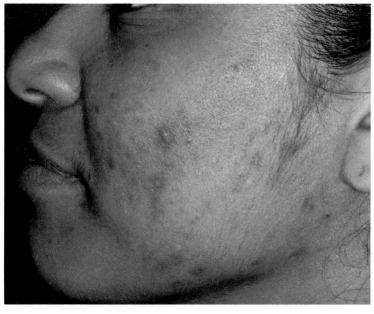

Fig. 4 Post-inflammatory hyperpigmented macules after acne treatment in a darker-skinned patient. Topical retinoids may help lighten and smooth out these changes.

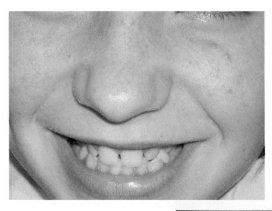

Fig. 5 Very mild acne in early adolescence with few small papules on the forehead.

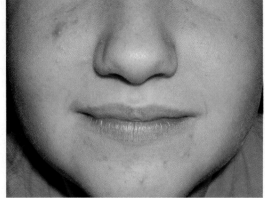

Fig. 6 Mild acne with papules and closed comedones on cheeks and chin.

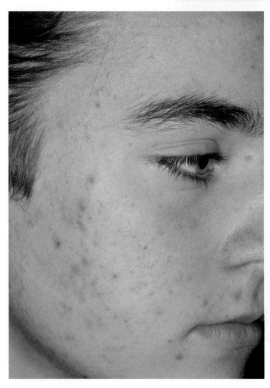

Fig. 7 Moderate inflammatory acne involving forehead, chin and cheeks.

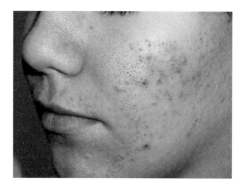

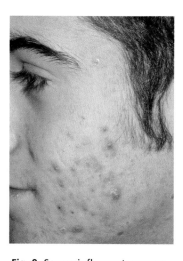

Fig. 8 Moderate acne with inflammatory papules and numerous open comedones.

Fig. 9 Severe inflammatory acne with prominent post-inflammatory erythema.

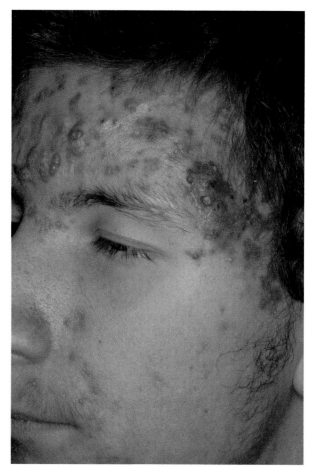

Fig. 10 Very severe, scarring inflammatory acne with large, coalescing nodules.

Table 2 The differential diagnosis of acne

Diagnosis	Clinical findings
Keratosis pilaris	• Small skin-coloured to pink follicular hyperkeratotic papules • Located on the extensor surfaces of the arms, thighs and cheeks • Autosomal dominant, usually presents in early childhood • Generally asymptomatic
Peri-oral/peri-orificial dermatitis	• Erythematous papules and pustules • Scaling variable • Symmetrically located around mouth, nose, and eyes (rarely groin) • Often associated with topical or inhaled corticosteroid use
Rosacea	• Persistent facial erythema, flushing, telangectasias, papules and pustules • Eye involvement common (ocular rosacea) • Located on the cheeks, chin and nasolabial areas • Most often seen in middle-aged adults but can present in the paediatric population • Associated with sensitivity to topical facial products and environmental factors (cold, heat, spicy foods)
Steroid acne	• Abrupt onset of monomorphous red papules or pustules • Upper trunk and arms • High doses of oral corticosteroids
Folliculitis	• *Staphylococcus aureus*, common cause of bacterial folliculitis • Pustules or papules involving the face (commonly the beard area), chest, back, buttocks and thighs • *Pityrosporum* folliculitis • Pruritic dome-shaped follicular papules and small pustules on the face, chest and back • Outbreaks tend to be chronic and do not respond well to typical acne medications • Confirm diagnosis with KOH preparation • Treat with topical or oral anti-fungal agent • Fungal folliculitis (majocchi granuloma) may be caused by *Trichophyton rubrum* or mentagrophytes • Perifollicular papules and nodules or deep pustular lesions resembling kerion or carbuncles are characteristic • Commonly located in the beard area, wrists or shins • Preceding trauma, topical steroid use or underlying immunosuppression are predisposing factors • Treatment with oral anti-fungal agents is often needed
Acniform drug reaction	• Monomorphic papules and pustules, abrupt in onset • Found in acneiform distribution and atypical areas • Causative agents include iodide- or bromide-containing medications, cyclosporine, anti-epileptic medications, lithium and epidermal growth factor inhibitors used in cancer treatment
Chemical acne	• Industrial chemicals such as chlorinated or polyhalogenated hydrocarbons or tars applied for medicinal purposes can also be culprits

Table 3 Acne-related disorders

Disorder	**Acne fulminans**
Cutaneous lesion	• Sudden onset of severe necrotising cysts and nodules • Suppurative as well as ragged painful ulcers • Scarring results
Systemic signs and symptoms	• Fever, leukocytosis, fatigue, anaemia, arthralgias, myalgias, arthritis, hepatospleno megaly, rare focal lytic bone lesions (sternoclavicular)
Epidemiology and incidence	• Rare • Teenage boys * Usually have preceding mild-to-moderate acne
Treatment	• First, prednisone for 4–6 weeks • Add low-dose oral isotretinoin around week 4 • Taper prednisone and continue oral isotretinoin until therapeutic doses attained • NSAIDs, warm compresses, topical steroids and antibacterial agents
Disorder	**Acne Conglobata**
Cutaneous lesion	• Slow onset of severe grouped comedones, abscesses, sinus tracts and large cysts • Heal with scarring • Chest, back, arms, shoulders. buttocks, face
Systemic signs and symptoms	• Rare musculoskeletal or arthritic symptoms • Associated PAPA syndrome
Epidemiology and incidence	• Uncommon • Young adults (aged 18–30 years) • Cases in infants rare but described
Treatment	• Oral isotretinoin (0.5–1.0 mg/kg for 4–6 months) • Prednisone may help • Dapsone for treatment-resistant cases • Case report with Infliximab treatment
Disorder	**SAPHO syndrome**
Cutaneous lesion	• Various skin findings described: acne conglobata, psoriasis, Sweet's syndrome, palmoplantar pustulosis, pyoderma gangrenosum
Systemic signs and symptoms	* Synovitis, pustulosis, hyperostosis, osteitis * Gradual onset of bone pain * No organism isolated
Epidemiology and incidence	• Rare • Children and young adults • Female predominance • Protracted course
Treatment	• NSAIDs, corticosteroids, bisphosphonates • Treatment response to oral antibiotics and immunosuppressants usually poor • Case report with Infliximab treatment
Disorder	**Gram-negative folliculitis**
Cutaneous lesion	• Superficial pustules, especially around nares • Fluctuant nodules
Systemic signs and symptoms	• No associated systemic findings • Culture can reveal *Klebsiella* spp. and *Proteus mirabilis, Escherichia coli, Pseudomonas aeruginosa, Serratia marcescans* or *Enterobacter* spp.
Epidemiology and incidence	• Occurs in patients on long-term antibiotic therapy or moderate inflammatory acne • Cessation of treatment response occurs
Treatment	• Oral isotretinoin is the treatment of choice • Second-line therapies: amoxicillin or trimethoprim-sulfamethoxazole

keloidal, and atrophic scars. Patients with the greatest potential for scarring are those with moderate-to-severe acne. However, any patient showing signs of scarring should be treated aggressively to prevent further disfigurement. While treatments such as acid peels and laser devices can improve scarring, the best treatment by far is prevention.

There are several mimickers of acne that clinicians will commonly encounter, and a few unusual imitators as well. Whenever a patient with facial papules and pustules presents atypically, clinical suspicion for an alternate diagnosis should arise. The differential diagnosis of acne is listed in Table 2. Additionally, there are a few systemic disorders that involve severe presentations of acne. While very rare, knowledge of their associations is necessary for accurate diagnosis and treatment. Severe cases of acne that involve systemic symptoms include acne conglobata, acne fulminans, PAPA syndrome (erosive pyogenic arthritis, pyoderma gangrenosum, and acne) and SAPHO syndrome (synovitis, acne, pustulosis, hyperostosis and osteomyelitis), among others (Table 3).

TREATMENT

Once the diagnosis of acne is made, the type of lesions and severity of disease will dictate an appropriate treatment regimen. A reasonable treatment plan involves taking into account the life-style of the patient, addressing realistic expectations and duration of treatment, and discussing the critical issue of compliance and expected side effects of the treatment medications. Table 4 outlines several strategies to increase compliance with acne treatments. The use of mild skin-care products is also important. Patients should use a mild cleanser twice daily and a non-comedogenic moisturiser to limit further irritation and dryness from many acne treatments. Leaving time for the skin to air-dry after cleansing (about 30 min) will help eliminate the burning or irritation that can occur from topical treatments applied immediately to damp skin. It is also essential to counsel patients that topical acne treatments should be applied to the entire face or affected area and not used as a 'spot' treatment.

Benzoyl peroxide is one of most frequently used topical treatments for acne. It is available both by prescription and over-the-counter in several preparations, including bars, washes, gels, and creams. It is generally well tolerated but side effects include dryness, erythema, itching and, uncommonly, contact dermatitis. Benzoyl peroxide is a potent antibacterial agent, highly effective against inflammatory lesions, and has keratolytic properties giving it a mild comedolytic effect. Also, *P. acnes* is unable to develop resistance to benzoyl peroxide, making it an extremely useful adjunctive therapy and the ideal antimicrobial preparation for long-term use. Although several strengths exist (2–10%), higher potency does not necessarily equate with greater efficacy and can often be more irritating. Importantly, benzoyl peroxide products should not be used together with topical tretinoin as the effectiveness of both medications is reduced. One important tip to warn patients and parents is that benzoyl peroxide will bleach towels and clothing. Suggesting patients use white towels and put their shirt on prior to applying benzoyl peroxide to prevent discoloration of either will help minimise unnecessary fustration.

Salicylic acid is a common β-hydroxy acid found in many over-the-counter preparations. It is available in 0.5–2% strengths in a variety of vehicles,

Table 4 Strategies to increase compliance with acne treatments

Assessment	Ask patients how the acne affects them physically and psychologically. Would they like to have their acne treated?
Education	Inform patients about why acne occurs and why you are choosing each medication as well as the common and potential severe side effects
Expectation	Make sure everyone has the same outcome in mind. Have realistic expectations from your patients. Complex regimens or taking medications on an empty stomach may not be feasible for all patients
Reinforcement	See patients back regularly, every 6–8 weeks if possible. Ask them specifically what they are using and how, using open-ended questions
Re-assurance	Let the patient know they are on the right track and doing a good job. Improvement takes time

including washes, creams and lotions. It exerts its action by promoting desquamation of the stratum corneum, mildly inhibiting comedogenesis and exhibiting anti-inflammatory properties. In general, it is very well tolerated, making it an ideal active ingredient for a wide audience.

The mainstay of treatment in the majority of patients with acne should be a topical retinoid. In general, retinoids work by influencing the proliferation and differentiation of keratinocytes, thus inhibiting microcomedone formation. While classically known for their comedolytic property, retinoids have anti-inflammatory and immunomodulatory activities as well.[19] These manifold effects make retinoids ideal for initial, as well as maintenance, therapy. In addition, retinoids will aid in the penetration of other medications and help improve the pigmentation changes and mild atrophic scars that can result after successful treatment.[2] Retinoid agents include tretinoin (0.025%, 0.05%, and 0.1%) and tazarotene (0.05% and 0.1%) in both cream and gel formulations. A unique microsphere gel formulation of tretinoin (Retin-A micro® 0.1% or 0.04% gel) has been shown to exhibit less photodegradation and irritation.[20] A synthetic topical retinoid, adapalene 0.1% gel, has similar efficacy to tretinoin 0.025% gel but is generally more tolerated by sensitive-skin patients than tretinoin due to less cutaneous side effects.[21] Topical tazarotene has shown to be a superior comedogenic and anti-inflammatory agent compared to tretinoin and adapalene but its use is often limited by its greater irritancy potential.[22] Possible side effects of topical retinoids include irritation, redness, dryness and peeling which are usually experienced during the first few weeks of therapy until a tolerance develops. Starting these medications every other day and the use of a mild, non-comedogenic moisturiser may ameliorate some of these side effects. Tretinoin can be degraded by sunlight and should be applied at bed-time. However, adapalene gel and the newer microsphere formulations of tretinoin can be used during day-time hours as these agents have been shown to be stable in ultraviolet light.[20,23] All agents are contra-indicated in pregnancy (class C). Tazarotene, specifically, is pregnancy category X and some practitioners advocate adequate contraceptive measures during treatment.

Several other less commonly used topical acne therapies are available that every practitioner should be familiar with and incorporated into their acne treatment protocols. Sulphur is often a part of several over-the-counter washes, preparations and bars and serves as a comedolytic agent with little irritation. However, its tolerability is somewhat clouded by its rather unpleasant odour. Lastly, azelaic acid, a prescription medication commonly used for the treatment of rosacea, has demonstrated comedolytic activity and some antimicrobial effects in acne vulgaris. Side effects include a transient burning sensation and mild irritation. Azelaic acid is also safe for use during pregnancy (category B). These agents have particular niches and are typically used together with other systemic and topical therapies. Their use as a single agent is limited to cases of mild acne or when other treatments are not tolerated.

Topical antimicrobial agents are also used for mild-to-moderate comedonal acne and mild inflammatory acne along with a topical retinoid. The most common agents used are clindamycin and erythromycin in creams, gels, lotions or in combination with benzoyl peroxide gel. These agents serve as antimicrobial and anti-inflammatory agents in the treatment of acne. Erythromycin and clindamycin are well tolerated, but *P. acnes* resistance to these agents is high, making their use as a single-agent therapy limited. The addition of benzoyl peroxide has been shown to enhance efficacy and reduce bacterial resistance of these medications.[24]

Antibiotics have been used for several decades against acne. Systemic antibiotics used in acne therapy include the tetracycline family (most commonly tetracycline, doxycycline and minocycline), trimethoprim-sulphamethoxazole and erythromycin. Oral antimicrobial agents are used for moderate and severe inflammatory acne, especially with extrafacial involvement, in combination with a retinoid and often a benzoyl peroxide formulation to limit bacterial resistance. These medications work not only due to their antimicrobial properties, but also their anti-inflammatory effects. Response to treatment may be seen as early as 6 weeks, but a full response should not be judged until 3 months.

Doxycycline (100–200 mg daily) and minocycline (100–200 mg daily) are often considered superior to tetracycline (500 mg twice daily) in efficacy for the treatment of acne, but all are commonly used.[24] The most frequent adverse events with doxycycline are photosensitivity and gastrointestinal upset including oesophagitis. Rare, but serious, side effects seen with minocycline are hepatitis, hypersensitivity reactions and systemic immune-mediated reactions, including a lupus erythematosus-like syndrome and a serum sickness-like reaction. Central nervous system effects include dizziness, vertigo and benign central hypertension with minocycline. Again, gastrointestinal upset can occur and hyperpigmentation or blue-grey discoloration can be experienced on mucous membranes, teeth, shins, nails and in acne scars. This is often reversible if the medication is stopped in a reasonable time and usually occurs with extended therapy or higher doses. Tetracycline side effects are similar to doxycycline and include gastrointestinal distress, photosensitivity, drug hypersensitivity and oesophagitis. Due to increased *P. acnes* resistance, erythromycin should only be used in pregnant patients, patients intolerant to tetracycline, or children under age 8 years. The most common side effect is gastrointestinal upset. Trimethoprim/sulphamethoxazole has also been used when the other agents have failed or are contra-indicated. This medication has been deemed relatively safe for use in long-term acne therapy with the main concerning side effect of drug hypersensitivity. Of note, all oral antibiotics may cause a vaginal candidiasis in females.

The relationship between antibiotic use and resistance of *P. acnes* has significantly changed since the 1970s when *P. acnes* was still widely susceptible to many therapeutic antimicrobial medications.[25] Antibiotics are now frequently part of acne treatment regimens and can be for several years. Several factors may contribute to bacterial resistance to antibiotics including non-compliance or inappropriate use, prolonged or inadequate therapy, high sebum excretion rate and carriage of resistant strains. This represents a world-wide problem as studies from European, Asian and the US have all documented emerging resistance to *P. acnes* with multiple antibiotics including topical and oral clindamycin and erythromycin and oral tetracyclines.[26]

It is important for practitioners to understand that *P. acnes* is a commensal bacterium in healthy skin; although treatment may reduce the number of organisms, they are never eliminated completely from the skin. Resistance by these organisms to commonly used antibiotics is demonstrably on the rise and becoming a therapeutic dilemma. Resistance to erythromycin and clindamycin are more common than to the oral tetracyclines. When resistance to tetracyclines is present, however, this is often associated with cross-resistance to erythromycin and clindamycin.[27] Several measures have been suggested to help prevent further resistance. Prescribing tips include always using a benzoyl peroxide agent with antimicrobial agents, limiting the duration of antibiotic exposure, and considering non-antibiotic options first (hormonal therapy, topical retinoids) in mild-to-moderate acne. Also, always use a combination therapy with topical retinoids and benzoyl peroxide when starting antibiotic therapy. Closely monitor all patients on antibiotics to evaluate for improvement. When patients are doing well, discontinue the antibiotic and initiate a maintenance regimen.

Oral isotretinoin, a potent vitamin A derivative, has been approved for severe, recalcitrant, nodulocystic acne since the early 1980s. It has been considered life-changing for many patients with severe, refractory and scarring acne and its efficacy has been well documented. Isotretinoin is the only acne medication to exhibit activity against all the major aetiological factors involved in acne production including reduction of sebum production, reduction of size and number of sebaceous glands, normalisation of keratinisation, and inhibition of growth of *P. acnes*, as well as direct anti-inflammatory activity.[19] Safe and close monitoring during the use of this medication is essential to limit and prevent unwanted and dangerous side effects. Before starting isotretinoin, a detailed discussion between the physician, patient and family is important for complete understanding of the risks, benefits, safety, cost and commitment required to take this medication. Guidelines for monitoring side effects and managing females of child-bearing potential vary in the US and Europe.

A typical course of isotretinoin is 20 weeks and the recommended starting dose is 0.5 mg/kg/day in Europe and the US.[28] The dose is usually adjusted the second month if tolerated to 1.0 mg/kg in two daily doses taken with food.

A cumulative dose of 100–120 mg/kg at the end of therapy is usually ideal to reduce further relapse.[29] After a course of isotretinoin, about 40% of patients remain free from acne, while another 40% may have a recurrence of acne with lower severity and a good response to previous acne medications.[2] A second course of treatment is needed in about 20% of patients, especially in younger patients, female patients, and those with more aggressive truncal acne.[19]

Common side effects of isotretinoin therapy include dry chapped lips, dry skin and eyes, secondary staphylococcal skin infections, gastrointestinal upset, headaches, arthralgias and myalgias. Severe persistent headaches with vision or hearing changes should raise concern for benign cranial hypertension, which can lead to permanent blindness if not recognised. Skeletal abnormalities have been reported with low-dose, long-term use, but are rare in patients receiving a standard course of therapy. Laboratory abnormalities include, most commonly, hypertriglyceridaemia and hypercholesterolaemia and, less likely, elevated liver enzymes. Rarely do these abnormalities require a decrease or cessation of therapy and a majority of cases normalise after the treatment course. Laboratory monitoring guidelines differ, but premedication baseline blood-work and after 1–2 months of therapy are generally recommended.

The most concerning side effect of isotretinoin is teratogenicity in females resulting in a large array of fetal malformations including cardiac, central nervous system, and facial abnormalities. The iPledge system in the US was developed to regulate isotretinoin in females of child-bearing potential strictly, imposing mandatory monthly pregnancy testing and strict time-lines for prescriptions with lockout periods. Two different forms of contraception for females are necessary. The European Directive dictates mandatory pregnancy testing pretherapy and at 5 weeks post-therapy; monthly pregnancy testing is recommended throughout the treatment.[28] The pregnancy prevention programme recommends that, whenever possible, patients should agree to at least one method of contraception, preferably two complimentary methods, including a barrier method before the start of treatment.[28] Dispensing restrictions in Europe do not apply to males on therapy and for females, include a 7-day window from the date of administration and a limited 30-day supply of medication.

Oral isotretinoin has also been associated with mood changes, depression and risk of suicide.[19] However, current and retrospective data do not support a causal relationship between the use of the medication and psychiatric illness.[30] Patients with a history of mood disorders and suicide attempts or those that may develop symptoms during treatment should also be under the care of a psychiatrist and cessation of treatment may be necessary. Often, improvement of acne with isotretinoin improves mood and depressive symptoms, resulting in a much happier patient.[31]

Hormonal treatment alone, or in combination, may benefit female acne patients with inflammatory acne. Hormonal therapies exert their effect through anti-androgen properties. While women with acne often have higher levels of serum DHEAS and testosterone than those without acne, their laboratory values still fall in the normal range.[32] An endocrine evaluation is recommended if these values are above normal, if the onset of acne is severe and sudden, if the patient has irregular menses or if there are any signs of hyperandrogenism.[32]

Oral contraceptive pills are the most commonly used hormonal therapy. They reduce ovarian hormone production and secretion, regulate the menstrual cycle as well as increase the production of sex-hormone binding globulin in the liver, thereby reducing circulating testosterone levels.[32] Two oral contraceptive pills are now FDA-approved for the treatment of acne in the US, norgestimate-ethinyl oestradiol (Ortho Tri-Cyclen®; Ortho-McNeil Pharmaceutical, Raritan, NJ, USA) and a low-dose oestrogen pill, norethindrone acetate-ethinyl oestradiol (Estrostep®; Parke Davis, Inc., Detroit, MI, USA), although several others have been studied and proven efficacious. Internationally, the combination of ethinyl oestradiol 0.035 mg and cyproterone acetate 2 mg (Diane-35) has displayed efficacy in multiple randomised controlled trials in acne therapy.[33,34] The use of drosperinone with its anti-androgenic and anti-mineralcorticoid activity in combination with ethinyl oestradiol 30 μg (Yasmin®; Schering AG) has also show significant efficacy in the treatment of acne.[35,36] Progesterone-only contraceptives should be avoided as these can worsen acne. Newer contraceptive formulations (such as the patch and ring form) have not been evaluated for acne treatment. Contra-indications to oral contraceptive pill use include uncontrolled hypertension, migraine headaches with central nervous symptoms, tobacco use, diabetes, hypercholesterolaemia, history of blood clots, systemic lupus, liver disease and pregnancy.[37] The risk of endometrial and ovarian cancer and the prevalence of anaemia is decreased with oral contraceptive pill use, while the risk of breast cancer may be increased.[37]

Androgen receptor blockers such as spironolactone, flutamide, and cyproterone acetate are also options for antihormonal therapy. Spironolactone is the most commonly prescribed agent in the US and has been found to decrease sebum excretion with recommended doses of 50–100 mg/day, although many women will respond to 25 mg twice daily. Breast tenderness and menstrual irregularities are common side effects; in some patients with underlying medical problems, serum electrolytes should be monitored. Pregnancy on spironolactone should be avoided. Flutamide, an anti-androgen used to treat prostate cancer has been used for acne in doses of 250 mg twice daily, but has fallen out of favour due to the risk of fatal hepatitis and monitoring of liver function tests. Cyproterone acetate inhibits ovulation and blocks the androgen receptor in doses of 2–100 mg/day. It is commonly used with an oral contraceptive pill and side effects at higher doses have included weight gain, breast tenderness, nausea, decreased libido and rarely, hepatitis. Like spironolactone, these medications are quite efficacious but should not be used if pregnancy is a concern.

COMBINATION AND MAINTENANCE THERAPY

Choosing a treatment plan should be based on the severity, extent and type of acne lesions present. Other factors to consider include the duration of disease, previous attempted treatments, presence of scarring and post-inflammatory changes as well as the psychological impact on the patient. Thus, acne therapy is highly individualised. A standard treatment algorithm is shown in Table 5. Noting the four major steps in the pathogenesis of acne, a combination of medications with different mechanisms of action (Table 6) is essential for maximum improvement. The most common regimen used is an antimicrobial

18

Table 5 Acne treatment algorithm

Classification	Mild → Mild-moderate		Moderate → Moderate-severe (mixed comedonal/inflammatory)		Severe
	Comedonal	(+) Papules/pustules	Comedones → Papules/pustules → Nodules		Conglobata/fulminans
First	Topical retinoid ± BPO	Topical retinoid + topical antimicrobial ± BPO	Topical retinoid ± BPO	Oral antibiotic + topical retinoid ± BPO	Oral isotretinoin ± oral corticosteroid
Second	Azelaic acid or salicylic acid ± BPO	Azelaic acid or salicylic acid ± BPO	Alternate topical retinoid, azelaic acid or salicylic acid ± BPO	Oral isotretinoin or alternate oral antibiotic + alternate topical retinoid ± BPO/azelaic acid	High-dose oral antibiotic + topical Retinoid + BPO
Female				+ Oral contraceptive/anti-androgen + BPO	+ Oral contraceptive/anti-androgen + BPO
Surgical options	Comedone extraction		Comedone extraction; chemical peel	Comedone extraction; Intralesional corticosteroid	Intralesional corticosteroid
Refractory to treatment	Culture to exclude Gram-negative folliculitis (especially on back) Females: exclude adrenal or ovarian dysfunction				
Maintenance	Topical retinoid ± BPO Females: oral contraceptive/anti-androgen				

BPO, benzoyl peroxide
Adapted from Gollnick.[39]

Table 6 Mechanism of action of common acne medications

Medication	Mechanism of action	Affect on lesion type
Topical retinoids	Normalises desquamation Anti-inflammatory	Comedones **** Inflammatory lesions***
Benzoyl peroxide	Potent antimicrobial	Inflammatory lesions***
Antibiotics	Decreases *P. acnes* Anti-inflammatory	Inflammatory lesions***
Oral contraceptives/ anti-androgens	Decreases sebum production	Inflammatory lesion***
Oral isotretinoin	Decreases sebum production Normalises desquamation Decreases *P. acnes* Anti-inflammatory	Comedones**** Inflammatory lesions****

agent in conjunction with a topical retinoid, as this combination targets the most steps in the pathogenesis of acne. Clinical trials studying combinations of acne medications resulted in significantly greater and faster improvement when using combination therapy versus a single agent alone.[38]

With acne incidence related to hormonal influence and sebum production during adolescence, treatment is often managed long term over several years. Often acne returns once therapy is tapered or discontinued. Therefore, maintenance therapy using a topical retinoid often with benzoyl peroxide is advocated by most experts.[39] This maintenance programme, being comedolytic and anti-inflammatory, will thus limit exposure to long-term antibiotic use and resistance to *P. acnes*. Females using oral contraceptives, or other anti-androgen therapy, may also maintain improvement with their continued use.

ACNE BEFORE ADOLESCENCE

Neonatal acne presents at birth or during the first few weeks of life and is commonly made up of a small number of erythematous papules and pustules on the cheeks and forehead. True comedones are rare and controversy exists regarding the designation of neonatal acne as a real acneiform process.[40] The role of *Malassezia* spp. and other yeast species, transient neonatal androgen production as well as the maternal androgen environment is thought to play a role in the pathogenesis. Up to 20% of newborns may experience acne with only a few severe enough to present to a dermatologist or paediatrician. It is important to emphasise that most neonatal acne is generally mild and spontaneously resolves without treatment and scarring in a few months.

An understanding of androgen production from birth until adulthood is important to explain the variation in sebum production and hormone levels which contribute to many forms of childhood acne. At birth, neonatal adrenal glands are hyperactive, consisting of an enlarged zona reticularis (androgen-producing zone) and produce significant quantities of β-hydroxysteroids. The sebaceous glands are hyperplastic accounting for increased sebum production. It is also hypothesised that stimulation by the maternal and infantile androgen milieu may be a contributing factor in neonatal acne. This hormonal environment often returns to baseline by age 6 months, although, in male infants, early levels of luteinizing hormone and testosterone can persist through age 6–12 months, explaining the male predominance of neonatal and infantile acne.[41,42] Between age 1 year and the onset of adrenarche, very little androgen is produced; thus, acne is rare during this period. Severe or persistent acne in this age group should prompt an investigation for hormonal abnormalities.

Infantile acne appears later than typical neonatal acne, usually between 3–9 months of age and has a male predominance as well. Again, most lesions are on the face, especially the cheeks. Most cases are mild to moderate and are composed of open and closed comedones as well as inflammatory lesions. The course of infantile acne can vary from 1–2 years or persist later into childhood or puberty. Severe cases, including acne conglobata, have been described and severe or persistent acne should prompt a work-up for hyperandrogenism. Treatment is similar to conventional acne; when oral antibiotics are indicated, erythromycin (125–250 mg twice daily) or trimethoprim (100 mg twice daily) may be tried.[43] Deep nodules may be injected with low doses of intralesional triamcinalone acetonide. If persistence of severity and scarring or, rarely, acne congloblata develop in an infant, oral isotretintoin is indicated (0.5 mg/kg for 4–5 months) with appropriate laboratory monitoring. In a retrospective series of 29 patients with infantile acne, scarring occurred in 17% of patients, thus illustrating the importance of early and effective treatment.[44]

Prepubescent or mid-childhood acne occurs between 1–7 years of age and is quite rare. When present, a work-up for hyperandrogenism should be done to rule out premature adrenarche, mild forms of congenital adrenal hyperplasia, gonadal or adrenal tumours, Cushing's syndrome and true precocious puberty.[42] Screening evaluation can include a growth chart and bone-age measurement as well as laboratory tests for DHEAS, luteinizing hormone, follicle stimulating hormone, prolactin, testosterone, and 17α-hydroxyprogesterone levels. Therapy for mid-childhood acne is similar to acne treatment at any age, although compliance is a difficult issue.

Key points for clinical practice

- Acne is a treatable condition. Neglect can cause significant physical and emotional distress; the sequelae from acne can affect a person for a life-time.

- Acne is a disorder of the pilosebaceous unit and involves four key steps in pathogenesis: increased sebum production, hyperkeratosis of the follicular infundibulum, the bacterium *Propionibacterium acnes*, and a cascade of inflammatory events.

- Treatments for acne should be based on knowledge of the pathogenesis.

- Retinoids should be considered first line for most cases of acne due to their efficacy against both comedonal and inflammatory acne.

Key points for clinical practice *(continued)*

- Combination therapy for acne vulgaris will result in faster clearance and efficacy and should be considered the gold standard in most forms of acne.

- Benzoyl peroxide is a great adjunctive therapy in almost all patients with acne and resistance of *Propionibacterium acnes* has not been documented.

- Drug resistance is an emerging problem in acne treatment. Therefore, antibiotics should be used until inflammatory lesions clear and then discontinued.

- In females, hormonal therapy, including oral contraceptive pills and anti-androgens, are an effective option for inflammatory acne, resulting in better long-term control and decreased use of antibiotics.

- Isotretinoin is a highly teratogenic oral retinoid that is indicated for severe nodulocystic, scarring, and refractory acne. Tight adherence to monitoring guidelines in females of child-bearing potential is essential.

- Infantile acne is treated as conventional acne with special regards to gentle formulations. Even fairly mild infantile acne can cause permanent scarring.

- Recognition of acne variants such as acne fulminans, acne conglobata and Gram-negative folliculitis is important to start early, appropriate treatment.

References

1. Fried RG, Wechsler A. Psychological problems in the acne patient. *Dermatol Ther* 2006; **19**: 237–240.
2. James WD. Clinical practice. Acne. *N Engl J Med* 2005; **352**: 1463–1472.
3. Purdy S, de Berker D. Acne. *BMJ* 2006; **333**: 949–953.
4. Thiboutot D. Regulation of human sebaceous glands. *J Invest Dermatol* 2004; **123**: 1–12.
5. Thiboutot D, Knaggs H, Gilliland K, Hagari S. Activity of type 1 5α-reductase is greater in the follicular infrainfundibulum compared with the epidermis. *Br J Dermatol* 1997; **136**: 166–171.
6. Lucky AW, Biro FM, Huster GA, Leach AD, Morrison JA, Ratterman J. Acne vulgaris in premenarchal girls. An early sign of puberty associated with rising levels of dehydroepiandrosterone. *Arch Dermatol* 1994; **130**: 308–314.
7. Sinclair W, Jordaan HF. Acne guideline 2005 update. *S Afr Med J* 2005; **95**: 881–892.
8. Downing DT, Stewart ME, Wirtz PW *et al.* Essential fatty acids and acne. *J Am Acad Dermatol* 1986; **14**: 221–225.
9. Eady EA, Ingham E, Walters CE, Cove JH, Cunliffe WJ. Modulation of comedonal levels of interleukin-1 in acne patients treated with tetracyclines. *J Invest Dermatol* 1993; **101**: 86–91.
10. Cunliffe WJ, Forster R. Androgen control of the pilosebaceous duct? *Br J Dermatol* 1987; **116**: 449.
11. Guy R, Green MR, Kealey T. Modeling acne *in vitro*. *J Invest Dermatol* 1996; **106**: 176–182.
12. Graham GM, Farrar MD, Cruse-Sawyer JE, Holland KT, Ingham E. Proinflammatory

cytokine production by human keratinocytes stimulated with *Propionibacterium acnes* and *P. acnes* GroEL. *Br J Dermatol* 2004; **150**: 421–428.

13. Ingham E, Eady EA, Goodwin CE, Cove JH, Cunliffe WJ. Pro-inflammatory levels of interleukin-1 alpha-like bioactivity are present in the majority of open comedones in acne vulgaris. *J Invest Dermatol* 1992; **98**: 895–901.

14. Leyden JJ, McGinley KJ, Mills OH, Kligman AM. *Propionibacterium* levels in patients with and without acne vulgaris. *J Invest Dermatol* 1975; **65**: 382–384.

15. Webster G, Indrisano J, Leyden JJ. Antibody titers to *Propionibacterium acnes* cell wall carbohydrate in nodulocystic acne patients. *J Invest Dermatol* 1985; **84**: 496–500.

16. Kim J, Ochoa M-T, Krutzik SR *et al*. Activation of Toll-like receptor 2 in acne triggers inflammatory cytokine responses. *J Immunol* 2002; **169**: 1535–1541.

17. Lee JK, Duong B, Ochoa M. *Propionibacterium acnes* induction of pro-inflammatory cytokines in polymorphonuclear cells occurs through Toll-like receptor 2: the role of innate immune response in acne vulgaris. *Abstr Soc Invest Dermatol*, 2002.

18. Holland DB, Jeremy AH, Roberts SG, Seukeran DC, Layton AM, Cunliffe WJ. Inflammation in acne scarring: a comparison of the responses in lesions from patients prone and not prone to scar. *Br J Dermatol* 2004; **150**: 72–81.

19. Thielitz A, Krautheim A, Gollnick H. Update in retinoid therapy of acne. *Dermatol Ther* 2006; **19**: 272–279.

20. Nighland M, Yusuf M, Wisniewski S, Huddleston K, Nyirady J. The effect of simulated solar UV irradiation on tretinoin in tretinoin gel microsphere 0.1% and tretinoin gel 0.025%. *Cutis* 2006; **77**: 313–316.

21. Cunliffe WJ, *et al*. A comparison of the efficacy and tolerability of adapalene 0.1% gel versus tretinoin 0.025% gel in patients with acne vulgaris: a meta-analysis of five randomized trials. *Br J Dermatol* 1998; **139 (Suppl 52)**: 48–56.

22. Haider A, Shaw JC. Treatment of acne vulgaris. *JAMA* 2004; **292**: 726–735.

23. Jain S. Topical tretinoin or adapalene in acne vulgaris: an overview. *J Dermatol Treat* 2004; **15**: 200–207.

24. Strauss JS, *et al*. Guidelines of care for acne vulgaris management. *J Am Acad Dermatol* 2007.

25. Leyden JJ. Antibiotic resistant acne. *Cutis* 1976; **17**: 593–596.

26. Ross JI, Snelling AM, Eady EA *et al*. Phenotypic and genotypic characterization of antibiotic-resistant *Propionibacterium acnes* isolated from acne patients attending dermatology clinics in Europe, the U.S.A., Japan and Australia [see comment]. *Br J Dermatol* 2001; **144**: 339–346.

27. Eady AE, Cove JH, Layton AM. Is antibiotic resistance in cutaneous propionibacteria clinically relevant? Implications of resistance for acne patients and prescribers. *Am J Clin Dermatol* 2003; **4**: 813–831.

28. Layton AM, Dreno B, Gollnik HPM, Zouboulis CC. A review of the European Directive for prescribing systemic isotretinoin for acne vulgaris. *J Eur Acad Dermatol Venereol* 2006; **20**: 773–776.

29. Stainforth JM, Layton AM, Taylor JP, Cunliffe WJ. Isotretinoin for the treatment of acne vulgaris: which factors may predict the need for more than one course? *Br J Dermatol* 1993; **129**: 297–301.

30. Strahan JE, Raimer S. Isotretinoin and the controversy of psychiatric adverse effects. *Int J Dermatol* 2006; **45**: 789–799.

31. Peck GL, Olsen TG, Butkus D et al. Isotretinoin versus placebo in the treatment of cystic acne. A randomized double-blind study. *J Am Acad Dermatol* 1982; **6 (Suppl)**: 735–745.

32. Thiboutot DM. Endocrinological evaluation and hormonal therapy for women with difficult acne. *J Eur Acad Dermatol Venereol* 2001; **15 (Suppl 3)**: 57–61.

33. Carlborg L. Cyproterone acetate versus levonorgestrel combined with ethinyl estradiol in the treatment of acne. Results of a multicenter study. *Acta Obstet Gynecol Scand Suppl* 1986; **134**: 29–32.

34. Colver GB, Mortimer PS, Dawber RP. Cyproterone acetate and two doses of oestrogen in female acne; a double-blind comparison. *Br J Dermatol* 1988; **118**: 95–99.

35. Thorneycroft H, Gollnick H, Schellschmidt I. Superiority of a combined contraceptive containing drospirenone to a triphasic preparation containing norgestimate in acne treatment. *Cutis* 2004; **74**: 123–130.

36. van Vloten WA, van Haselen CW, van Zuuren EJ, Gerlinger C, Heithecker R. The effect of 2 combined oral contraceptives containing either drospirenone or cyproterone acetate on acne and seborrhea. *Cutis* 2002; **69 (Suppl)**: 2–15.

37. Poulin Y. Practical approach to the hormonal treatment of acne. *J Cutan Med Surg* 2004; **8 (Suppl 4)**: 16–21.

38. Leyden JJ. A review of the use of combination therapies for the treatment of acne vulgaris. *J Am Acad Dermatol* 2003; **49 (Suppl)**: S200–S210.

39. Gollnick H. Management of acne: a report from a Global Alliance to Improve Outcomes in Acne. *J Am Acad Dermatol* 2003; **49 (Suppl)**: S1.

40. Niamba P, Weill FX, Sarlangue J, Labrèze C, Couprie B, Taieb A. Is common neonatal cephalic pustulosis (neonatal acne) triggered by *Malassezia sympodialis*? Arch Dermatol 1998; **134**: 995–998.

41. Katsambas AD, Katoulis AC, Stavropoulos P. Acne neonatorum: a study of 22 cases. *Int J Dermatol* 1999; **38**: 128–130.

42. Lucky AW. A review of infantile and pediatric acne. *Dermatology* 1998; **196**: 95–97.

43. Herane MI, Ando I. Acne in infancy and acne genetics. *Dermatology* 2003; **206**: 24–28.

44. Cunliffe WJ, Baron SE, Coulson IH. A clinical and therapeutic study of 29 patients with infantile acne. *Br J Dermatol* 2001; **145**: 463–466.

45. Jeremy AHT, Holland DB, Roberts SG, Thomson KF, Cuncliffe WJ. Inflammatory events are involved in acne lesion initiation. *J Invest Dermatol* 2003; **121**: 20–27.

Hermann Feldmeier Thomas Wilcke

2

Scabies in childhood

Scabies has been a scourge of human society for at least 2500 years. Its clinical appearance puzzled doctors in ancient times and although the parasite was referred to in medical texts by the 12th century, its biology and host-seeking behaviour remained elusive until recently. Treatment has always been difficult and treatment options currently at hand are suboptimal, since no single therapy is easy to use, highly effective, cosmetically acceptable and non-toxic for scabies patients of all age groups.

MITE BIOLOGY AND LIFE CYCLE

When placed on human skin, the female *Sarcoptes scabiei* mite looks for a suitable place to burrow into the epidermis. It is assumed that mites prefer skin areas with little keratinisation and a constant temperature. Fertilised female mites live 4–6 weeks and produce 2–4 eggs per day which are deposited in the tunnel. Larvae hatch 2–4 days after the eggs have been laid, and adult mites can be observed 10–14 days later. Parasites accumulate only temporarily in the skin and then decrease in number over time (partly due to protective immune responses mounted by the host, partly because scratching destroys burrows and eliminates mites); on average, no more than 10 mites are found after 6 months of infestation.[1]

Off-host mites are able to survive and remain capable of carrying infection for 24–36 h at 21°C and 40–80% relative humidity. Lower temperatures and higher relative humidity prolong survival.[2] At temperatures below 20°C, mites

Hermann Feldmeier MD PhD (for correspondence)
Professor of Tropical Medicine, Institute of Microbiology and Hygiene, Charité University Medicine,
Campus Benjamin Franklin, Hindenburgdamm 27, 12203 Berlin, Germany
E-mail: hermann.feldmeier@charite.de

Thomas Wilcke MD
Paediatrician, Department of Paediatrics, Barnim Klinikum, Eberswalde, Germany

are unable to move and cannot penetrate into the skin. Infestivity decreases the longer mites are off-host.

During evolution, *S. scabiei* has adapted to various mammalian hosts with limited cross-infestivity between different host species. Humans are the only suitable host for *S. scabiei* var. *hominis*, although Sarcoptes mites from pets occasionally infest humans. The resulting clinical pattern is different from human scabies, the infestation is self-limiting, and usually requires no treatment.[3]

EPIDEMIOLOGY AND TRANSMISSION

Scabies occurs as a sporadic disease, in epidemics, and endemically. Sporadic cases are typically observed in industrialised countries; in resource-poor communities in the developing world, scabies is endemic. In Europe, epidemics have been described in day-care centres, schools, shelters for the homeless, prisons, nursing homes and hospitals (in the latter two settings, patients infect personnel and *vice versa*).

World-wide, it has been estimated that 300 million individuals are infested with *S. scabiei* at any time and that children are disproportionally affected. As most of the disease burden occurs in developing countries, and since in the developing world children less than 15 years constitute 50% or more of the total population, on a global view scabies is essentially a paediatric disease. This assumption is confirmed by data from European countries. In Poland, for example, between 1990 and 1998, 44% of all cases occurred in children aged 6–15 years, and 12% in children < 6 years of age.[4] Similarly, in Birmingham, the incidence was highest in children aged 5–14 years, and children constituted roughly one-third of all recorded scabies cases between 1994 and 2003.[5] Whereas in the UK, a preponderance in females was observed (female:male ratio 1.25), in Poland only in rural areas were females disproportionally more affected.[4,5] These data presumably reflect differences in culturally determined behaviour of mothers as to intensity and duration of body contact with their children.

A simplified description of the epidemiology of scabies in the UK was given by Mellanby.[6]

> *Recondite research on Sarcoptes*
> *Has revealed that infection begin*
> *At home with your wives and your children*
> *Or when you are living in sin*
> *Excepted in the case of the clergy*
> *Who accomplish remarkable feats*
> *And catch scabies and crabs*
> *From doorhandles and cabs*
> *and from blankets and lavatory seats.*

The poem nicely illustrates that the role of poor hygiene is overestimated by the layman. Mites burrowed in the epidermis are resistant to water and soap and continue to be viable even after daily hot baths.[7] Correspondingly, lack of hygiene has not been found to be associated with scabies.[8] Environmental and behavioural factors associated with increased occurrence of scabies in a community are poor housing, crowding, sharing of bedstalls and intimate body contact.[8] In Brazil, scabies was twice as prevalent in an urban slum with a high population density than in a resource-poor fishing community, where families lived on more ample compounds.[9] In Poland, where housing is still rather poor in the countryside, the incidence of scabies was 1.3 times higher in rural than urban areas.[4] Data collected from countries in temperate zones indicate that there the incidence is higher in autumn/winter than in spring/summer, probably due to increased host crowding during the cold season and prolonged off-host survival at lower temperatures.[4,10,11]

It has been hypothesised that, world-wide, the incidence of scabies ondulates in cycles of 30 years and that, at present, the infestation is on the rise. However, as reliable incidence data do not exist, this assumption is entirely speculative. Data from general practitioners in Birmingham indicate that the occurrence of scabies cases decreased from 470 per 100,000 inhabitants in 2000 to 233 in 2003.[5] These data make it unlikely that the incidence of scabies has increased during recent years, at least in the UK.

Scabies is highly contagious and is spread from person to person by direct skin contact. A single female mite may suffice to initiate disease in a new host.[1] In a classical experiment performed in Great Britain in 1940, Mellanby[12] showed that transmission almost exclusively occurs by body contact and that, under normal conditions, fomites such as clothes or bedding are unlikely to transmit the infectious agent. In contrast, bedding and clothing may serve as important fomites when used by patients with crusted ('Norwegian') scabies, in whom mites multiply in their millions.[7,13]

Mites dislodged from an infested individual use odour and thermal stimuli to find a new host. For these stimuli to be present in sufficient intensity, close skin contact must occur. This explains why a child usually gets infested through contact with an infested sibling or the mother. Grandmothers, who have prolonged and intimate contact with a grandchild, can also be the source of an infestation.[14] If children are adopted from a developing country, the diagnosis is sometimes only made when the child has transmitted scabies to the adoptive mother.[15] Intimate mother-to-child contact is also reflected by the topographic site at which scabies develops in the child, such as in a mother with scabies of the nipples who transmitted the disease to her 3-month-old child during breast-feeding.[16] The infant initially developed facial papules and later a generalised dermatitis.

IMMUNOLOGICAL HOST–PARASITE INTERACTIONS

Little is known about immunological host–parasite interactions in scabies. As pruritus and papular rash take 4 weeks or more to develop after primary infestation, but become evident within 24–48 h after secondary infestation, a delayed-type hypersensitivity response to mite antigens is indicated. Both experimental studies and clinical observations suggest that protective immune responses may develop in immunocompetent hosts. The development of a partially protective immunity would explain why experimental re-infestation fails in previously sensitised patients and why in individuals experiencing a second infestation, the parasite load is usually rather low.[17] The importance of the immune system in containing the propagation of the mites is confirmed by observations in patients with innate or secondary immunodeficiency. In individuals infected with HIV or HTLV-1, for example, scabies progresses in an uncontrolled manner. Even the temporary topical application of cortico-steroids can make scabies worse.[18]

The immunological host–parasite interactions seem to be different in normal, as compared to crusted, scabies. The latter patients show extremely high levels of IgE and IgG_4.[13,19] Both types of immunoglobulins are Th2-helper cell dependent and are co-expressed through sequential switching.

Histopathological examination of skin biopsies has shown that mites are surrounded by inflammatory cell infiltrates comprising eosinophils, lymphocytes and histiocytes. Whether, in crusted scabies, an intense allergic sensitisation to mite antigens is the immunological basis of skin alterations, such as hyperkeratosis and parakeratosis, remains elusive.[20] It is tempting to speculate that scabies is a spectral disease with some similarities to leprosy. At one end of the spectrum, an immunocompetent host limits the propagation of the parasite effectively (nodular scabies); at the other end of the spectrum, immunocompromised individuals cannot contain the infestation and develop crusted scabies. 'Normal' scabies would then be a reaction type located in the middle of the spectrum.

CLINICAL ASPECTS

Scabies can mimic a broad range of skin diseases (Table 1). Excoriations as a consequence of scratching, haemorrhagic crusts forming on the top of vesicles and secondary infection produce a complex clinical picture. When a patient uses cosmetics extensively, such as teenage girls are likely to do, typical lesions may even be absent (scabies incognito). The systemic or topical administration of corticosteroids also masks the typical clinical picture.

The burrow consists of a short, wavy line and is most commonly encountered on the fingers, wrists and penis. Papules are small and erythematous. They may be sparse or numerous and closely set. Over time, papules may change into vesicles and, rarely, into bullae. Burrows, papules and vesicles frequently develop into secondary scabies lesions – excoriations, crusts, eczematisation and secondary infection. In the latter case, the clinical picture is often similar to pyoderma. Very young children often have a wide-spread eczematous erythema, particularly on the trunk.[21]

Table 1 Differential diagnosis

Normal scabies	Eczema, atopic dermatitis, lupus erythematosus
Bullous scabies	Acropustolosis, pemphigoid, pemphigus, arthropod bites, bullous impetigo, dystrophic bullous epidermolysis, drug reaction
Nodular scabies	Insect bites, urticaria pigmentosa, pseudolymphoma, Langerhans' cell histiocytosis
Crusted scabies	Psoriasis, seborrhoeic dermatitis, lichen planus, Darier disease, ichthyosis, exfoliative dermatitis, chronic eczema

It is generally assumed that predilection sites are different as compared to older individuals. In fact, in a population-based study, it was shown that wrists, feet, genitals, scalp, neck and face were significantly more often involved in children aged < 7 years than in older patients.[22] Vesicles and superinfection s were also significantly more common in very young patients.[22]

Crusted or 'Norwegian' scabies is a hyperinfestation with myriads of mites present in exfoliating scales (up to 4700 mites per gram of scales). These patients are highly contagious. The condition occurs in individuals with a compromised immune responsiveness such as in AIDS, in HTLV-1 infection, after immunosuppressive therapies, malignancies, and congenital immune defects. Cases have been reported in patients with leprosy and tuberculosis, endocrinopathies (diabetes mellitus and hypoparathyroidism), rheumatic conditions (systemic lupus erythematosus and dermatomyositis), or after treatment with corticosteroids.[23] Children with neuropsychiatric, cognitive disorders or with Down syndrome are also prone to develop crusted scabies because they may be unable to eliminate mites through scratching. Neonates and infants may also develop the crusted form.

As a reaction to the massive infestation, the stratum corneum thickens, forming crusts and warty hyperkeratotic lesions, particularly at topographic sites where the horny layer usually is comparatively thin such as the face.[18] Typically, individual lesions become confluent, so that hyperkeratosis affects large areas. A variable degree of erythema is common.

Nodular scabies is a clinical variant in which extremely pruritic nodules are present on covered or soft skin areas such as in the axillae and groin and on the buttocks and genitals. It is a common presentation in infants. Nodules are firm, dull-red or brownish masses that may persist for months and probably represent an intense hypersensitivity reaction to the mite or its products. Nodules do not contain mites. Infection and secondary eczematous changes are common and might make the diagnosis even more difficult.[23]

Bullous scabies is a distinct subtype of scabies that may arise in young children.[23] The thinness of the stratum corneum and the loose adherence of the epithelial layers favour the appearance of erythematous vesiculopustular lesions. The condition probably represents a particular hypersensitivity reaction. Bullae persist for months.

Pruritus is intense and consistently more severe at night resulting in sleep disturbance.[22] It has been suggested that the perception of itch is more intense when the skin temperature is maintained at a higher level during the night by bedding.[18] However, patients living in the tropics report that the intensity of itch also increases at night, although they do not use bedding and sleep without pyjamas or night-gowns. As in many dermatoses, the intensity of itch is significantly higher during the first 3 h of sleep,[24] we suggest that in scabies, as with other parasitic skin diseases, the threshold of itch is down-regulated at night. This means that the patient only perceives the itch as more intensive at night which, in turn, augments scratching during sleep.[24]

Breaks in the epidermis, scratching by the patient and subsequent excoriations serve as an entry point for pathogenic bacteria. Pyoderma is, therefore, a common complication, particularly in children.[22] Infection with group A streptococci can lead to post-streptococcal glomerulonephritis.[25] Currie and Brewster[26] suggested that the high burden of group A streptococci on the skin of Australian Aboriginals together with a high prevalence of scabies contributed to the exceptionally high incidence of acute rheumatic fever observed in this population. In addition, pyoderma is the predominant source of GAS invasive disease. In crusted scabies, a generalised lymphadenopathy is common and secondary sepsis may lead to death.[27]

Scabies causes considerable distress in the patient and carers. The ectoparasitosis is still considered to be related to poor hygiene and is, in one way or another, associated with impoverished living conditions. This explains why the disease is stigmatised and patients may face ostracism.

DIAGNOSIS

Clinical diagnosis requires a high index of suspicion. Pruritus is the hallmark of scabies regardless of age. The diagnosis is confirmed when a burrow is detected at a typical predilection site and the lesion is severely itching. In this case, even a single burrow is pathognomonic. However, in practice, burrows are often obliterated by bathing, scratching, formation of crusts or superinfection. In severely affected communities in developing countries such as in Brazil, burrows are observed very rarely.[9,22]

A history of itching in several family members over the same period is almost pathognomonic. Authors of dermatology text books claim that the confirmation of the diagnosis of scabies requires the microscopic detection of the mite, ova or faecal pellets in a skin scraping. Various methods for the preparation of skin scrapings exist but, unfortunately, their sensitivity has never been determined systematically. The method, though, is very specific and a mite or eggs seen in the microscope are diagnostic. Treatment should be started if scabies is suspected clinically, even if it cannot be confirmed by microscopy.

Confocal microscopy, epiluminescence microscopy, or high-resolution videodermatoscopy seem to be promising tools,[28–30] but sound studies comparing sensitivity and specificity of clinical diagnosis and microscopical examinations of the skin are lacking. The high costs of the equipment and the considerable experience needed by the examiner make these techniques accessible only in specialised settings.

Recently, a simple diagnostic method was described in which a strong transparent adhesive tape was firmly applied onto skin lesions and then transferred directly on a slide for microscopy.[31] Accidentally, the diagnosis is established when a skin scraping is examined microbiologically. Wong et al.[32] observed a serpiginous track on the surface of dextrose agar used for fungal culture which turned out to be the track of a sarcoptes mite.

TREATMENT

Immediate treatment of the patient with an effective drug and rigorous treatment of close contacts are the principles of case management. As individuals may be infested without having symptoms, contacts should be treated, independently if clinical symptoms are present or not.[33] For many years, the topical application of acaricides of different nature was the only remedy available for scabies patients; with the advent of ivermectin, the ectoparasitosis may also be treated orally.

TOPICAL AGENTS

Based on the rationale that the mite is confined to the superficial layers of the epidermis, topical agents have been used for many years. Initially, they held the promise of a high efficacy without the risk of systemic adverse events. Problems associated with topical therapies, however, soon emerged. The efficacy of the compounds varied from setting to setting and the development of resistance became obvious.[33] Topical therapies are laborious to use, require time-consuming applications, and some are even messy.[34] Some experts demand that nails are cut and that the patient wears gloves during the application.[18] The patient has to ensure that the compound remains on the skin for the required time, must carefully wash off remaining cream or lotion and eventually should apply a body cosmetic to counteract the irritating effect of the topical acaricide.[18] Moreover, because Sarcoptes shares biochemical pathways with humans, and since several acaricides are actually pesticides with a neurotoxic mode of action, drug safety has become a matter of concern. As excoriations are common and diminish the barrier function of the epidermis, the acaricide may penetrate into the blood circulation and cause systemic adverse events. In infants and small children, the risk of toxic reactions is higher than in older individuals, because their body surface area is comparatively large and the scabicide may be licked off by the patient.

Lindane

For more than 40 years, lindane has been the mainstay of therapy against scabies. Toxic effects have raised concern about the use of lindane since the 1970s. Adverse events occur particularly when the manufacturer's instructions are not followed rigorously, such as the application on altered skin or the use with a frequency greater than recommended.[35] Toxic effects include neurotoxic symptoms such as numbness, restlessness, anxiety, tremor and convulsions.[36] Accidental oral ingestion may lead to nervous system damage and death.[37]

The danger of neurotoxic adverse events is particularly high in infants and young children.[38,39] Because of its side-effects, lindane had always been contra-indicated in infants, pregnant women, nursing mothers, and patients with seizures or other neurological diseases. In the EU, lindane has been banned from use in agriculture since 2001, because of safety concerns for people who have to handle it. Lindane has to be withdrawn from the EU pharmaceutical market by the end of 2007.

Permethrin

Permethrin, a synthetic pyrethroid, is used in many countries as first-line therapy. The toxicity of permethrin is considered low.[33,35] The recommended use is a single 10-h application of a 5% cream. Permethrin is approved for use in infants older than 2 months of age and is considered to be safe in newborns.[35,40] Permethrin can cause a burning sensation, exanthema, pruritus and folliculitis.[41] Like other natural or synthetic pyrethroids, permethrin has an allergic potential. Given its wide use in agriculture and gardening, previous sensitisation of a child with scabies may have occurred. In this case, permethrin is contra-indicated. Neuromuscular adverse reactions may occur after inappropriate occupational exposure to permethrin-containing insecticides. Recently, Coleman et al.[42] reported a case of severe neck dystonia after topical application of 5% permethrin cream. Even at a concentration as low as 0.5% (as used for the treatment of headlice), permethrin enters the circulation and its metabolites can be detected in urine for 100 h.[43] Permethrin applied in a thermolabile foam formulation seem to be better tolerated and reduce itching more rapidly than permethrin cream.[44] Resistance to permethrin is well recognised.[33]

Malathion

Malathion exists as a 0.5% alcoholic or aqueous solution. It is an organo-phosphate and inhibits acetylcholinesterase irreversibly. The odour is quite objectionable, and inhaling the fumes can result in severe headaches.[36] In the US, it has be withdrawn from the market because of poor cosmetic acceptance.

Benzyl benzoate

Benzyl benzoate was first known as a component of 'balsam of Peru'. A high efficacy of benzyl benzoate 25% has been reported by some authors, but was questioned by others and comparison with other compounds has seldomly been done. The substance requires repeated applications (twice daily for 2–3 days; repeat after 10 days). It is a skin irritant and may produce a burning sensation, pruritus and keratosis, thereby greatly reducing compliance.[37]

Sulphur *in petrolatum*

Sulphur *in petrolatum* has been used for centuries and it is still considered a first-line treatment in resource-poor settings although its efficacy has never been evaluated. The substance needs to be applied for three consecutive nights and to be washed off thoroughly 24 h after the last application. It is far from being cosmetically acceptable since it has a foul odour, it is messy and it stains clothing and bedding. It can also produce an irritant dermatitis. It has been considered safe, appropriate for infants younger than 2 months of age, for pregnant women or lactating mothers.[45] Recently, Haustein[37] questioned the safety of sulphur *in petrolatum* and considered the drug obsolete due to its potential liver and kidney toxicity in infants and small children.

Crotamiton

Crotamiton (10% in a cream/lotion) is applied for 24 h on two consecutive days. Since the compound is not very effective, some authors have suggested a 5-day application. It has an antipruritic effect but can induce an irritation of the skin and contact dermatitis.[46,47] Otherwise, Crotamiton is considered safe for use in children and infants.

Surprisingly, there are very few appropriately controlled studies comparing the effectiveness of topical compounds currently on the market.[48] As a consequence, treatment recommendations vary from one country to another (Table 2), and the selection of a drug is often based on the personal preference of the physician, local availability and cost, rather than on medical evidence. Superinfection should be treated with a topical antibiotic effective against Staphylococcus aureus and streptococci.

Four weeks after treatment, the patient has to be re-examined. Even after successful elimination of all mites, pruritic papules and nodules may persist

Table 2 Treatment guidelines according to country and age

Age group	UK[a]	Germany[b]	USA[c]	Canada[d]	Australia[e]
Newborns					
First line	No recommendation	Permethrin	No recommendation	Sulphur *in petrolatum*	Sulphur *in petrolatum*
Second line		Crotamiton			Crotamiton
Infants					
First line	Permethrin	Permethrin	Permethrin	Permethrin	Permethrin
Second line	Malathion	Crotamiton	Crotamiton		Benzyl benzoate
Children					
First line	Permethrin	Permethrin	Permethrin	Permethrin	Permethrin
Second line	Malathion	Benzyl benzoate/ Crotamiton	Crotamiton		Benzyl benzoate

[a]Synthesis: National Guidelines on the Management of Scabies and Control of Communicable Disease: Scabies Guidelines (Department of Public Health, 2004).
[b]Synthesis: Empfehlungen und Leitlinien der Deutschen Dermatologischen Gesellschaft,[18] and Fölster-Holst et al.[37].
[c]Red Book: *Scabies*, American Academy of Pediatrics, 2006.
[d]Indian and Inuit Health Committee, Canadian Pediatric Society. *Scabies Management*, 2005.
[e]Blue Book: *Guidelines for the Control of Infectious Diseases*, revised edn, 2005. <www.health.vic.gov.au/bluebook/Scabies.htm>.

for months. Another explanation of persisting itch and eczema after effective therapy is the development of a contact dermatitis due to the topical acaricide.[18]

Presumably, the majority of relapses are due to the lack of adherence to treatment protocols and a low compliance. Frequently, not all body parts are covered and the head, the genitals or the periungual area are, particularly, left untreated. In the case of treatment failure, a different compound should be used in order to avoid the development of resistance and/or cumulative toxicity.

PLANT EXTRACTS

As many scabicides are potentially hazardous molecules, patients and carers often seek less toxic alternatives. Essential oils showed an impressive effect against mites *in vitro* as well as in preliminary clinical studies. For example, tea tree (*Melaleuca alternifolia*) oil has been shown to be highly effective *in vitro*[49] and a paste composed of an extract of neem (*Azadirachta indica*) and *Curcuma longa* (turmeric) cured 97% of patients with scabies.[50] In a randomised, controlled study in Brazil, a commercially available repellent based on coconut and jojoba oil showed a similar efficacy as permethrin (J. Heukelbach, unpublished observation, 2006). Appropriately designed clinical studies are urgently needed to determine the true efficacy of plant-based acaricides and the safety of the various compounds.

Oral treatment: ivermectin

The advent of ivermectin, a macrolytic lactone, has opened a new area in the treatment of scabies.[51] Since the mid-1980s, ivermectin has been administered to humans, and several hundred million individuals have been treated with this drug in onchocerciasis and lymphatic filariasis control programmes in Africa and South America. Comparative trials have shown that the efficacy and effectiveness of oral ivermectin (200 µg/kg; repeat after 8–10 days) is similar or even better than that of topically applied lindane,[52] benzyl benzoate[53] and permethrin.[54] In developing countries, ivermectin has been used to control scabies at the community level and to reduce effectively scabies-associated morbidity.[55] In crusted scabies, ivermectin is the drug of choice. Usually, 5–7 doses of oral ivermectin are given. Some authors suggest a combination with keratolytic therapy and topical permethrin.[13] Ivermectin is also the drug of choice in scabies patients with innate or acquired immunodeficiency. Adverse events are rare, of minor importance and only of transient nature. Ivermectin is considered to be a drug with an excellent safety profile.[56] At present, oral ivermectin is – except in a few countries such as France and Brazil – only approved for the treatment of nematode infections. However, off-label use for parasitic skin diseases is common world-wide.[8]

So far, resistance to oral ivermectin has been reported in two cases from Australia. These patients, Aboriginals with extremely severe crusted scabies, had received 30–58 doses of ivermectin over a period of 4 years.[57]

Whether or not ivermectin should be considered as the drug of choice in all forms of scabies is still a matter of debate.[37,45] Its safety and efficacy in very young children has still to be determined.

CLOTHING AND BED LINEN

The treatment of clothing and bed linen (washing at 60°C, treatment with an antiscabietic lotion or putting it in a hermetically sealed bag for several days) has been recommended. However, this practice should be restricted to patients with crusted scabies, since the risk of a re-infestation through fomites is negligible in other forms of scabies.

The different treatment options currently available are summarised in Table 3. As evidence data are scarce, recommendations are based on reasonable best practice.

SCABIES IN THE DEVELOPING WORLD

In contrast to industrialised countries, in the developing world scabies is a public health threat of considerable importance. Here, scabies is common in resource-poor urban and rural communities with prevalences reaching up to 10% in the general population and 50% in children.[9,58,59] In an urban squatter settlement in Bangladesh, the incidence in children less than 6 years of age was 952 per 1000 per year which means that virtually all children experienced at least one infestation with *S. scabiei* per year.[60]

Poverty with its typical consequences – disastrous living conditions, over-crowding and a low level of education – appears to be a major driving force for keeping incidence and prevalence at high levels.[8] The best evidence for the predominant role of poverty in determining the occurrence of scabies in a community comes from Bangladesh, where family members in households with scabies significantly less frequently owned the house, had their house more often constructed from waste material, less frequently had electricity and had a lower monthly income than households without scabies.[60]

In the tropics, the topographical distribution of scabies lesions is different from the developed world, and commonly includes also the face, neck, scalp and

Table 3 Recommendations for treatment of scabies in newborns, infants, children, during pregnancy and lactation[a]

	Benzyl benzoate	Crotamiton	Permethrin	Malathion	Ivermectin
Newborn	Not recommended	Treatment only under strict medical supervision[b]	Treatment only under strict medical supervision[b]	Not recommended	Not recommended[c]
Infants	Treatment only under strict medical supervision[b]	Recommended[d]	Recommended[d]	Not recommended[c]	Not recommended[c]
Children	Recommended[e]	Recommended[d]	Recommended[d]	Second-line treatment[f]	Recommended
Pregnancy	Recommendation disputed[g]	Only in exceptional cases	Treatment only under strict medical supervision	Not recommended	Not recommended[h]
Lactation	Treatment only under strict medical supervision[i]	Not recommended	Not recommended[j]	Not recommended	Not recommended[h]

aLindane not mentioned as banned from the pharmaceutical market by the end of 2007; sulphur in *petrolatum* not mentioned due to safety concerns.[37]

bPreferably in hospital setting.

cManufacturer does not recommend treatment in children less than 5 years of age or weighing less than 15 kg.

dOnly if skin is not excoriated or denudated; permethrin contra-indicated if child is allergic to pyrethrins/pyrethroids.

eIf child older than 6 years.

fAn aqueous preparation should be used, because alcoholic prepations sting and cause wheeze.

gManufacturer allows prescription; however, in the US, use is prohibited as embryo may be at risk of gasping syndrome.[18,36]

hBy manufacturer. However, no adverse events were observed in thousands of women inadvertently treated during pregnancy and lactation in onchocerciasis control programmes.

iDo not apply to the breasts and nipples.

jPermethrin is present in breast milk.

post-auricular fold. Thus, mass treatment with topical drugs is rather difficult as the whole body surface has to be covered with a malodourous compound unlikely to be missed by the neighbours. This, in turn, will reinforce stigmatisation. Oral treatment with ivermectin is more easily accepted and administration can be directly observed by auxiliary personnel.

Key points for clinical practice

- Scabies is an extremely itchy parasitic skin disease caused by the mite *Sarcoptes scabiei*.

- Transmission occurs mainly through direct contact from person to person. Fomites play only a negligible role, except in patients with crusted scabies.

- The incubation period varies between 3–6 weeks, but symptoms appear rapidly in individuals who have experienced scabies previously.

- In industrialised countries, scabies is predominantly an infestation of children and institutionalised elderly.

- Scabies mimics many clinical conditions. The clinical manifestations depend on the age and the immunocompetence of the host.

- Children with primary or secondary immunodeficiency are prone to develop crusted (Norwegian) scabies, a form in which millions of mites are present in hyperkeratotic skin and exfoliating scales.

- Topical application of corticosteroids also causes mites to proliferate uncontrolled.

- Superinfection is common, and *Staphylococcus aureus* and group A streptococci are frequently isolated.

- Diagnosis is based on a high index of suspicion and is usually made clinically. Skin scrapings have a low sensitivity.

- Emerging diagnostic techniques, such as confocal microscopy, epiluminescence microscopy, or high-resolution videodermatoscopy, require expensive equipment and considerable experience.

- Treatment guidelines vary considerably between countries and depend on age of the patient.

- Topical compounds are sulphur *in pretolatum*, benzyl benzoate, crotamiton, permethrin, and malathion. Lindane will be banned from the pharmaceutical market by the end of 2007. All compounds require strict adherence to treatment protocols and are potentially hazardous. Resistance is emerging and is likely to increase in the future.

- Ivermectin (200 µg/kg twice 8–10 days apart) is an excellent alternative and is the drug of choice in crusted scabies. However, drug safety in children less than 5 years of age or weighing less than 15 kg awaits confirmation.

- In order to interrupt transmission, all contacts have to be treated on the same day.

References

1. Burgess IF. *Sarcoptes scabiei* and scabies. *Adv Parasitol* 1994; **33**: 235–292.
2. Arlian LG. Biology, host relations, and epidemiology of *Sarcoptes scabiei*. *Annu Rev Entomol* 1989; **34**: 139–161.
3. Arlian LG, Runyan RA, Estes SA. Cross infestivity of *Sarcoptes scabiei*. *J Am Acad Dermatol* 1984; **10**: 979–986.
4. Buczek A, Pabis B, Bartosik K, Stanislawek IM, Salata M, Pabis A. Epidemiological study of scabies in different environmental conditions in central Poland. *Ann Epidemiol* 2006; **16**: 423–428.
5. Pannell RS, Fleming DM, Cross KW. The incidence of molluscum contagiosum, scabies and lichen planus. *Epidemiol Infect* 2005; **133**: 985–991.
6. Mellanby K. Biology of the parasite. In: Orkin M, Maibach HI. (eds) *Cutaneous infestations and insect bites*. New York: Marcel Dekker, 1985; 9–18.
7. Andrews JR, Tonkin SL. Scabies and pediculosis in Tokelau Island children in New Zealand. *J R Soc Health* 1989; **109**: 199–203.
8. Heukelbach J, Feldmeier H. Scabies. *Lancet* 2006; **367**: 1767–1774.
9. Heukelbach J, Wilcke T, Winter B, Feldmeier H. Epidemioloy and morbidity of scabies and pediculosis capitis in resource-poor communities in Brazil. *Br J Dermatol* 2007; **153**: 150–156.
10. Mimouni D, Ankol OE, Davidovitch N, Gdalevich M, Zangvil E, Grotto I. Seasonality trends of scabies in a young adult population: a 20-year follow-up. *Br J Dermatol* 2003; **149**: 157–159.
11. Downs AM. Seasonal variation in scabies. *Br J Dermatol* 2004; **150**: 602–603.
12. Mellanby K. The transmission of scabies. *BMJ* 1941; **2**: 405–406.
13. Roberts LJ, Huffam SE, Walton SF, Currie BJ. Crusted scabies: clinical and immunological findings in seventy-eight patients and a review of the literature. *J Infect* 2005; **50**: 375–381.
14. Fox GN, Usatine RP. Itching and rash in a boy and his grandmother. *J Fam Pract* 2006; **55**: 679–684.
15. Haas N, Stuttgen G. Scabies in an adopted infant from Brazil. *Monatsschr Kinderheilkd* 1987; **135**: 171–172.
16. Haas N, Stuttgen G. Facial involvement in scabies in infancy. *Hautarzt* 1987; **38**: 622–623.
17. Lalli PN, Morgan MS, Arlian LG. Skewed Th1/Th2 immune response to *Sarcoptes scabiei*. *J Parasitol* 2004; **90**: 711–714.
18. Empfehlungen und Leitlinien der Deutschen Dermatologischen Gesellschaft (DDG): Skabies. 2007. <http://www.uni-duesseldorf.de/AWMF/11/013-052.htm> [assessed 3 March 2007].
19. Dougall A, Holt DC, Fischer K, Currie BJ, Kemp DJ, Walton SF. Identification and characterization of *Sarcoptes scabiei* and *Dermatophagoides pteronyssinus* glutathione S-transferases: implication as a potential major allergen in crusted scabies. *Am J Trop Med Hyg* 2005; **73**: 977–984.
20. van Neste D, Lachapelle JM. Host-parasitic relationships in hyperkeratotic (Norwegian) scabies: pathological and immunological findings. *Br J Dermatol* 1981; **105**: 667–678.
21. Dias AL. Scabies in very small children (babies). *BMJ* 2005; **331**: 619–622.
22. Jackson A, Heukelbach J, Ferreira da Silva Filho A, Barros Campelo Jr E, Feldmeier H. Clinical features and associated morbidity of scabies in a rural community in Alagoas, Brazil. *Trop Med Int Health* 2007; **12**: 1–11.
23. Cestari TF, Martignago BF. Scabies, pediculosis, bedbugs, and stinkbugs: uncommon presentations. *Clin Dermatol* 2005; **23**: 545–554.
24. Hon KL, Lam MC, Leung TF, Chik KW, Leung AK. A malignant itch. *J Natl Med Assoc* 2006; **98**: 1992–1994.
25. Feldmeier H, Chatwal GS, Guerra H. Pyoderma, group A streptococci and parasitic skin disease – a dangerous relationship. *Trop Med Int Health* 2005; **10**: 713–716.
26. Currie B, Brewster DR. Rheumatic fever in Aboriginal children. *J Paediatr Child Health* 2002; **38**: 223–225.
27. Hulbert TV, Larsen RA. Hyperkeratotic (Norwegian) scabies with Gram-negative bacteremia as the initial presentation of AIDS. *Clin Infect Dis* 1992; **14**: 1164–1165.
28. Longo C, Bassoli S, Monari P, Seidenari S, Pellacani G. Reflectance-mode confocal microscopy for the *in vivo* detection of *Sarcoptes scabiei*. *Arch Dermatol* 2005; **141**; 1336.
29. Micali G, Lacarrubba F, Tedeschi A. Videodermatoscopy enhances the ability to monitor efficacy of scabies treatment and allows optimal timing of drug application. *J Eur Acad Dermatol Venereol* 2004; **18**: 153–154.

30. Haas N, Sterry W. The use of ELM to monitor the success of antiscabietic treatment. Epiluminescence light microscopy. *Arch Dermatol* 2001; **137**: 1656–1657.

31. Katsumata K, Katsumata K. Simple method of detecting *Sarcoptes scabiei* var. *hominis* mites among bedridden elderly patients suffering from severe scabies infestation using an adhesive-tape. *Intern Med* 2006; **45**: 857–859.

32. Wong SS, Woo PC, Yuen KY. Unusual laboratory findings in a case of Norwegian scabies provided a clue to diagnosis. *J Clin Microbiol* 2005; **43**: 2542–2544.

33. Johnston G, Sladden M. Scabies: diagnosis and treatment. *BMJ* 2005; **331**: 619–622.

34. Orion E, Matz H, Ruocco V, Wolf R. Parasitic skin infestations II, scabies, pediculosis, spider bites: unapproved treatments. *Clin Dermatol* 2002; **20**: 618–625.

35. Fölster-Host R, Rufli T, Christophers E. Die Skabiestherapie unter besonderer Berücksichtigung des frühen Kindesalters, der Schwangerschaft und Stillzeit. *Hautarzt* 2000; **51**: 7–13.

36. Meinking TL. Infestations. *Curr Probl Dermatol* 1999; **11**: 73–120.

37. Haustein UF. Behandlung der Skabies. Permethrin ist Mittel der Wahl. *JDDG* 2006; **4**: 387–390.

38. Boffa MJ, Brough PA, Ead RD. Lindane neurotoxicity. *Br J Dermatol* 1995; **133**: 1013.

39. Singal A, Thami GP. Lindane neurotoxicity in childhood. *Am J Ther* 2006; **13**: 277–280.

40. Quarterman MJ, Lesher JL. Neonatal scabies treated with permethrin 5% cream. *Pediatr Dermatol* 1994; **11**: 264–266.

41. Hamm H. Milben, Läuse und Flöhe. *Hautarzt* 2005; **56**: 915–924.

42. Coleman CI, Gillespie EL, White CM. Probable topical permethrin-induced neck dystonia. *Pharmacotherapy* 2005; **25**: 448–450.

43. Tomalik-Scharte, Lazar A, Meins J, Bastian B, Ihrig M, Wachall B *et al.* Dermal absorption of permethrin following topical administration. *Eur J Clin Pharmacol* 2005; **61**: 399–404.

44. Amerio P, Capizzi R, Milani M. Efficacy and tolerability of natural synergised pyrethrins in a new thermolabile foam formulation in topical treatment of scabies: a prospective, randomised, investigator-blinded, comparative trial vs. permethrin cream. *Eur J Dermatol* 2003; **13**: 69–71.

45. Buffet M, Dupin N. Current treatments for scabies. *Fundam Clin Pharmacol* 2003; **17**: 217–225.

46. Hara H, Masuda T, Yokoyama A, Asaki H, Okada T, Suzuki H. Allergic contact dermatitis due to crotamiton. *Contact Dermatitis* 2007; **49**: 219.

47. Oiso N, Fukai K, Ishii M. Concomitant allergic reaction to cetyl alcohol and crotamiton. *Contact Dermatitis* 2003; **49**: 261.

48. Walker GJ, Johnstone PW. Interventions for treating scabies. *Cochrane Database Syst Rev* 2000; 2: CD000320.

49. Walton SF, McKinnon M, Pizzutto S, Dougall A, Williams E, Currie BJ. Acaricidal activity of *Melaleuca alternifolia* (tea tree) oil: *in vitro* sensitivity of *Sarcoptes scabiei* var. *hominis* to terpinen-4-ol. *Arch Dermatol* 2004; **140**: 563–566.

50. Charles V, Charles SX. The use and efficacy of *Azadirachta indica* ADR ('Neem') and *Curcuma longa* ('Turmeric') in scabies. A pilot study. *Trop Geogr Med* 1992; **44**: 178–181.

51. Burkhart KM, Burkhart CN, Burkhart CG. Our scabies treatment is archaic, but ivermectin has arrived. *Int J Dermatol* 1998; **37**: 76–77.

52. Madan V, Jaskiran K, Gupta U, Gupta DK. Oral ivermectin in scabies patients: a comparison with 1% topical lindane lotion. *J Dermatol* 2001; **28**: 481–484.

53. Glaziou P, Cartel JL, Alzieu P, Briot C, Moulia-Pelat JP, Martin PM. Comparison of ivermectin and benzyl benzoate for treatment of scabies. *Trop Med Parasitol* 1993; **44**: 331–332.

54. Usha V, Gopalakrishnan Nair TV. A comparative study of oral ivermectin and topical permethrin cream in the treatment of scabies. *J Am Acad Dermatol* 2000; **42**: 236–240.

55. Heukelbach J, Winter B, Wilcke T, Muehlen M, Albrecht S, Oliveira FA *et al.* Selective mass treatment with ivermectin to control intestinal helminthiases and parasitic skin diseases in a severely affected population. *Bull World Health Organ* 2004; **82**: 563–571.

56. Elgart GW, Meinking TL. Ivermectin. *Dermatol Clin* 2003; **21**: 277–282.

57. Currie BJ, Harumal P, McKinnon M, Walton SF. First documentation of *in vivo* and *in vitro* ivermectin resistance in *Sarcoptes scabiei*. *Clin Infect Dis* 2004; **39**: e8–e12.

58. Kristensen JK. Scabies and pyoderma in Lilongwe, Malawi. Prevalence and seasonal fluctuation. *Int J Dermatol* 1991; **30**: 699–702.

59. Terry BC, Kanjah F, Sahr F, Kortequee S, Dukulay I, Gbakima AA. *Sarcoptes scabiei* infestation among children in a displacement camp in Sierra Leone. *Public Health* 2001; **115**: 208–211.

60. Stanton B, Khanam S, Nazrul H, Nurani S, Khair T. Scabies in urban Bangladesh. *J Trop Med Hygiene* 1987; **90**: 219–226.

Antony E. Wiskin R. Mark Beattie

3

Crohn's disease

About 25% of inflammatory bowel disease (IBD) presents in childhood; Crohn's disease more commonly than ulcerative colitis. Crohn's disease is characterised by a chronic relapsing disease course. Growth failure is common. The pathology is a transmural inflammation anywhere along the gastrointestinal tract. Management in children is different to the adult population with growth and pubertal development being key priorities.

This review will focus on the epidemiology and pathogenesis of Crohn's disease including the recent advances in genetics. It will also examine the importance of nutritional management, review the current evidence for pharmacological therapies and give practical guidance on diagnosis and management.

EPIDEMIOLOGY

Crohn's disease is most commonly diagnosed in adolescents or young adults with 10%–15% of disease beginning in children aged less than 16 years. The incidence is thought to be increasing in children although the population prevalence in developed countries has now stabilised following increases reported in the 1980s and 1990s.[1] In the UK in 13 months from June 1998, a total of 431 children aged < 16 years were diagnosed with Crohn's disease, (approximately 3 per 100,000) compared to 211 children with ulcerative colitis (approximately 1.5 per 100,000).[2]

Crohn's disease has traditionally been considered a disease of the developed world with the highest prevalence in Caucasians from North America, UK and

Antony E. Wiskin MRCPCH
Academic Clinical Fellow, Paediatric Medical Unit, Southampton General Hospital, Tremona Road, Southampton SO16 6YD, UK

R. Mark Beattie FRCPCH MRCP (for correspondence)
Consultant Paediatric Gastroenterologist, Paediatric Medical Unit, Southampton General Hospital, Tremona Road, Southampton SO16 6YD, UK
E-mail: mark.beattie@suht.swest.nhs.uk

Northern Europe, particularly Jewish families. While this group still represents by far the largest number of affected individuals, there is evidence that other populations are also affected. There has, for example, been an increase in incidence amongst African-Americans and in Asians particularly second generation South Asians who have migrated to more developed countries.[3]

PATHOGENESIS

The precise aetiology is not known although many factors are thought to contribute. The contribution each element plays may vary between individuals and this may explain the dramatic heterogeneity of clinical manifestations. The innate immune response is fundamental; how this response is altered by genetic expression, and how this expression is affected by changes in environment, intestinal flora and nutritional state is also important. Modern techniques have allowed considerable investigation into the genetics of inflammatory bowel disease. There are, however, many unanswered questions regarding potential environmental triggers. Tobacco smoking is a risk factor. There is debate over the role of potential infective and dietary triggers including the role of breast feeding and the significance of perinatal or early childhood infections. The relationship with measles infection, the MMR vaccine, and Crohn's disease has caused significant debate in the past. Most recently, a systematic review by Gosh et al.[4] concluded there was no proven causative association between the development of Crohn's disease and the MMR vaccine, and no evidence of persistence of measles virus infection in the intestine of patients with Crohn's disease.

GENETICS

It is accepted that Crohn's disease is caused by environmental stimuli in genetically susceptible individuals. This is supported by familial disease, twin concordance and ethnic differences. A positive family history is one of the best established risk factors; between 6% and 32% of patients with inflammatory bowel disease have an affected relative.[5] Concordance rates are higher in monozygotic than dizygotic twins.[6] Genome scans have identified many potential areas of genetic linkage, seven of which, designated IBD-1-7, meet the strict criteria required.[7] One area of particular interest is the gene encoding caspase activating recruitment domain (CARD)-15 also known as nucleotide oligomerisation domain (NOD)-2 found in the IBD-1 locus on chromosome 16. Variants in this gene are found in different populations although their contribution to developing Crohn's disease is variable. However, CARD-15 mutations show preponderance to an ileal disease phenotype. CARD-15 mRNA is found in highest quantities in Paneth cells (found in high numbers in the ileum) which produce defensins – antibacterial proteins.[8] It is hypothesised that mutant CARD-15 genes lead to weakness in defence against intraluminal bacteria and results in inflammation. Other areas of interest include genes for cell-surface Toll-like receptors (TLRs). Mutations in various TLR genes have shown increased and decreased susceptibility to colitis. The IBD-3 locus on chromosome 6p is implicated in coding for the major histocompatibility

Table 1 Presenting features of Crohn's disease

Presenting features	Frequency
Abdominal pain	72%
Weight loss	58%
Diarrhoea	56%
Diarrhoea and weight loss	45%
Lethargy	27%
Anorexia	25%
Abdominal pain, weight loss and diarrhoea	25%
Bleeding	22%

Data from the British Paediatric Surveillance Unit survey 1998/1999.[10]

complex. Mutations in this locus can lead to differences in the capacity to respond to antigens and seem particularly associated with a colonic inflammatory bowel disease phenotype.[9] Developments in understanding of the genetic basis of Crohn's disease raise the possibility of specific genotype–phenotype groups which could potentially allow tailored treatment options and a better prediction of the disease course.

CLINICAL FEATURES

The classical triad of presenting features are abdominal pain, diarrhoea and weight loss. In the British Paediatric Surveillance Unit survey by Sawczenko and Sandhu,[10] this triad was seen in only 25% of children. Abdominal pain was the commonest symptom occurring in 75%, nearly 60% had weight loss preceding diagnosis, 56% of children had diarrhoea while only 45% reported both diarrhoea and weight loss. The data are shown in Table 1. The median age of onset of symptoms was 11.8 years with a median age at diagnosis of 12.9 years. These data highlight the difficulty in making a diagnosis of Crohn's disease as many children complain of vague symptoms, such as lethargy or anorexia, and only mild abdominal discomfort in the months prior to presentation with either these, or more florid symptoms.[10]

Specific positive examination findings include pallor, clubbing, lip swelling and aphthous ulceration. Signs of poor nutrition include weight loss, reduced subcutaneous fat and reduced muscle mass. Poor growth and delayed puberty may be present. Of particular importance is the peri-anal examination. This does not need to include a rectal examination. The presence of skin tags, fistulae or abscesses are suggestive of Crohn's disease. It is crucial, therefore, in children with gut symptoms to do a peri-anal examination. Extra-intestinal manifestations include erythema nodosum, pyoderma gangrenosum, uveitis, hepatobiliary disease and arthropathy.

A combination of recurrent abdominal symptoms and the clinical signs above, especially if there is growth impairment and delayed puberty, should prompt investigation for inflammatory bowel disease.

GROWTH FAILURE AND NUTRITION IMPAIRMENT

Two-thirds of children with Crohn's disease have weight loss at presentation[10] and historical data show that up to one-third of patients suffer permanent growth impairment.[11] The aetiology of growth failure and the factors that contribute to the nutritional deficit are poorly understood, partly because of the wide variance in the constituent factors between individuals in both health and disease, and partly as a consequence of the heterogeneous nature of the disease process. Aetiological factors include nutritional impairment, the systemic consequences of gut inflammation, disturbances of the growth hormone/insulin-like growth factor axis,[12,13] and the side effects of corticosteroids when used.[14]

The inflammatory response has direct effects on growth through specific cytokines and their interactions with insulin-like growth factor (IGF).[15] Interleukin-16 (IL-6) is a cytokine that induces C-reactive protein (CRP) production. Expression of IL-6 is increased in Crohn's disease and circulating levels parallel disease activity.[16] Work on transgenic mice has shown that mice which over-express IL-6 are growth retarded mediated by decreased IGF-1 levels.[17] Sawczenko et al.[18] reported in rats with 2,4,6-trinitrobenzenesulphonic acid-induced colitis that administration of IL-6 antibody restored linear growth and increased IGF-1 but did not improve nutrient intake or reduce intestinal inflammation when compared with untreated disease controls, demonstrating that altering the inflammatory response alone can produce significant improvements in growth. Different genotypes have been described relating to IL-6 activity in individuals. Growth retardation at diagnosis and circulating CRP levels were higher at diagnosis in children with the IL-6 GG genotype compared with the GC or CC genotypes in the study by Sawczenko et al.[18]

Evidence for high energy requirements in both active disease and remission highlights the importance of understanding energy balance in this population. Azcue et al.[19] demonstrated that patients with anorexia had significantly lower resting energy expenditure than similarly malnourished children with Crohn's disease. Varille and colleagues[20] found that resting energy expenditure fell in Crohn's patients after surgery but still remained higher than controls. Hart and co-workers[21] established that children with Crohn's disease in remission (many of whom were exhibiting catch-up growth) had higher overall energy needs than predicted. It is possible, therefore, that in active Crohn's disease, resting energy expenditure fails to down-regulate as one would expect with malnutrition, due to the additional demands placed on the body by the inflammatory process. As the disease enters remission, the demands placed by the inflammatory process diminish but are replaced by the demands to replenish body stores and allow tissue growth and repair and increased physical activity levels with improved health. These altered requirements are likely to vary markedly between patients due to differences in disease severity, degree of malnutrition and inherent metabolic phenotype and would contribute, at least in part, to the variation in energy requirements reported in the literature.[22]

There are few long-term studies that examine adult growth outcomes of childhood inflammatory bowel disease. The recent increased use of immunosuppressive agents including monoclonal antibody therapy is not yet reflected in outcome studies. The impact of corticosteroids on growth is well known. Markowitz et al.[14] analysed the records of 48 adults who had been diagnosed with IBD in early adolescence and, depending on the criteria used, reported permanent growth failure in 19–35% with a positive correlation between corticosteroid use and permanent growth impairment. A cohort of 135 patients from The Netherlands were reported in 2001, all of whom had onset of Crohn's disease before puberty. Longer courses of corticosteroids during puberty resulted in a reduced final adult height compared to shorter courses.[23] A recent study by Sawczenko et al.[24] has shown the length of the interval between symptom onset and diagnosis correlates negatively with height SD scores (Standard Deviation Scores using the 1990 UK standards) at diagnosis and that height SD scores at diagnosis were related to final height SD scores independent of mid-parental height.

BONE DISEASE

Metabolic bone disease is common. Metabolic bone disease reflects altered calcium homeostasis as a result of inflammation or malnutrition and also complications of treatments such as steroids. Bone mineral density (BMD) is commonly assessed by dual energy X-ray absorptiometry (DXA). However, there is considerable debate over how best to interpret DXA results. Boot and colleagues[25] performed DXA on 55 children, 22 with Crohn's disease and 33 with ulcerative colitis. BMD was decreased in children with Crohn's disease compared to previously published controls. Ahmed et al.[26] have suggested that BMD may, in fact, be misleading. In their study of 47 children with IBD, they found that using BMD for age, 65% of their population had osteopenia. They observed that the standards being used are created from healthy normally grown children. Many of the children studied have growth failure and, therefore, less bone mass. Variations in bone mass will, of course, alter bone density. They adjusted the results for bone area and found only 22% had osteopenia.[26] Treatment with corticosteroids has a negative impact on bone density. In a study by Abitbol et al.,[27] osteopenia was observed in 52% of patients treated with steroids and 28% of those without. Similarly, Silvennionen and co-workers[28] demonstrated, in 152 IBD patients, that those whose life-time steroid exposure was greater than 10 g had significantly lower bone density compared to groups with no steroid or less than 5 g exposure. Osteopenia is of considerable clinical significance in later life. Of 156 adult Crohn's patients with osteopenia studied by Klaus et al.,[29] 34 (22%) had vertebral fractures and approximately one-third of these patients were aged less than 30 years, while in the Abitbol et al.[27] study of 84 patients, 7% had vertebral crush fractures.

INVESTIGATION

Children with recurrent abdominal pain are common in clinical practice. The presence of other symptoms such as weight loss, diarrhoea, fever, nausea, aching joints, and vomiting that are also recurrent (> 2 episodes in 6 months) or persistent (> 4 weeks) should raise suspicion of inflammatory bowel disease.[30] These children should have initial screening blood tests including a

Table 2 Differential diagnosis of Crohn's disease

- Infection
    - Bacterial (*Campylobacter, Shigella, Salmonella, Yersinia* spp.)
    - Tuberculosis
    - Protozoal (*Cryptosporidium, Entamoeba histolytica, Giardia*)
- Appendicular abscess
- Eosinophilic gastroenteritis
- Cows' milk/allergic colitis
- Immunodeficiency states (*e.g.* chronic granulomatous disease)
- Intestinal lymphoma
- Graft versus host disease

full blood count, erythrocyte sedimentation rate (ESR), C-reactive protein (CRP), urea and electrolytes, and liver function.[31] Typical findings are of a low haemoglobin and albumin with raised platelet count, ESR and CRP, although initial blood tests can be normal. Stool samples should be sent for microscopy (including ova, cysts and parasites) and culture to exclude an infective colitis. Important differentials are listed in Table 2. Further investigation is by endoscopy. A positive family history should lower the threshold for endoscopy.

Blood investigations are not always predictive of endoscopic findings either at diagnosis or subsequently and there has been interest in finding specific serological and faecal markers that accurately predict active disease and could decrease the need for invasive investigation. A recent retrospective study has reviewed the role of serological testing for inflammatory bowel disease compared to the combination of ESR and haemoglobin. Antibodies against the yeast *Saccharomyces cerevisiae* (ASCA IgA and IgG), perinuclear cytoplasmic immunofluorescent antibodies (p-ANCA) and antibodies to outer membrane porin of *Escherichia coli* (anti-OmpC) were measured. A 60% sensitivity and 92% specificity for these antibodies compared to 83% sensitivity and 96% specificity for elevated ESR and anaemia was found.[32] Faecal markers of non-specific gastrointestinal inflammation include lactoferrin and calprotectin, both proteins secreted by polymorphonuclear cells; these have been used in clinical practice and research and correlate reasonably with disease activity, although are not sufficiently sensitive or specific for routine use.[33]

Initial positive blood results or persistent clinical suspicion should prompt further diagnostic investigations. The most appropriate tests and how to interpret the results have been reviewed by consensus groups from both the European Crohn's and Colitis Organisation[34] and the European Society for Paediatric Gastroenterology, Hepatology and Nutrition.[30] Upper and lower gastrointestinal endoscopy including intubation of the terminal ileum with multiple biopsies are indicated in all cases as this will increase the diagnostic yield and better assess disease extent. Disease activity is most commonly in the terminal ileum and right colon but can occur at any site in the gastrointestinal tract (Table 3).

An area of considerable interest is how best to image the small bowel not visualised by standard endoscopic techniques. The importance of this is to map disease extent and identify complications such as strictures or fistulae. Barium studies as either a small bowel enema or small bowel meal are the

Table 3 Disease activity by site

Site	Percentage of cases with disease activity
Mouth	22
Oesophagus	16
Gastroduodenum	52
Jejunum	18
Ileum	71
Right colon	71
Transverse colon	64
Left colon/sigmoid	59
Rectum	49
Peri-anal	45

Data from the British Paediatric Surveillance Unit survey 1998/1999.[10]

standard techniques employed,[30] although they involve a high dose of radiation. Consequently, other options have been trialed including ultrasonography, magnetic resonance imaging (MRI), computed tomography (CT) which also employs a high radiation dose, and capsule endoscopy. Ultrasonography has a good positive predictive value although a negative study does not exclude small bowel disease. Comparisons of capsule endoscopy, MRI and barium studies have been published; although they have relatively small numbers, they suggest that capsule endoscopy has a high diagnostic yield similar to MRI – both are better than barium studies.[36,37] The main problem with capsule endoscopy is capsule retention, particularly in the presence of stricturing disease, which should be excluded prior to the study. Pelvic MRI is useful for imaging peri-anal Crohn's disease particularly the assessment of peri-anal fistulas and planning of surgery.[38] Until further studies can confirm superiority of these other tests, the gold standard to establish diagnosis and disease extent is barium radiography of the small bowel combined with upper and lower gastrointestinal endoscopy including intubation of terminal ileum.[30,34]

MANAGEMENT STRATEGY

Crohn's disease runs a chronic relapsing and remitting course and is life-long. The management should be led by a team with specific expertise in paediatric inflammatory bowel disease, as part of a clinical network, in conjunction with the child and family. The team should include paediatric dietitians with experience in the use of enteral nutrition, specialist nurses who are vital as a point of contact for patients and families, education and mental health support. The specialist nurse provides practical support, for example, facilitating rapid access to toilets in the school setting. Many different medical specialists are involved including paediatric gastroenterologists, general paediatricians, paediatric and adult surgeons, radiologists and histopathologists.

The aims of management are to induce disease remission and to optimise growth avoiding treatment toxicity if possible. In order to monitor growth, height and weight should be measured at diagnosis and 3–4 monthly thereafter; pubertal assessment should be made at diagnosis and then 6 monthly. These results should be interpreted in the light of the child's predicted growth potential based on parental height. Children with impaired growth while on apparently effective treatment may need further investigation to exclude disease that may not be obvious clinically or on biochemical criteria (*e.g.* stricture). Steroid-sparing agents should be used where possible and surgery may be indicated for refractory disease.

There is a limited body of evidence for pharmacological interventions in paediatric Crohn's disease and much clinical practice is based on consensus and evidence derived from adult studies.[34,39–41]

PSYCHOLOGICAL ISSUES

The disease typically affects adolescents. Normal concerns concerning body image are amplified by the disease morbidity associated with impaired nutrition, growth and pubertal delay and pharmacological interventions, especially side-effects of corticosteroids. Low mood at disease presentation is common secondary to persistent abdominal discomfort, anorexia and fatigue. Quickly establishing a diagnosis and producing an early remission provokes a rebound of energy and positive attitude. Careful attention to nutritional management will help to optimise growth and pubertal development, which is one of the major concerns of this patient group.

Compliance can be a problem in adolescents with any chronic disease and young people with Crohn's disease often need to take several medications every day. Oliva-Hemker *et al.*,[42] using a validated formula from pharmacy records, found compliance rates of 50% for thiopurines and 66% for mesalamine in American children with Crohn's disease.

TRANSITION

An important time for adolescents is the transition from paediatric to adult services. This has to ensure smooth transfer of care but also has to manage the problems of adolescence and chronic disease. These include ensuring adequate patient knowledge of their disease and how to seek help when unwell, the ability to manage their own medications and how this fits into changing life-styles at work or college. This needs to be facilitated by a gradual reduction in parental support. Prior involvement of the child in treatment plans will enable this to run smoothly. Joint clinics for adolescents run by adult and paediatric physicians involving both multidisciplinary teams help this process.

SPECIFIC MANAGEMENT

INDUCTION OF REMISSION

This can be with either exclusive enteral nutrition or corticosteroids.[30,34]

Exclusive enteral nutrition

The use of exclusive enteral nutrition (elemental or polymeric diets) as treatment for Crohn's disease was first reported in the 1970s. Early studies examining enteral nutrition in paediatric patients demonstrated significant improvements in growth accompanying disease remission.[43,44] By the middle of the 1980s, elemental diets were widely used in the UK as primary therapy in children with Crohn's disease. There have been numerous trials that suggest polymeric diets are as effective as elemental diets in adult patients[45-47] and there has been a Cochrane review with nine studies included comparing elemental diet (n = 170) with non-elemental diet (n = 128) with no significant difference in outcome.[48] A review of published data that included the 5 paediatric, randomised, controlled studies with data from 194 patients suggested that enteral nutrition in children was as effective as corticosteroids in the induction of remission.[49] Recent data, principally from cohort studies, suggest remission rates of up to 80% can be achieved using exclusive enteral nutrition to induce remission in active disease.[50,51] A recent Cochrane review of growth failure in childhood Crohn's disease has examined the impact of different treatments on growth.[52] It concluded that there was some evidence that exclusive enteral nutrition has additional benefits on growth when compared to steroids. The evidence for effectiveness is supported by the clinical experience of advocates of enteral nutrition who see it as well-tolerated, non-toxic and acceptable to patients. A 6–8-week course is generally used. The amount required is gradually increased to about 120% of recommended nutritional intake over 3 days.[50] The feed is most palatable chilled and can be flavoured. Compliance as a consequence of multidisciplinary and family support is good and most children do not require a nasogastric tube. Gradual food introduction is supervised by dietitians at the end of treatment while weaning enteral nutrition to allow identification of potential food triggers. Subsequent courses of enteral nutrition for relapses are successful at inducing remission although tend to be less well tolerated.

Corticosteroids

Traditionally, corticosteroids have been used for the initial treatment of Crohn's disease. Prednisolone remains the corticosteroid of choice and is widely used. Recent guidance suggests that budesonide is as effective for induction of remission in mild-to-moderate ileocaecal disease,[34] although there are still reservations about its efficacy. Intravenous hydrocortisone is reserved for children who are systemically unwell with acute toxic colitis. In this instance, intravenous antibiotics, fluid resuscitation and blood transfusion may also be required.

5-Aminosalicylates

Many children receive 5-aminosalicylate-derived compounds in addition to corticosteroids or enteral nutrition although there are no randomised, controlled studies of their efficacy in children. In adults, a meta-analysis of three placebo-controlled, multicentre trials showed overall significant mean reduction of disease activity score compared to placebo.[53]

MAINTENANCE

Crohn's disease is, by its nature, a chronic relapsing and remitting condition. Most children will relapse within 12 months even if early remission is achieved. Repeated courses of induction therapy are often required with many children becoming steroid dependent.

Corticosteroids
There is no evidence that corticosteroids are an effective maintenance therapy. A recent Cochrane review examined three studies performed in adults and concluded that corticosteroids did not reduce the risk of relapse over a 24-month period of follow-up.[54] Despite its lower side-effect profile, budesonide has similar results.[55]

5-Aminosalicylates
5-Aminosalicylate-derived compounds have historically been employed as maintenance therapy and are still frequently used. There are no randomised controlled studies of their use in children. However, in a meta-analysis of seven adult studies which compared 5-aminosalicylate to placebo over 12 or 24 months, there was no evidence that 5-aminosalicylate was superior to placebo for the maintenance of remission long term.[56]

Thiopurine derivatives
The thiopurine group of medicines – azathioprine and 6-mercaptopurine – are widely used as maintenance therapy and highly effective. They are indicated in children with frequently relapsing disease and those with steroid toxicity, but have a slow onset of action. They should be considered at diagnosis in children with severe and/or pan-enteric disease. Five adult studies of azathioprine use in adults were reviewed by the Cochrane collaboration and demonstrated good evidence for efficacy.[57] The decision as to whether all children should have thiopurines at diagnosis is not straight-forward. A multicentre study in children demonstrated relapse rates of 9% at 18 months in those who received 6-mercaptopurine plus initial steroids at diagnosis versus 47% in those who received steroids alone. However, this study was small ($n = 55$) and has not been replicated elsewhere. It is worth noting that 53% of children who only received prednisolone at diagnosis were in remission at 18 months, suggesting that azathioprine is not necessary for all patients. Thiopurines have potential to suppress bone marrow and to cause pancreatitis. In children receiving azathioprine, genetically determined thiopurine methyltransferase (TPMT) activity may be a substantial regulator of the cytotoxic effect of 6-mercaptopurine, an effect which in turn could be important in predicting toxicity and influencing the outcome of therapy.[59] Regular full blood count monitoring is essential and this should also be performed if a child becomes acutely unwell. Children being treated with thiopurine derivatives should not receive live vaccines.

Additional immunosuppressants
There is very little evidence available in the paediatric population for second-line immunosuppressant drugs such as methotrexate and cyclosporine. In a small cohort of 14 children with Crohn's disease, nine (who were unable to tolerate or failed to respond to azathioprine) clinically improved with methotrexate at 4 weeks.[60] An analysis of four randomised, double-blind, placebo-controlled trials of cyclosporine in adults concluded that low-dose cyclosporine is not effective for treatment of active Crohn's disease.[61]

Nutrition

Nutrition remains a priority once disease is in remission with either continued nutritional supplements or close dietetic follow-up to ensure nutritional intake is adequate. Multivitamins and calcium supplements may be instituted particularly in severe disease and during periods of rapid growth. The role of enteral nutrition as maintenance therapy is still unclear. Johnson *et al.*[62] suggested that, while partial enteral nutrition may result in some symptomatic improvements, it does not alter the inflammatory process and thus has no long-term role in maintaining disease remission. However Wilschanski and colleagues,[63] in a retrospective study, showed significant improvements in both growth velocity and time to relapse in children who continued supplementary nocturnal enteral nutrition compared to those who did not. Other studies have shown a similar trend towards lower relapse rates in patients that continued a small amount of enteral nutrition in addition to normal diet.

Probiotics

The potential aetiological relationship between intestinal flora and the gut mucosa has led several investigators to examine the effect of probiotics. The effect is thought to be mediated through alterations in growth and activity of intraluminal bacteria. Seven studies were examined as part of a Cochrane review. Studies varied in choice of probiotic and in treatment protocol. All had small numbers. Three placebo studies showed no benefit of probiotics, while two studies showed no difference in relapse rates between those on probiotics and those on mesalazine.[64]

REFRACTORY DISEASE

Refractory disease refers to disease that fails to respond to the standard therapies described above.

INFLIXIMAB

Tumour necrosis factor-α (TNF-α) is a pro-inflammatory cytokine produced in lymphocytes and macrophages that has been implicated in the pathogenesis of Crohn's disease. There are several therapeutic modalities that antagonise the effects of TNF-α. These include anti-TNF-α antibodies (mouse–human-derived Infliximab, and the fully humanised Adalimumab), an engineered TNF-α receptor fusion protein (Etanercept), integrin-specific humanised monoclonal antibody (Natalizumab) and thalidomide and its analogues. Infliximab is a monoclonal immunoglobulin (Ig)G_1 antibody to TNF and is able to inhibit TNF-α activity. Its initial published use was in a child with refractory Crohn's colitis.[65] Since then, there have been few controlled trials of its use in children but several studies show it can be successful at reducing clinical disease severity. Recent consensus guidance suggests that Infliximab is effective for induction of remission in refractory paediatric Crohn's disease, including refractory fistulating disease.[34] A study to evaluate the safety and efficacy of Infliximab in children with moderate-to-severe active disease has recently been published. A total of 112 children were treated with Infliximab at 1, 2 and 6 weeks. At 10 weeks, 88.4% had responded with improved clinical score and 58.9% achieved clinical remission. The children who responded were then allocated to receive maintenance Infliximab at 8 or 12 week intervals. Those receiving 8 weekly infusions had improved remission rates.[66] Infliximab, however, is not without side effects some of which can be significant. Re-activation of latent tuberculosis has been reported and an increased risk of lymphoma has been shown in patients receiving Infliximab in combination with other immunosuppressive agents.[67] The US Food and Drug Administration's adverse event reporting system has received data on eight cases of hepatosplenic T-cell lymphoma (to October 2006) associated with Infliximab use for Crohn's disease mainly in adolescents.[68] All patients were also taking a thiopurine derivative. This type of lymphoma is rare (about 100 published cases world-wide) but uniformly fatal and why there is an increased incidence in this group is unknown.[69] A further problem with Infliximab is antibody formation which may produce hypersensitivity or a progressively reduced clinical response. This can be reduced by prophylaxis with hydro-cortisone prior to each infusion.[67] Assessing the risk–benefit balance using a decision analysis model for Infliximab in refractory Crohn's disease suggests the benefits generally outweigh the risks, with fewer operative interventions and a better quality of life for patients, despite an increase in serious infections and lymphoma. However, these conclusions are not necessarily applicable to paediatric populations who have potential for more years to be affected by adverse reactions, infections or malignancy.[70] The National Institute for Health and Clinical Excellence (NICE) recommends that Infliximab use in adults is restricted to patients with severe active disease with very poor general health, where treatment with immunomodulators and corticosteroids has not worked and where surgery is not appropriate. This guidance can reasonably be applied to children.

SURGERY

A complete discussion of the role of surgery in paediatric Crohn's disease is beyond the scope of this chapter; however, it remains an important treatment option for patients with refractory disease. Surgical options range from removal of isolated disease segments or strictures to extensive panproctocolectomy and the possibility of permanent stoma formation. Surgical resection of active disease can lead to rapid increases in growth and a prolonged period of disease remission; therefore, timing of surgery relative to the pubertal growth spurt is crucial.

Key points for clinical practice

- The incidence of paediatric Crohn's disease is increasing particularly in migrant populations to the UK.

- A greater awareness of the importance of vague abdominal symptoms and clinical signs in children including accurate growth data are important to prevent delays in diagnosis.

- Impaired nutrition and delayed growth is common at presentation.

Key points for clinical practice *(Continued)*

- Investigation and early management should occur at a centre with a multidisciplinary team specialised in the care of children with inflammatory bowel disease.

- The gold standard to establish diagnosis and disease extent is barium radiography of the small bowel combined with upper and lower gastrointestinal endoscopy including intubation of terminal ileum.

- The treatment priority is to induce disease remission with minimal toxicity and, thereby, facilitate normal growth and pubertal development.

- Enteral nutrition should be considered as first-line treatment for most children with Crohn's disease and definitely for those with ileocolonic disease.

- Early introduction of azathioprine should be considered in those with severe disease.

- Careful consideration should be given prior to starting Infliximab although this should not preclude its use when other treatments have been tried and disease remains active.

- Continuous nutritional support should be offered to all children.

- The impact of disease on the child's education and social development should be carefully considered.

References

1. Edward V, Loftus JR. Clinical epidemiology of inflammatory bowel disease: incidence, prevalence and environmental influences. *Gastroenterology* 2004; **126**: 1504–1517.
2. Sawczenko A, Sandhu BK, Logan RF et al. Prospective survey of childhood inflammatory bowel disease in the British Isles. *Lancet* 2001; **357**: 1093–1094.
3. Hanauer SB. Inflammatory bowel disease: epidemiology, pathogenesis, and therapeutic opportunities. *Inflamm Bowel Dis* 2006; **12**: S3–S9.
4. Ghosh S, Armitage E, Wilson D et al. Detection of persistent measles virus infection in Crohn's disease: current status of experimental work. *Gut* 2001; **48**: 748–752.
5. Ahmad T, Satsangi J, McGovern D et al. The genetics of inflammatory bowel disease. *Aliment Pharmacol Ther* 2001; **15**: 731–748.
6. Orholm M, Binder V, Sorensen TIA et al. Concordance of inflammatory bowel disease among Danish twins: results of a nationwide survey. *Scand J Gatroenterol* 2000; **35**: 1075–1081.
7. Ahmad T, Tamboli CP, Jewell D, Colombel J. Clinical relevance of advances in genetics and pharmacogenetics of IBD. *Gastroenterology* 2004; **126**: 1533–1549.
8. Gaya DR, Russell RK, Nimmo ER, Satsangi J. New genes in inflammatory bowel disease: lessons for complex diseases? *Lancet* 2006; **367**: 1271–1284.
9. Russell RK, Wilson DC, Satsangi J. Unravelling the complex genetics of inflammatory bowel disease. *Arch Dis Child* 2004; **89**: 598–603.
10. Sawczenko A, Sandhu BK. Presenting features of inflammatory bowel disease in Great Britain and Ireland. *Arch Dis Child* 2003; **88**: 995—1000.
11. Markowitz J, Daum F. Growth impairment in pediatric inflammatory bowel disease. *Am J Gastroenterol* 1994; **89**: 319–326.

12. Thomas AG, Holly JM, Taylor F, Miller V. Insulin like growth factor-1, insulin like growth factor binding protein-1, and insulin in childhood Crohn's disease. *Gut* 1993; **34**: 944–947.

13. Beattie RM, Camacho-Hubner C, Wacharasindhu S *et al.* Responsiveness of IGF-I and IGFBP-3 to therapeutic intervention in children and adolescents with Crohn's disease. *Clin Endocrinol* 1998; **49**: 483–489.

14. Markowitz J, Grancher K, Rosa J *et al.* Growth failure in pediatric inflammatory bowel disease. *J Pediatr Gastroenterol Nutr* 1993; **16**: 373–380.

15. Murch SH, Lamkin VA, Savage MO *et al.* Serum concentrations of tumour necrosis factor alpha in childhood chronic inflammatory bowel disease. *Gut* 1991; **32**: 913–917.

16. Bannerjee K, Camacho-Hubner C, Babinska K *et al.* Anti-inflammatory and growth stimulating effects precede nutritional restitution during enteral feeding in Crohn's disease. *J Pediatr Gastroenterol Nutr* 2004; **38**: 270–275.

17. De Benedetti F, Alonzi T, Moretta A *et al.* Interleukin 6 causes growth impairment in transgenic mice through a decrease in insulin-like growth factor-1: a model for stunted growth in children with chronic inflammation. *J Clin Invest* 1997; **99**: 643–650.

18. Sawczenko A, Azooz O, Paraszczuk J *et al.* Intestinal inflammation-induced growth retardation acts through IL-6 in rats and depends on the –174 IL-6 G/C polymorphism in children. *Proc Natl Acad Sci USA* 2005; **102**: 13260–13265.

19. Azcue M, Rashid M, Griffiths A, Pencharz PB. Energy expenditure and body composition in children with Crohn's disease: effect of enteral nutrition and treatment with prednisolone. *Gut* 1997; **41**: 203–208.

20. Varille V, Cézard JP, de Lagausie P *et al.* Resting energy expenditure before and after surgical resection of gut lesions in pediatric Crohn's disease. *J Pediatr Gastroenterol Nutr* 1996; **23**: 13–19.

21. Hart JW, Bremner AR, Wootton SA, Beattie RM. Measured versus predicted energy expenditure in children with inactive Crohn's disease. *Clin Nutr* 2005; **24**: 1047–1055.

22. Wiskin AE, Wootton SA, Beattie RM. Nutrition issues in pediatric Crohn's disease. *Nutr Clin Pract* 2007; **22**: 214–222.

23. Alemzadeh N, Rekers-Mombarg LTM, Mearin ML *et al.* Adult height in patients with early onset of Crohn's disease. *Gut* 2001; **51**: 26–29.

24. Sawczenko A, Ballinger AB, Savage MO, Sanderson IR. Clinical features affecting final adult height in patients with pediatric-onset Crohn's disease. *Pediatrics* 2006; **118**: 124–129.

25. Boot AM, Bouquet J, Krenning EP, Muinck Keizer-Schrama SM. Bone mineral density and nutritional status in children with chronic inflammatory bowel disease. *Gut* 1998; **42**: 188–194.

26. Ahmed SF, Horrocks IA, Patterson T *et al.* Bone mineral assessment by dual energy X-ray absorptiometry in children with inflammatory bowel disease: evaluation by age or bone area. *J Pediatr Gastroenterol Nutr* 2004; **38**: 276–281.

27. Abitbol V, Roux C, Chaussade S *et al.* Metabolic bone assessment in patients with inflammatory bowel disease. *Gastroenterology* 1995; **108**: 417–422.

28. Silvennoinen JA, Karttunen TJ, Niemela SE *et al.* A controlled study of bone mineral density in patients with inflammatory bowel disease. *Gut* 1995; **37**: 71–76.

29. Klaus J, Armbrecht G, Steinkamp M, *et al.* High prevalence of osteoporotic vertebral fractures in patients with Crohn's disease. *Gut* 2002; **51**: 654–658.

30. Inflammatory bowel disease in children and adolescents: recommendations for diagnosis – The PORTO Criteria. *J Pediatr Gastroenterol Nutr* 2005; **41**: 1–7.

31. Beattie RM, Walker-Smith JA, Murch SH. Indications for investigation of chronic gastrointestinal symptoms. *Arch Dis Child* 1995; **73**: 354–355.

32. Sabery N, Bass D. Use of serologic markers as a screening tool in inflammatory bowel disease compared with elevated erythrocyte sedimentation rate and anemia. *Pediatrics* 2007; **1**: e193–e199.

33. Amati L, Passeri ME, Seicato F *et al.* New insights into the biological and clinical significance of fecal calprotectin in inflammatory bowel disease. *Immunopharmacol Immunotoxicol* 2006; **28**: 665–681.

34. European evidence-based consensus on the diagnosis and management of Crohn's disease. *Gut* 2006; **55**: 1–58.

35. Bremner AR, Pridgeon J, Fairhurst J, Beattie RM. Ultrasound scanning may reduce the need for barium radiology in the assessment of small bowel Crohn's disease. *Acta Paediatr* 2003; **93**: 479–481.

36. Hara AK, Leighton JA, Heigh RI *et al.* Crohn disease of the small bowel: preliminary comparison among CT enterography, capsule endoscopy, small-bowel follow-through, and ileoscopy. *Radiology* 2006; **238**: 128–134.

37. Albert JG, Martiny A, Krummenerl A *et al.* Diagnosis of small bowel Crohn's disease: a prospective comparison of capsule endoscopy with magnetic resonance imaging and fluoroscopic enterolysis, *Gut* 2005; **54**: 1721–1727.

38. Essary B, Kim J, Anupindi S *et al.* Pelvic MRI in children with Crohn disease and suspected perianal involvement. *Pediatr Radiol* 2007; **32**: 201–208.

39. Escher JC, Taminiau JAJK, Nieuwenhuis EES *et al.* Treatment of inflammatory bowel disease in childhood: best available evidence. *Inflamm Bowel Dis* 2003; **9**: 34–58.

40. Beattie RM, Croft NM, Fell JM *et al.* Inflammatory bowel disease. *Arch Dis Child* 2006; **91**: 426–432.

41. Carter MJ, Lobo AJ, Travis SPL. Guidelines for the management of inflammatory bowel disease in adults. *Gut* 2004; **53**: v1–v16.

42. Oliva-Hemker M, Abadom V, Cuffari C, Thompson RE. Nonadherence with thiopurine immunomodulator and mesalamine medications in children with Crohn disease. *J Pediatr Gatroenterol Nutr* 2007; **44**: 180–184.

43. Kirschner BS, Klich JR, Kalman SS *et al.* Reversal of growth retardation in Crohn's disease with therapy emphasising oral nutritional restitution. *Gastroenterology* 1981; **80**: 10–15.

44. O'Morain C, Segal AM, Levi AJ, Valman HB. Elemental diet in acute Crohn's disease. *Arch Dis Child* 1983; **58**: 44–47.

45. Griffiths AM, Ohlsson A, Sherman PM, Sutherland LR. Meta-analysis of enteral nutrition as a primary treatment of active Crohn's disease. *Gastroenterology* 1995; **108**: 1056–1067.

46. Fernandez-Banares F, Cabre E, Esteve-Comas M, Gassull MA. How effective is enteral nutrition in inducing clinical remission in active Crohn's disease? A meta-analysis of the randomized clinical trials. *J Parenteral Enteral Nutr* 1995; **19**: 356–364.

47. Wight N, Scott BB, Wright N. Dietary treatment of active Crohn's disease. *BMJ* 1997; **314**: 454–455.

48. Zachos M, Tondeur M, Griffiths AM. Enteral nutritional therapy for induction of remission in Crohn's disease. Cochrane Database Syst Rev 2007, Issue 1. CD000542.

49. Heuschkel RB, Menache CC, Megerian JT, Baird AE. Enteral nutrition and corticosteroids in the treatment of acute Crohn's disease in children. *J Pediatr Gastroenterol Nutr* 2000; **31**: 8–15.

50. Fell JM, Paintin M, Arnaud-Battandier F *et al.* Mucosal healing and a fall in mucosal pro-inflammatory cytokine mRNA induced by a specific oral polymeric diet in paediatric Crohn's disease. *Aliment Pharmacol Ther* 2000; **14**: 281–289.

51. Gavin J, Anderson CE, Bremner AR, Beattie RM. Energy intakes of children with Crohn's disease treated with enteral nutrition as primary therapy. *J Hum Nutr Diet* 2005; **18**: 337–342.

52. Newby EA, Sawczenko A, Thomas AG, Wilson D. Interventions for growth failure in childhood Crohn's disease. Cochrane Database Syst Rev 2005, Issue 3. CD003873.

53. Haneuer SB, Stromberg U. Oral pentasa in the treatment of active Crohn's disease: a meta-analysis of double-blind, placebo-controlled trials. *Clin Gastroenterol Hepatol* 2004; **2**: 379–388.

54. Steinhart AH, Ewe K, Griffiths AM, Modigliani R, Thomsen OO. Corticosteroids for maintenance of remission in Crohn's disease. Cochrane Database Syst Rev 2003, Issue 4. CD000301.

55. Simms L, Steinhart AH. Budesonide for maintenance of remission in Crohn's disease. Cochrane Database Syst Rev 2001, Issue 1. CD002913.

56. Akobeng AK, Gardener E. Oral 5-aminosalicylic acid for maintenance of medically-induced remission in Crohn's Disease. Cochrane Database Syst Rev 2005, Issue 1. CD003715.

57. Pearson DC, May GR, Fick G, Sutherland LR. Azathioprine for maintenance of remission in Crohn's disease. Cochrane Database Syst Rev 1998, Issue 4. CD000067.

58. Markowitz J, Grancher K, Kohn N *et al*. A multi-centre trial of 6-mercaptopurine and prednisolone in children with newly diagnosed Crohn's disease. *Gastroenterology* 2000; **119**: 895–902.

59. Lennard L, Lilleyman JS, Van Loon J, Weinshilboum RM. Genetic variation in response to 6-mercaptopurine for childhood acute lymphoblastic leukaemia. *Lancet* 1990; **336**: 225–229.

60. Mack DR, Young R, Kaufman SS *et al*. Methotrexate in patients with Crohn's disease after 6-mercaptopurine. *J Pediatr* 1998; **132**: 830–835.

61. McDonald JWD, Feagan BG, Jewell D *et al*. Cyclosporine for induction of remission in Crohn's disease. Cochrane Database Syst Rev 2005, Issue 2. CD000297.

62. Johnson T, Macdonald S, Hill SM *et al*. Treatment of active Crohn's disease in children using partial enteral nutrition with liquid formula: a randomised controlled study. *Gut* 2006; **55**: 356–361.

63. Wilschanski M, Sherman P, Pencharz P *et al*. Supplementary enteral nutrition maintains remission in paediatric Crohn's disease. *Gut* 1996; **38**: 543–548.

64. Rolfe VE, Fortun PJ, Hawkey CJ, Bath-Hextall F. Probiotics for maintenance of remission in Crohn's disease. Cochrane Database Syst Rev 2006, Issue 4. CD004826.

65. Derkx B, Taminiau J, Radema S *et al*. Tumour-necrosis-factor antibody treatment in Crohn's disease. *Lancet* 1993; **342**: 173–174.

66. Hyams J, Crandell W, Kugathasan S *et al*. Induction and maintenance Infliximab therapy for the treatment of moderate-to-severe Crohn's disease in children. *Gastroenterology* 2007; **132**: 863–873.

67. Rutgeerts P, Van Assche G, Vermeire S. Optimizing anti-TNF treatment in inflammatory bowel disease. *Gastroenterology* 2004; **126**: 1593–1610.

68. Mackey AC, Grenn L, Liang L *et al* Hepatosplenic T cell lymphoma associated with Infliximab use in young patients treated for inflammatory bowel disease. *J Pediatr Gastroenterol Nutr* 2007; **44**: 265–267.

69. Rosh JR, Oliva-Hemker M. Infliximab use and hepatosplenic T cell lymphoma: questions to be asked and lessons learned. *J Pediatr Gastroenterol Nutr* 2007; **44**: 165–167.

70. Siegel CA, Hur C, Korzenik JR *et al*. Risks and benefits of Infliximab for the treatment of Crohn's disease. *Clin Gastroenterol Hepatol* 2006; **4**: 1017–1024.

Girish L. Gupte Ian W. Booth

4

Intestinal failure

Until the 1970s, long-term intestinal failure was inevitably a death sentence. During the 1980s and 1990s, the provision of long-term parenteral nutrition enabled children with intestinal failure to remain alive, with a reasonable quality of life until the inevitable development of life-threatening complications. Over the last 15 years, small bowel transplantation has been developed, offering these children the prospect of long-term survival.[1]

DEFINITION OF INTESTINAL FAILURE

The most accepted definition seems to be 'a critical reduction of functional gut mass below the minimal amount necessary for adequate digestion and absorption to satisfy body nutrient and fluid requirements for maintenance in adults and children'.[1] This definition stresses that intestinal failure can be present in individuals with a normal, but dysfunctional, length of bowel. Intestinal failure can also be defined in relation to objective measurements of intestinal function, *e.g.* absorption of essential nutrients and electrolytes.[1]

EPIDEMIOLOGY

The exact incidence of intestinal failure in the developed world is not known and so home parenteral nutrition has been used as a proxy to estimate the incidence of intestinal failure. About 40,000 North American patients (children

Girish L. Gupte MD(India) DNB MRCPI (for correspondence)
Consultant Paediatric Hepatologist, Liver Unit, Birmingham Children's Hospital, Steelhouse Lane, Birmingham B4 6NH, UK
E mail: girish.gupte@bch.nhs.uk

Ian W. Booth BSc MSc MD FRCP FRCPCH
Leonard Parsons Professor of Paediatrics and Child Health, Institute of Child Health, University of Birmingham, Birmingham B4 6NH, UK

and adults) were documented to be receiving home parenteral nutrition. The British Artificial Nutrition Survey (2005) reported that 71 children were registered for home parenteral nutrition at the end of 2003.[2] A survey conducted by seven European centres in 2001 estimated an incidence of paediatric home parenteral nutrition of 2–6.8 per million population.[2] Recent increases in the incidence of gastroschisis in the UK, advances in neonatal intensive care and surgical techniques, long-term survival on home parenteral nutrition and the prospect of improved survival following small bowel transplantation are all likely to result in an increased incidence of intestinal failure in the future. A British Intestinal Failure Registry has been started to document the incidence of intestinal failure within the UK, with the aim of planning future services more effectively.

AETIOLOGY

The causes of intestinal failure can be divided into three categories – enteropathies, motility disorders, and short bowel syndrome.

ENTEROPATHIES

NEONATAL ENTEROPATHIES

Microvillous inclusion disease (microvillous atrophy)

This disorder is a common cause of severe protracted diarrhoea beginning in the newborn period. It appears to be transmitted as an autosomal recessive disorder and, characteristically, presents with severe watery diarrhoea in the first few days of life.[3] In some cases, onset may be delayed to a few months of age. Stool volumes are usually high (up to 300 ml/kg/day) and may have both an osmotic and a secretory component. The disorder is fatal without long-term parenteral nutrition. Diagnosis depends on the demonstration of hypoplastic villous atrophy with the accumulation of PAS-positive secretory granules within the atypical cytoplasm of enterocytes. On electron microscopy, microvilli are almost completely absent, and the enterocytes contain microvillous inclusions and numerous cytoplasmic vesicular bodies.[3]

Epithelial dysplasia (tufting enteropathy)

This disorder, which has characteristic histological appearances, also presents in the first week of life with intractable watery diarrhoea requiring long-term parenteral nutrition. About 40% have consanguineous parents and/or affected siblings who died during the first few months of life with severe diarrhoea. Variable villous atrophy is present, together with disorganisation of surface enterocytes producing so-called tufting.[4] Crypts are often dilated and pseudo-cystic. Early biopsies may show villous atrophy only; therefore, repeated duodenal biopsies are often needed to make the diagnosis.

Phenotypic (syndromic) diarrhoea

Patients present with diarrhoea in the first 6 months of life. Many are small for gestational age and have dysmorphic features, hypertelorism and woolly,

A

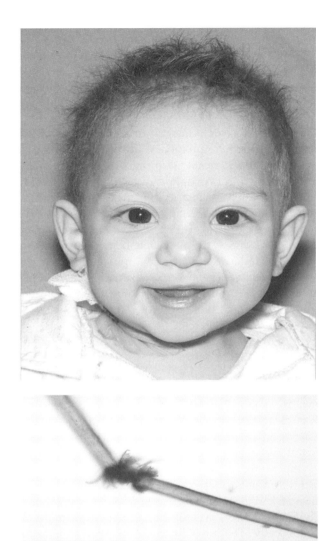

B

Fig. 1. Phenotypic diarrhoea. (A) Characteristic facies; (B) trichorrhexis nodosa.

easily removed hair with trichorrhexis nodosa (Fig. 1).[5] Antibody responses are often defective. Small bowel biopsy shows moderate-to-severe villous atrophy. The diarrhoea, which is of unknown cause, is intractable and intestinal failure-associated liver disease is common. Death before the age of 5 years is frequent but not invariable.

IPEX SYNDROME

IPEX (immune dysregulation, polyendocrinopathy, enteropathy, X-linked) is a rare disorder presenting most commonly in infancy with protracted diarrhoea, icthyosiform dermatitis, insulin-dependent diabetes mellitus, thyroiditis and haemolytic anaemia.[6] The disorder is caused by mutations in the *FOXP3* gene, which is essential for the development of regulatory T-cells. The *FOXP3* gene encodes a DNA-binding protein of the fork head/winged-helix family, and is central to the control of the development of CD4[+] CD25[+] regulatory T-cells, a deficiency of which causes increased immunological reactivity and autoimmunity.

Presentation is usually at birth or in the first few weeks of life, with type 1 diabetes mellitus and an enteropathy, manifesting as a secretory diarrhoea or ileus. Diabetes probably results from inflammatory destruction of islet cells, rather than islet cell agenesis. Growth retardation, which may begin antenatally, and malnutrition are prominent features. Sepsis is common and the disorder is usually fatal. A variety of immunosuppressive regimens have been used (high-dose steroids, cyclosporin A, tacrolimus and serolimus) with varying success in addition to supportive measures such as parenteral nutrition, insulin, and blood transfusion.

Given the immunological basis of IPEX, bone marrow transplantation has been advocated as a treatment. An allogeneic bone marrow transplantation from an HLA-identical family member in a 4-month-old patient resulted in complete remission which was sustained for 2 years before the patient died of an unexplained, rapidly progressive haemophagocytic syndrome.[7] Successful bone marrow transplant in four patients using reduced-intensity conditioning has recently been reported.[8]

AUTOIMMUNE ENTEROPATHY

Goulet et al.[5] described 24 infants with intractable diarrhoea and persistent villous atrophy, in whom gut auto-antibodies were present. A severe enteropathy was characteristic, with infiltration of the lamina propria by mononuclear cells and crypt hyperplasia.[5] Several patients had a protein losing enteropathy and gastric/colonic involvement was common. Half the patients had symptomatic evidence of extra-intestinal disease – arthritis, diabetes, dermatitis, thrombocytopenia, and renal disease.

There was a variable, and sometimes absent, response to immunosuppressive treatment including steroids, cyclosporin, cyclophosphamide, Infliximab, tacrolimus or azathioprine. The use of immunosuppressive treatment needs to be balanced against the increased risk of infection as many of the patients remain on long-term parenteral nutrition.

MOTILITY DISORDERS

CHRONIC INTESTINAL PSEUDO-OBSTRUCTION

This is a heterogeneous group of disorders in which functional, rather than mechanical, obstruction is present as a result of enteric neuronal diseases involving lengthy segments of gut.[9] The underlying pathology can be a smooth muscle myopathy or enteric neuropathy. Associated malrotation, congenital shortening of the small intestine or involvement of the urinary tract are common.

Most children present in the newborn period, although a quarter develop symptoms after 1 year of age. Intestinal failure requiring long-term parenteral nutrition is common, particularly in patients with malrotation, short small bowel, urinary tract abnormalities or a myopathic histology.

Table 1 Causes of short bowel syndrome

Necrotising enterocolitis	27%
Congenital atresias	23%
Volvulus	23%
Gastroschisis	14%
Hirschsprung's disease	4%
Other	4%

Adapted from Koffeman *et al. Best Pract Res Clin Gastroenterol* 2003; **17**: 879–893.

Intestinal aganglionosis

An important sub-group of patients with pseudo-obstruction have total intestinal aganglionosis, resulting from a failure of migration of new neural crest cells into the gut during embryonic life. It presents with severe pseudo-obstruction and without parenteral nutrition support is rapidly fatal. Whilst it is currently incurable, the ability to transplant the enteric nervous system is becoming a realistic possibility. In the experimental animal, autologous transplantation can be used to treat aganglionosis by implanting stem cells derived from the neural crest.[10]

SHORT BOWEL SYNDROME

Short bowel syndrome can be defined as the intestinal failure which results from massive resection of the small intestine. Implicit in the definition is severe nutrient, water and electrolyte malabsorption and a dependence on parenteral nutrition. Most cases originate in the newborn period (Table 1) and result from congenital anomalies or severe necrotising enterocolitis requiring extensive resection. For reasons that are poorly understood, gastroschisis has increased in frequency over the last 15 years, with most of the increase in babies born to younger mothers (CMO Report 2004 <http://www.dh.gov.uk/cmo>).

The epidemiology of neonatal short bowel syndrome has recently been defined.[11] In a careful study from Toronto, the overall incidence of short bowel syndrome was 22.1 per 1000 neonatal intensive care unit admissions and 24.5 per

Table 2 Factors determining clinical effects of small intestinal resection

Jejunal versus ileal resection
        Less jejunal than ileal adaptation
        Large volume, isotonic losses following ileal resection
        Greater reduction in transit time following ileal resection
        Specialised sites of absorption in ileum
Loss of ileocaecal valve
        Adversely affects prognosis
Co-existent small intestinal disease
        Post-necrotising enterocolitis injury
        Crohn's disease
Disease/resection of colon
Co-existent liver or pancreatic disease

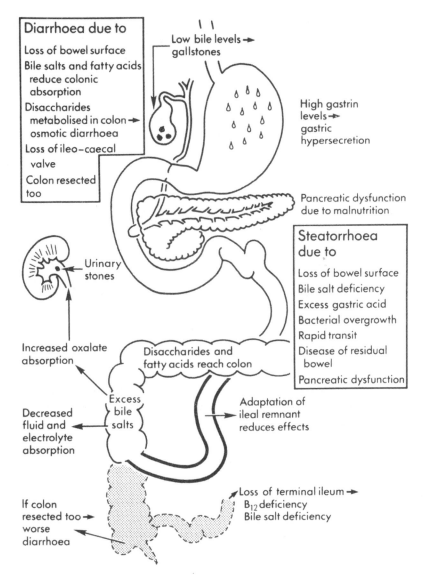

Fig. 2. Consequences of massive small intestinal resection. Reproduced, with permission, from Green *et al. Nutrition* 1992; **8**: 186–190.

100,000 live births. As expected, the incidence was much higher in premature infants. Necrotising enterocolitis accounted for about one-third of cases.

Short bowel syndrome is a disorder associated with high morbidity, is potentially lethal, and often requires months, sometimes years, in hospital on parenteral nutrition. A number of factors will determine the overall clinical effect (Table 2). Moreover, massive small bowel resection causes wide-spread disruption to normal gastrointestinal physiology (Fig. 2).

Fortunately, the small intestine has a large functional reserve, and 40–50% can usually be resected without major metabolic or nutritional sequelae.[12] However, if more than 75% is lost, nutritional status and growth can only usually be maintained with parenteral nutrition. In practice, prolonged parenteral nutrition is uncommon when more than 80 cm of small intestine remains following surgery in the newborn period. Even when less than 40 cm is present, long-term survival without parenteral nutrition occurs in 94% of infants.[13] The major effects of short bowel syndrome are summarised in Table 2.

Post-resection adaptation

Adaptation is the term applied to the progressive recovery from intestinal failure that follows a loss of intestinal length. There is a gradual increase in the tolerance of enteral nutrition allowing intravenous nutritional support to be slowly reduced whilst still maintaining adequate growth. During adaptation, the intestine dilates, lengthens and thickens. The villi become longer and the crypts deepen with more cells in the proliferative zone.

A number of factors promote intestinal adaptation, most notably the presence of nutrients in the intestinal lumen. More recently, experimental interventions using growth-promoting peptides and hormones have been tried as a means of enhancing adaptation. Of these, glucagon-like peptide 2 (GLP-2) appears to be the most promising.[14] In addition to marked effects in the experimental animal, GLP-2 has beneficial effects in humans with short bowel syndrome.

Recently, R-spondin-1 has been identified as a potent stimulant to intestinal growth in the experimental animal.[15] R-spondin-1 knock-in mice have dramatically enlarged intestines, and administration of R-spondin-1 abrogates the deleterious effects of parenteral fluorouracil on the gut. Elaboration of the balance between promotion of gastrointestinal epithelial growth and healing on the one hand, and neoplasia and access growth on the other, is required before the therapeutic effects of R-spondin-1 can be tested in man.

MANAGEMENT OF SHORT BOWEL SYNDROME

The place of a multidisciplinary nutritional care team

The observation that patients with intestinal failure have better outcomes when cared for by a nutritional care team is not a new observation. Recent data confirm our earlier observation that children with intestinal failure referred for consideration of small bowel transplant are in better condition and have a significantly better prognosis when referred from a nutritional care team.[16]

The role of enteral nutrition

A defined formula comprising a protein hydrolysate, glucose polymer and a long/medium chain triglyceride mixture is usually started if there is no supply of breast milk (*e.g.* Pregestimil Mead Johnson; Pepdite 0-2 [SHS]). The volume is increased to the limit of tolerance, which is usually defined by the onset of diarrhoea or large nasogastric aspirates.

Carbohydrate intolerance

The onset of diarrhoea following increases in the hourly volume of defined formula is usually caused by glucose polymer intolerance.[17] This reflects the absence of pancreatic amylase in the first 6–12 months of life, and insufficient small intestinal mucosal glucomylase activity to hydrolyse glucose polymer. It is more common when: (i) only 15–50 cm of small intestine remain; (ii) following necrotising enterocolitis, when mucosal damage may be severe; or (iii) when the colon is resected or not in continuity.

Modular feeds

When feed intolerance, particularly carbohydrate intolerance, is a problem, a modular feed may be successful in avoiding parenteral nutrition, as it allows the individual components of the feed to be varied independently and tailored to the tolerances of the individual patient. For example, in glucose polymer intolerance, alternative carbohydrates may be substituted which use different hydrolytic mechanisms and absorptive pathways. Thus, patients who develop sugary-osmotic diarrhoea on a feed containing 8 g/100 ml glucose polymer, may tolerate a modular feed containing 6 g/100 ml polymer plus 2 g/100 ml sucrose.

PROGNOSIS IN SHORT BOWEL SYNDROME

Accurate definition of the prognosis is difficult because of marked differences between studies in defining the population at risk and in defining the cases. A recent study from Toronto tends to confirm the suspicion that survival rates reported from tertiary gastroenterology centres may be artificially high; some babies with short bowel syndrome do not survive for long enough to be referred to a tertiary centre.[18] In a study enrolling neonatal subjects for 3 years in the late 1990s and followed up for 18 months after entry to the study closed, the overall mortality rate was 37.5%.[19] This figure contrasts sharply with long-term survival figures reported from tertiary centres of well over 80%.[20]

Goulet et al.[21] have recently reported long-term outcomes in 87 children who underwent extensive neonatal small bowel resection. They point out that

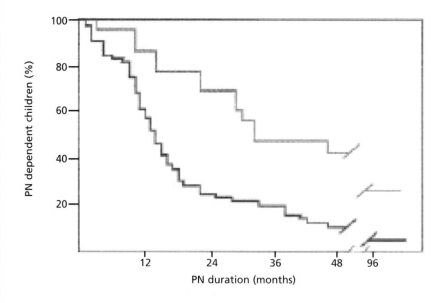

Fig. 3 Presence of ileocaecal valve is associated with a shorter duration of parenteral nutrition. Reproduced, with permission, from Goulet et al. Eur J Pediatr Surg 2005; **15**: 95–101.

Table 3 Non-transplant surgical techniques in the management of short bowel syndrome.

Adequate length of bowel and who have stomas and/or on-going primary pathology

    Maximal use of existing bowel
        Closure of stomas
        Closure of enterocutaneous fistula
        Relief of obstruction or blind loop

    Improving propulsion of dilated bowel
        Tapering procedure
        Intestinal plication

Dilated segments of bowel with preserved hepatic function

    Delaying transit
        Reversing intestinal segments
        Colon interposition between a divided proximal jejunum

    Bowel lengthening procedures
        Longitudinal intestinal lengthening procedure or Bianchi procedure
        Serial transverse enteroplasty procedure

---

the prognosis has improved substantially over the last 20 years. Indeed, of their cohort born between 1995 and 1991, overall survival was 90% (72% pre-1985; 96% survival after 1985). They also emphasised the importance of the ileocaecal valve and the length of residual small intestine in determining the duration of parenteral nutrition that is required (Fig. 3).

NON-TRANSPLANT SURGERY

A variety of innovative techniques for improving intestinal adaptation by performing non-transplant surgery have been described. Current surgical approach aims to maximise residual function of the bowel by the simplest procedure. The non-transplant surgical techniques can be divided into four categories depending on the length of residual bowel (Table 3).[22,23]

The timing of the successful surgical intervention is crucial in the overall management of short bowel syndrome.[23] A careful evaluation of the severity of liver disease and portal hypertension is necessary before any non-transplant surgical procedure. Children with intestinal failure and advanced liver disease, portal hypertension, ascites and coagulopathy are best treated with liver–small bowel transplantation, as non-transplant surgery may accelerate the progression of intestinal failure associated liver disease.

Bianchi et al.[23] described the cumulative experience of longitudinal intestinal lengthening technique or Bianchi procedure in various centres (Fig. 4).[23] Of particular relevance is the observation that an intestinal lengthening procedure does not reverse the progression of liver damage due to intestinal failure associated liver disease and, in fact, might cause progression leading to early onset liver failure and death if not transplanted.

The serial transverse enteroplasty procedure recently described[24] is a novel technique of increasing intestinal length (Fig. 5). The suggested advantages to serial transverse enteroplasty are: (i) reduced risk of bowel complications, as

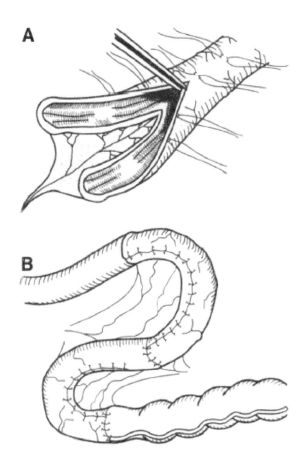

Fig. 4 Longitudinal intestinal lengthening technique or Bianchi procedure.(A) Because the mesenteric blood vessels enter the small bowel loop along its lateral aspects, it is possible to divide the dilated bowel longitudinally in the midline along the mesenteric and antemesenteric borders and to create two fully vascularised isopropulsive hemiloops. (B) The two bowel loops are anastomosed isoperistaltically. Reproduced, with permission, from Bianchi A. *Gastroenterology* 2006; **130**: S138–S146.

the staple lines are not continuous and the dissection along the anti-mesenteric border is avoided; (ii) there is no anastomosis between the segments and hence less chance of strictures; (iii) it can be performed when smaller segments require dilatation; and (iv) it can be performed on segments of bowel which have become dilated following a Bianchi procedure. Importantly, long-term data regarding the serial transverse enteroplasty procedure are not yet available.

The largest, single-centre experience with the Bianchi (n = 40) and serial transverse enteroplasty procedure (n = 31) is from Omaha between 1982 to 2006 (Deb Sudan, personal communication). Survival at a median follow-up of 3.7 years is 94% overall (Bianchi, 93%; serial transverse enteroplasty procedure, 97%). Of patients, 60% were off total parenteral nutrition at most recent follow-up. Intestinal transplantation salvage was required in 10% of patients at a median of 3.1 years (range, 1.3–5.6 years) after lengthening.

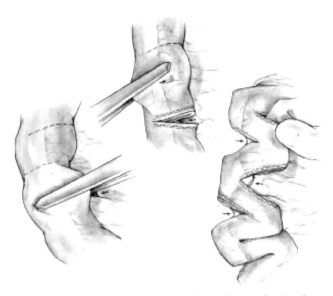

Fig. 5 The serial transverse enteroplasty procedure relies on the simple anatomical principle that the blood supply to the small bowel travels from the mesentery and traverses the bowel perpendicular to its long axis. In the procedure, special devices are used to cut and staple the bowel simultaneously in a direction parallel to this plane. Immediately after the serial transverse enteroplasty procedure, the small bowel has a 'zigzag' appearance from these staples lines. Reproduced from Kim HB et al. *J Pediatr Surg* 2003; **38**: 881–885 © 2003 Elsevier with permission.

COMPLICATIONS RELATED TO PARENTERAL NUTRITION

Impaired venous access

The use of central venous catheters, though useful in the long-term administration of parenteral nutrition, are associated with mechanical complications, infection and thrombosis. The associated morbidity, mortality, risks and quality of life issues associated with the complications necessitate the need for involvement of a specialised nutritional care team.[25] The role of the nutritional care team is not only in minimising the incidence of catheter-related blood-stream infections, but in delivering effective treatment and deciding about the timing of line removal and insertion.[26]

The Seldinger technique of line insertion under ultrasound guidance by an interventional radiologist/skilled paediatric surgeon/transplant anaesthetist is the preferred technique at our institution to a venotomy in maintaining long-term central venous access.[27] There is not enough evidence in the literature, at present, to support the use of prophylactic anticoagulation therapy to minimise thrombosis.[28] When conventional sites of venous access are lost, techniques of accessing the superior vena cava using intra-atrial and trans-lumbar line insertion have been described.[29]

Intestinal failure associated liver disease

The term intestinal failure associated liver disease replaces the old terminology of parenteral nutrition associated liver disease or total parenteral nutrition liver disease. It is a more appropriate term as it emphasises that liver disease

Table 4 Risk factors responsible for intestinal failure associated liver disease

Prematurity and low birth-weight

Multiple laparotomies

Duration of parenteral nutrition

Lack of enteral feeding

Recurrent central venous catheter infections

Components of parenteral nutrition
        Choline deficiency
        Taurine deficiency
        Carnitine deficiency
        Glutamine deficiency
        Aluminium overlaod
        High dextrose concentrations (> 16 g/kg/day)
        Excess lipids (> 3 g/kg/day)

in children with intestinal failure is due to a combination of factors, rather than due to parenteral nutrition alone. Intestinal failure associated liver disease is defined as 'the development of hepatobiliary dysfunction as a consequence of medical and surgical management strategies for intestinal failure which can variably progress to end-stage liver disease or can be stabilised or reversed with promotion of intestinal adaptation'.

The exact incidence of intestinal failure associated liver disease is not known, but a 15–85% incidence has been variably quoted in the literature. Cavicchi *et al.*[30] have described the incidence of chronic cholestasis and complicated liver disease in 90 patients (aged 6–77 years; median age, 45 years) as 55% and 26% at 2 years, 64% and 39% at 4 years and 72% and 50% at 6 years, respectively. The exact reason for development of liver disease in children with long-term parenteral nutrition is not known, but is believed to be multifactorial (Table 4). Beath *et al.*[31] analysed 74 post-surgical neonates started on parenteral nutrition following birth to determine the risk factors for developing liver disease. Episodes of catheter sepsis, low gestational age and exposure to parenteral nutrition were found to be significant factors.[31] Each episode of catheter sepsis produced a 30% rise in serum bilirubin. Sondheimer *et al.*[32] described the importance of early line infection as a contributing factor to end-stage liver disease. Small bowel bacterial overgrowth may also be a contributing factor to the development of intestinal failure associated liver disease. Bacterial endotoxin and inducible pro-inflammatory mediators such as tumour necrosis factor probably stimulate *de novo* fatty acid and triglyceride synthesis resulting in steatosis and liver disease.[33] The gold standard for the diagnosis of small bowel bacterial overgrowth is culture of jejunal secretions, but may not be always possible and other surrogate tests are not as useful in establishing the diagnosis. A high index of clinical suspicion and a trial with a cyclical course (treatment course of 3 weeks followed by 1–2 weeks of no treatment) of oral selective decontamination agents in various combinations (*e.g.* colistin [1.5 megaunits PO tds]; gentamicin [2.5 mg/kg/dose tds]; tobramycin [20–80 mg four times a day]; amphotericin [100,000 units tds]) to assess improvement should, therefore, be considered.[34]

Table 5 Medical and surgical management strategies for children with intestinal failure associated liver disease

---

Encourage enteral feeding

Adjustment of the calories and the lipid intake in parenteral nutrition

Cycling of parenteral nutrition

Early discharge on home parenteral nutrition

Treatment of small bowel bacterial overgrowth

Meticulous care of the catheter to prevent catheter-related blood-stream infections

Treatment with ursodeoxycholic acid (20–30 mg/kg/day)

Barium studies to exclude obstruction or assess the motility and distension of the bowel
> Reversal of the stoma
> Non-transplant surgery, e.g. intestinal lengthening procedures, serial transverse enteroplasty procedure to promote intestinal adaptation

Transplantation
> Isolated liver transplantation
> Intestinal transplantation

Abdominal ultrasound to assess the direction of portal flow along with the degree of splenomegaly is an important non-invasive investigation in determining the progression of intestinal failure associated liver disease. In our experience, oesophageal varices are frequently absent even in children with advanced intestinal failure associated liver disease, unlike children with advanced primary liver disease. Prompt recognition of advancing intestinal failure associated liver disease (progressive rise in serum bilirubin, progressive splenomegaly, development of ascites) is necessary for an early referral to an intestinal transplant centre. Isolated liver transplantation can be considered: (i) in a select subgroup of children with intestinal failure associated liver disease and small bowel syndrome, where the residual bowel has the potential to adapt; (ii) when adequate evidence that progression of intestinal failure associated liver disease and portal hypertension has prevented intestinal adaptation is documented; and (iii) there is a lack of recurrent episodes of catheter sepsis.[35] The management strategies for intestinal failure associated liver disease are outlined in Table 5.

INTESTINAL TRANSPLANTATION

Intestinal transplantation is no longer an experimental treatment, but has evolved in the last decade as a well-established treatment for children and adults with complications of intestinal failure. The Intestinal Transplant Registry (a central database collecting information on all the intestinal transplants performed world-wide in children and adults) documents that more than 1500 small bowel transplants have been performed world-wide. The indications and contra-indications for intestinal transplantation are outlined in Tables 6 and 7.[36]

TYPE OF TRANSPLANT

Children with intestinal failure and mild intestinal failure associated liver disease can be offered an isolated intestinal transplant, while children with

Table 6 Indications for intestinal transplantation

Irreversible intestinal failure and **one of the following**
- Impaired venous access (reduced to two suitable veins for placement of feeding catheters)
- Progressive liver disease with coagulopathy, ascites and encephalopathy
- Life-threatening episodes of catheter sepsis

Table 7 Contra-indications to intestinal transplantation

Absolute contra-indications
- Profound neurological disabilities
- Life-threatening and other irreversible disease not related to the digestive system
- Non-resectable malignancies

Relative contra-indications
- Severe congenital or acquired immunological deficiencies
- Multisystem autoimmune diseases
- Insufficient vascular patency to guarantee vascular access for up to 6 months after transplant
- Chronic lung disease of prematurity

intestinal failure and moderate-to-severe intestinal failure associated liver disease can be offered a combined liver and small bowel transplant. Children with foregut dysmotility will need inclusion of donor stomach or a partial gastrectomy with a jejunogastrostomy.[36]

PROGNOSIS OF INTESTINAL TRANSPLANTATION

The poor outcome following intestinal transplantation in the 1990s was due to the complications of acute rejection and opportunistic infections (cytomegalovirus, Epstein-Barr virus related post-transplant lymphoproliferative disease, *etc.*). In the past, acute rejection was reported in approximately 90% of the intestinal transplant recipients. With the greater use of tacrolimus and introduction of newer induction agents like IL-2 blockers (monocolonal antibodies to CD25) and rabbit antithymocyte globulin, the incidence of acute rejection has dramatically decreased.[2] The easy availability of techniques such as polymerase chain reaction to monitor viral load, has resulted in early diagnosis and treatment of opportunistic infections.

Constant improvements in the surgical techniques during the last two decades have also contributed to the improved outcome (Fig. 6).[37] There is a high mortality of children (predominantly less than 10 kg in weight) on the waiting list for a transplant due to the shortage of size-matched donor organs. Reduction techniques (excision of the right lobe of the liver and mid-small bowel) and pretransplant abdominal expanders are some of the techniques used in our unit so that organs from older donors can be transplanted into children. Living-related intestinal transplantation has recently been practised in some centres, but does not offer any immunological benefits over cadaveric transplantation.

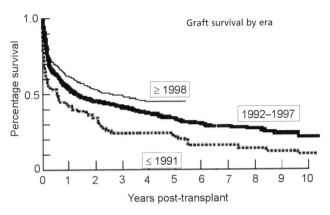

Fig. 6 Graft survival rates after intestine transplantation have significantly improved over time (*P* < 0.001) as per data from the Intestinal Transplant Registry. Reproduced, with permission, from Grant *et al. Ann Surg* 2005; **241**: 607–613.

In a study on quality of life in children following intestinal transplantation, the children rated their quality of life as comparable to that of healthy, school-going children, whereas the parents of transplanted children exhibited a higher level of anxiety as compared to the parents of healthy children.[38]

The catch-up growth following intestinal transplantation is less than that seen following liver transplantation. This is probably due to the severity of the illness in the pretransplant period and the high intensity of immunosuppression seen in the post-transplant period.[2]

In the UK, the Birmingham Children's Hospital is the single designated centre for paediatric intestinal transplantation and 46 intestinal transplants have been performed with 23 transplants being done in the last 4 years. Results have improved with current 1-year survival of 70% and 4-year survival of 62%.

Key points for clinical practice

- Recent increases of gastroschisis in the UK, advances in neonatal intensive care and surgical techniques, long-term survival on home parenteral nutrition and the prospect of improved survival following small bowel transplantation are all likely to result in an increased incidence of intestinal failure in the future.

- The causes of intestinal failure can be divided into three categories – enteropathies, motility disorders, and short bowel syndrome.

- Short bowel syndrome can be defined as the intestinal failure which results from massive resection of the small intestine. Most cases originate in the newborn period and result from congenital anomalies or severe necrotising enterocolitis requiring extensive resection.

- The small intestine has a large functional reserve, and 40–50% can usually be resected without major metabolic or nutritional sequelae. However, if more than 75% is lost, nutritional status and growth can only usually be maintained with parenteral nutrition.

Key points for clinical practice *(continued)*

- Children with short bowel syndrome have the greatest potential to wean from long-term parenteral nutrition.

- Children with short bowel syndrome demonstrating poor feed tolerance should have a trial of modular feeds under the supervision of a experienced paediatric dietitian.

- Exciting discoveries of new humoral and mucosal growth factors in the promotion of intestinal adaptation will play a crucial role in the future in weaning the children from parenteral nutrition.

- Multidisciplinary team management of children with intestinal failure is essential to decide about the optimal timing of non-transplant surgery and prevention of complications related to intestinal failure.

- Early recognition of progressive intestinal failure associated liver disease (serum bilirubin > 100 µmol/l sustained for few weeks) should prompt referral for intestinal transplantation.

- Intestinal transplantation is a well-established treatment option for children with complications related to management of irreversible intestinal failure.

References

1. Goulet O, Ruemmele F. Causes and management of intestinal failure in children. *Gastroenterology* 2006; **130**: S16–S28.
2. Gupte GL, Beath SV, Kelly DA, Millar AJ, Booth IW. Current issues in the management of intestinal failure. *Arch Dis Child* 2006; **91**: 259–264.
3. Murch SH. Toward a molecular understanding of complex childhood enteropathies. *J Pediatr Gastroenterol Nutr* 2002; **34 (Suppl 1)**: S4–S10.
4. Goulet O, Ruemmele F, Lacaille F, Colomb V. Irreversible intestinal failure. *J Pediatr Gastroenterol Nutr* 2004; **38**: 250–269.
5. Goulet OJ, Brousse N, Canioni D, Walker-Smith JA, Schmitz J, Phillips AD. Syndrome of intractable diarrhoea with persistent villous atrophy in early childhood: a clinicopathological survey of 47 cases. *J Pediatr Gastroenterol Nutr* 1998; **26**: 151–161.
6. Wildin RS, Freitas A. IPEX and FOXP3: clinical and research perspectives. *J Autoimmun* 2005; **25 (Suppl)**: 56–62.
7. Baud O, Goulet O, Canioni D *et al*. Treatment of the immune dysregulation, polyendocrinopathy, enteropathy, X-linked syndrome (IPEX) by allogeneic bone marrow transplantation. *N Engl J Med* 2001; **344**: 1758–1762.
8. Rao A, Kamani N, Filipovich A *et al*. Successful bone marrow transplantation for IPEX syndrome after reduced-intensity conditioning. *Blood* 2007; **109**: 383–385.
9. Connor FL, Di Lorenzo C. Chronic intestinal pseudo-obstruction: assessment and management. *Gastroenterology* 2006; **130**: S29–S36.
10. Gershon MD. Transplanting the enteric nervous system: a step closer to treatment for aganglionosis. *Gut* 2007; **56**: 459–461.
11. Wales PW, De Silva N, Kim J, Lecce L, To T, Moore A. Neonatal short bowel syndrome: population-based estimates of incidence and mortality rates. *J Pediatr Surg* 2004; **39**: 690–695.
12. Jeejeebhoy KN. Therapy of the short-gut syndrome. *Lancet* 1983; **1**: 1427–1430.
13. Goulet OJ, Revillon Y, Jan D *et al*. Neonatal short bowel syndrome. *J Pediatr* 1991; **119**: 18–23.
14. Jeppesen PB. Clinical significance of GLP-2 in short-bowel syndrome. *J Nutr* 2003; **133**: 3721–3724.

15. Abraham C, Cho JH. Inducing intestinal growth. *N Engl J Med* 2005; **353**: 2297–2299.
16. Gupte GL, Beath SV, Protheroe S *et al*. Improved outcome of referrals for intestinal transplantation in the UK. *Arch Dis Child* 2007; **92**: 147–152.
17. Ameen VZ, Powell GK, Jones LA. Quantitation of fecal carbohydrate excretion in patients with short bowel syndrome. *Gastroenterology* 1987; **92**: 493–500.
18. Wales PW, De Silva N, Kim JH, Lecce L, Sandhu A, Moore AM. Neonatal short bowel syndrome: a cohort study. *J Pediatr Surg* 2005; **40**: 755–762.
19. Beath SV, Needham SJ, Kelly DA *et al*. Clinical features and prognosis of children assessed for isolated small bowel or combined small bowel and liver transplantation. *J Pediatr Surg* 1997; **32**: 459–461.
20. Keller J, Panter H, Layer P. Management of the short bowel syndrome after extensive small bowel resection. *Best Pract Res Clin Gastroenterol* 2004; **18**: 977–992.
21. Goulet O, Baglin-Gobet S, Talbotec C *et al*. Outcome and long-term growth after extensive small bowel resection in the neonatal period: a survey of 87 children. *Eur J Pediatr Surg* 2005; **15**: 95–101.
22. Sudan D, Dibaise J, Torres C *et al*. A multidisciplinary approach to the treatment of intestinal failure. *J Gastrointest Surg* 2005; **9**: 165–177.
23. Bianchi A. From the cradle to enteral autonomy: the role of autologous gastrointestinal reconstruction. *Gastroenterology* 2006; **130**: S138–S146.
24. Modi BP, Javid PJ, Jaksic T *et al*. First Report of the International Serial Transverse Enteroplasty Data Registry: Indications, Efficacy, and Complications. *J Am Coll Surg* 2007; **204**: 365–371.
25. Agostoni C, Axelson I, Colomb V *et al*. The need for nutrition support teams in pediatric units: a commentary by the ESPGHAN committee on nutrition. *J Pediatr Gastroenterol Nutr* 2005; **41**: 8–11.
26. Gupte GL, Beath SV, Protheroe S *et al*. Improved outcome of referrals for intestinal transplantation in the UK. *Arch Dis Child* 2007; **92**: 147–152.
27. Gann Jr M, Sardi A. Improved results using ultrasound guidance for central venous access. *Am Surg* 2003; **69**: 1104–1107.
28. Linenberger ML. Catheter-related thrombosis: risks, diagnosis, and management. *J Natl Compr Cancer Netw* 2006; **4**: 889–901.
29. Mehta C, De Giovanni J, Sharif K, Gupte GL. Stereotactic technique of catheter placement in the stump of the superior vena cava in children with impaired venous access. *J Vasc Intervent Radiol* 2006; **17**: 2005–2009.
30. Cavicchi M, Beau P, Crenn P, Degott C, Messing B. Prevalence of liver disease and contributing factors in patients receiving home parenteral nutrition for permanent intestinal failure. *Ann Intern Med* 2000; **132**: 525–532.
31. Beath SV, Davies P, Papadopoulou A *et al*. Parenteral nutrition-related cholestasis in postsurgical neonates: multivariate analysis of risk factors. *J Pediatr Surg* 1996; **31**: 604–606.
32. Sondheimer JM, Asturias E, Cadnapaphornchai M. Infection and cholestasis in neonates with intestinal resection and long-term parenteral nutrition. *J Pediatr Gastroenterol Nutr* 1998; **27**: 131–137.
33. Kaufman SS, Loseke CA, Lupo JV *et al*. Influence of bacterial overgrowth and intestinal inflammation on duration of parenteral nutrition in children with short bowel syndrome. *J Pediatr* 1997; **131**: 356–361.
34. Quigley EM, Quera R. Small intestinal bacterial overgrowth: roles of antibiotics, prebiotics, and probiotics. *Gastroenterology* 2006; **130**: S78–S90.
35. Botha JF, Grant WJ, Torres C *et al*. Isolated liver transplantation in infants with end-stage liver disease due to short bowel syndrome. *Liver Transpl* 2006; **12**: 1062–1066.
36. Kaufman SS, Atkinson JB, Bianchi A *et al*. Indications for pediatric intestinal transplantation: a position paper of the American Society of Transplantation. *Pediatr Transplant* 2001; **5**: 80–87.
37. Grant D, Abu-Elmagd K, Reyes J *et al*. 2003 report of the intestine transplant registry: a new era has dawned. *Ann Surg* 2005; **241**: 607–613.
38. Sudan D, Horslen S, Botha J *et al*. Quality of life after pediatric intestinal transplantation: the perception of pediatric recipients and their parents. *Am J Transplant* 2004; **4**: 407–413.

5

The dangers of re-feeding

Re-feeding a malnourished patient may appear to be straight forward – just give them the calories they need and they will start to put on weight. However, there is real danger in re-feeding as the body adjusts from its patho-physiological starved or semi-starved state. This chapter will highlight these dangers and suggest approaches to prevent the potentially fatal complications of re-feeding syndrome.

WHAT IS RE-FEEDING SYNDROME?

Re-feeding syndrome represents a number of different metabolic complications that sometimes result when feeding a malnourished patient. Although hypophosphataemia is the most common complication of re-feeding syndrome, it is now acknowledged that the syndrome encompasses many other metabolic consequences including abnormalities of potassium, magnesium, glucose and fluid balance. A broader definition is, therefore:

> *Re-feeding syndrome is a potentially lethal condition defined as severe electrolyte and fluid shifts with metabolic abnormalities in malnourished patients undergoing re-feeding orally, enterally or parenterally.*
>
> Crook et al.[1]

EVIDENCE FOR THE EXISTENCE OF RE-FEEDING SYNDROME

Evidence for the existence of the syndrome first came to light from prisoners of the Japanese and victims of the Leningrad and Dutch famines during World War II. When liberated prisoners and civilians were provided with food after a

Loveday Jane Jago MBBS MRCPCH
Paediatric Gastroenterology Specialist Registrar, Booth Hall Children's Hospital, Charlestown Road, Blackley, Manchester M9 7AA, UK
E-mail: loveday@doctors.org.uk

period of prolonged starvation, many suffered from hypertension, peripheral oedema, cardiac failure, and sudden death.[2]

In 1950, Keys et al.[3] conducted 'the Minnesota experiment', which looked at the effect of drastic food restriction and subsequent oral re-feeding in previously healthy subjects. They found that, in subjects who had undergone 6 months of starvation, there was no evidence of dyspnoea, increased venous pressure or cardiac dilatation. However, during the recovery phase, as the volunteers were re-fed the cardiovascular reserve was diminished to the point where cardiac failure occurred in some.

As total parenteral nutrition was introduced in the 1970s, severe complications of re-feeding were rediscovered. A pivotal paper in 1981 by Weinsier and Krumdieck[4] described how the overzealous administration of total parenteral nutrition in two chronically malnourished, but stable, patients led to the precipitation of deterioration in their clinical status. Both patients were given aggressive total parenteral nutrition support, which was rapidly followed by acute cardiopulmonary decompensation associated with severe hypophosphataemia and other metabolic abnormalities. Despite attempts at correction, progressive multiple-systems failure led to death.

Reports of re-feeding syndrome in children are rare; in the industrialised world most cases are adolescents with anorexia nervosa.

Afzal et al.[5] performed a systematic literature review of the cases of re-feeding syndrome reported with enteral nutrition in children. This revealed eight published case reports with a total of 27 children (aged < 18 years) with a diagnosis of re-feeding syndrome made by a fall in phosphate levels after the onset of enteral re-feeding. The underlying diagnoses were kwashiorkor ($n = 14$) anorexia nervosa ($n = 5$) neurological disease and neglect ($n = 3$) and not recorded ($n = 5$). They also reported what they believed to be the first case of re-feeding syndrome in an adolescent with newly diagnosed Crohn's disease, which developed within a few days of starting exclusive polymeric enteral nutrition.

In our paediatric gastroenterology unit, we have seen several children with Crohn's disease who have presented significantly under weight for height and have demonstrated electrolyte disturbances consistent with re-feeding syndrome during the first week of commencing enteral feeds.

WHO IS AT RISK OF THE RE-FEEDING SYNDROME?

Generally, any patient who has been chronically deprived of adequate nutrition is at risk of re-feeding syndrome. This includes any patient unfed in 7–10 days with evidence of stress and depletion, prolonged fasting and prolonged intravenous hydration. There are certain other categories of patients who should be considered especially 'at risk'. Table 1 lists some of the categories of patients who are considered to be especially at risk of re-feeding syndrome.

MALNUTRITION

Malnutrition remains one of the most common causes of morbidity and mortality among children throughout the world. Approximately 9% of

Table 1 Categories of patients at risk of re-feeding syndrome

•   Chronic malnutrition-underfeeding
•   Marasmus
•   Kwashiorkor
•   Anorexia nervosa
•   Chronic alcoholism
•   Morbid obesity with massive weight loss

children below 5 years of age suffer from wasting (weight for height below –2 standard deviations of National Centre for Health Statistics/World Health Organization [WHO] reference ranges) and are at risk of death or severe impairment of growth and psychological development.[6] Severe malnutrition in infants is common in areas with insufficient food, inadequate knowledge of feeding techniques or poor hygiene. Malnutrition can be divided into three clinical subtypes: (i) marasmus; (ii) kwashiorkor; and (iii) marasmus/kwashiorkor.

Marasmus results from insufficient calorie intake and is characterised by emaciation. Kwashiorkor results from severe deficiency of protein and energy intake and is also known as immunosuppressive or hypoalbuminaemic malnutrition. Oedema is characteristic of kwashiorkor. Children may also present with a mixed picture of marasmus and kwashiorkor. The WHO now uses the more general term of protein-energy malnutrition, as distinctions between the clinical subtypes are probably unnecessary as the approach to treatment is similar.

Malnourished children in both developing and developed countries are at risk of re-feeding syndrome. Manary et al.,[7] in 1998, studied 68 children (aged < 10 years) with kwashiorkor admitted to a hospital in Malawi. Severe hypophosphataemia (serum concentration < 0.32 mmol/l) occurred in 8 (12%) within 48 h of admission. Five out of these 8 children died compared with 13 of 60 (22%) without severe hypophosphataemia.

Malnutrition in the developed world is often multifactorial and may be intentional or unintentional. Kellogg et al.[8] described the clinical findings and legal outcomes of 12 prosecuted cases of infant and child starvation. All survivors manifested complications with re-feeding. All required phosphate supplements during hospitalisation. Children who required more than 10 days' hospitalisation had difficulties with diarrhoea, hyperglycaemia resulting from insulin suppression, and fluid overload manifested by oedema or congestive heart failure.

ANOREXIA NERVOSA

Anorexia nervosa is one of the most common forms of malnutrition observed in Western societies in individuals without physical disease, with an average mortality of 20% in young people aged 15–25 years.[9] Adolescents with anorexia undergo intentional starvation and extreme weight loss. Re-feeding syndrome is well described in adolescents with anorexia nervosa; studies indicate that re-feeding syndrome can result from the use of oral, parenteral or enteral nutrition.[10]

Table 2 National Collaborating Centre for Acute Care criteria for determining adults at high risk of developing re-feeding problems

> Patient has one or more of the following
> - Body mass index (BMI) less than 16 kg/m^2
> - Unintentional weight loss > 15% within the last 3–6 months
> - Little or no nutritional intake for > 10 days
> - Low levels of potassium, phosphate or magnesium prior to feeding
>
> Or, patient has two or more of the following
> - BMI less than 18.5 kg/m^2
> - Unintentional weight loss > 10% within last 3–6 months
> - Little or nutritional intake for > 5 days
> - A history of alcohol abuse or drugs including insulin, chemotherapy, antacids or diuretics

CHRONIC ALCOHOLISM AND MORBID OBESITY WITH MASSIVE WEIGHT LOSS

Chronic alcoholism and morbid obesity with massive weight loss are not common problems in paediatrics but re-feeding syndrome has been reported in both these conditions in adults.[11,12]

ADULTS AT RISK FOR RE-FEEDING SYNDROME

The National Collaborating Centre for Acute Care[13] has produced nutrition support guidelines in adults and outlined criteria for determining adults at high risk of developing re-feeding problems (Table 2). There are no similar published guidelines for determining children at high risk of developing re-feeding syndrome.

PATHOGENESIS

IN STARVATION

To understand the pathogenesis of re-feeding syndrome, it is important to comprehend the physiological processes that take place during starvation.

Initially, in starvation or inadequate dietary intake, the body relies on the breakdown of hepatic glycogen to glucose for energy. Glycogen stores in the liver are small; therefore, gluconeogenesis is soon necessary to maintain glucose levels. Endogenous proteins are utilised to provide amino acids for gluconeogenesis and loss of muscle bulk eventually occurs. Lipolysis, the breakdown of the body's fat stores, also occurs. These processes are inhibited by insulin but the level of this hormone falls as starvation continues. Triglycerides are hydrolysed by lipase to glycerol which is used for gluconeogenesis and non-esterified fatty acids which are used directly as a fuel or oxidised in the liver to ketone bodies.

As the body adapts to starvation, there is a decrease in metabolic rate and total body energy expenditure. The central nervous system fuel changes from glucose to ketone bodies and ketone bodies become the major energy source. Gluconeogenesis in the liver decreases with a consequent reduction of protein breakdown, both being inhibited directly by ketone bodies. Most of the energy at this stage comes from adipose tissue with some gluconeogenesis from amino acids.

DURING RE-FEEDING

During re-feeding, a shift from fat to carbohydrate metabolism occurs. A glucose load evokes insulin release causing increased cellular uptake of glucose, phosphate, potassium, magnesium and water and protein synthesis.[1]

Re-introduction of carbohydrate into the system (orally, enterally or parenterally) can inhibit fat metabolism and promotes glucose metabolism causing an increase in the use of phosphate to produce phosphorylated intermediates of glycolysis, adenosine triphosphate (ATP) and 2,3-diphospho-glycerate (2,3-DPG). This results in the hypophosphataemia of re-feeding. Additionally, the high glucose load induces hyperinsulinaemia which is postulated to be the cause of the increased intracellular water that accompanies re-feeding.[14]

Carbohydrate re-feeding causes increased cellular thiamine utilisation and thiamine deficiency is postulated as having a contributory role in re-feeding syndrome, especially in those patients whose thiamine stores are already depleted.[15]

CLINICAL FEATURES OF RE-FEEDING SYNDROME

The metabolic consequences of the re-feeding syndrome include abnormalities of fluid balance and glucose metabolism, hypophosphataemia, hypokalaemia, hypomagnesaemia and thiamine deficiency. Re-feeding syndrome can, therefore, affect multiple organ systems and produce varied clinical features.

Below, the clinical features are outlined according to the individual metabolic consequence to help further understand the pathophysiology of re-feeding syndrome. Also included are the normal physiological roles of the electrolyte or vitamin involved so that it becomes easier to comprehend the clinical manifestations that result as a consequence of their deficiency.

ABNORMALITIES OF FLUID BALANCE

1. Re-feeding with carbohydrate results in reduction of sodium and water excretion; with concurrent sodium ingestion, this can lead to rapid expansion of the extracellular fluid volume.

2. Weight gain can be directly attributed to gains in total body water and extracellular fluid volume; this may predispose patients to fluid overload.

3. Enhanced fluid retention may be exacerbated by loss of tissue mass present in starvation.

4. Re-feeding with predominantly protein or lipid can result in weight loss and urinary sodium excretion leading to a negative nitrogen balance.

Table 3 Clinical features associated with abnormal fluid balance in re-feeding

Cardiac	Congestive heart failure, hypotension, sudden death
Haemodynamic	Dehydration, fluid overload
Renal	Uraemia, pre-renal failure
Metabolic	Hypernatraemia, metabolic acidosis

5. High protein feeding can result in hypernatraemia associated with hypertonic dehydration uraemia and metabolic acidosis.

Table 3 outlines the clinical features associated with abnormal fluid balance in re-feeding syndrome.

ABNORMALITIES OF GLUCOSE METABOLISM

1. Glucose ingestion suppresses gluconeogenesis and the utilisation of amino acids leading to a less negative nitrogen balance.

2. Further administration of glucose can lead to hyperglycaemia which can subsequently cause hyperosmolar non-ketotic coma, ketoacidosis, osmotic diuresis and dehydration.

3. Further delivered glucose is converted to fat (lipogenesis) resulting in hypertriglyceridaemia, fatty liver, abnormal liver function tests, a higher respiratory quotient with increased carbon dioxide production, hypercapnia and possible respiratory failure.

Table 4 outlines the clinical features associated with abnormal glucose metabolism in re-feeding syndrome.

HYPOPHOSPHATAEMIA

Hypophosphataemia is one of the predominant features of re-feeding syndrome. The combination of depletion of total body phosphorous stores during catabolic starvation and increased cellular influx of phosphorous during anabolic re-feeding leads to severe extracellular hypophosphataemia.

1. Phosphate is essential for cell function, being an important intracellular buffer and buffering hydrogen ions in the urine. It has a structural role as

Table 4 Clinical features associated with abnormal glucose metabolism in re-feeding syndrome

Cardiac	Hypotension
Respiratory	Carbon dioxide retention, respiratory depression
Neurological	Hyperosmolar non-ketotic coma
Gastrointestinal	Fatty liver
Metabolic	Hyperglycaemia, ketoacidosis, metabolic acidosis
Renal	Osmotic diuresis, hypernatraemia, uraemia
Haemodynamic	Dehydration

Table 5 Normal blood concentrations for phosphorous in children

Age group	Phosphorous (mg/dl)
Newborn	4.2–9.0
1 year	3.8–6.2
2–5 years	3.5–6.8

a major component of phospholipids, nucleoproteins and nucleic acids and a central role in cellular metabolic pathways, *e.g.* glycolysis and oxidative phosphorylation.

2. Phosphate helps to make 2,3-DPG, a by-product of glycolysis, which regulates the dissociation of oxygen from haemoglobin and subsequent delivery of oxygen to the tissues.

3. Phosphate is important in excitation stimulus response coupling and nervous system conduction.

4. Phosphate also has an important role in the phagocytic and chemotactic properties of white blood cells and clot retraction in platelets.

It is important to note that normal serum phosphate levels are different in children compared to adults and the diagnosis of hypophosphataemia is, therefore, based on different reference ranges. Normal blood concentrations for phosphorous in children are shown in the Table 5.[16] The lower limits are cut-off points for the diagnosis of hypophosphataemia.

Hypophosphataemia in children older than 5 years is classified in the same way as in adults and is summarised in Table 6.

Clinical conditions associated with hypophosphataemia and, therefore, possible differential diagnoses of re-feeding syndrome include alkalosis, sepsis, alcoholism, surgery, diarrhoea, vomiting, uncontrolled diabetes, cirrhosis, drugs (*e.g.* corticosteroids, insulin, diuretics), hypercalcaemia and Fanconi syndrome.[17]

Mild hypophosphataemia is usually tolerated without adverse affects; however, moderate and severe hypophosphataemia are often symptomatic. In anorexia nervosa, for example, loss of appetite, fatigue and muscle weakness is often reported but may be important early signs of phosphate depletion and hypophosphataemia. Starvation, vomiting, laxative abuse and exercise all contribute to a negative phosphate balance.[18]

Untreated, severe hypophosphataemia leads to depletion of phosphorylated compounds and may result in neuromuscular, haematological and respiratory compromise.

Table 6 Classification of hypophosphataemia in children older than 5 years

Hypophosphataemia	Phosphorous (mg/dl)
Mild	2.0–2.5
Moderate	1.0–2.0
Severe	< 1.0

Table 7 Clinical features that are the sequelae of severe hypophosphataemia in re-feeding syndrome

Respiratory	Diaphragmatic weakness, dyspnoea, respiratory failure
Cardiac	Hypotension, shock, altered myocardial function – decreased stroke volume, decreased mean arterial pressure, decreased left ventricular stroke volume, increased wedge pressure, arrhythmia, congestive heart failure, sudden death
Neuromuscular	Weakness, paresthesias, delirium, confusion, cranial nerve palsies, acute areflexic paralysis, seizures, coma, rhabdomyolysis
Haematological	Altered red blood cell morphology, haemolytic anaemia, white blood cell dysfunction, thrombocytopenia, depressed platelet function, haemorrhage
Hepatic	Liver dysfunction (especially in cirrhotics)
Skeletal	Osteopaenia (in long-term hypophosphataemia)
Renal	Acute tubular necrosis, tubular defects

Table 7 illustrates the clinical features that are the sequelae of severe hypophosphataemia in re-feeding syndrome.

HYPOKALAEMIA

1. Potassium is the predominant intracellular cation and is essential for maintaining the cell membrane action potential.

2. Potassium is an important component of normal cellular metabolism.

During re-feeding, potassium moves into the newly formed cells and serum levels may fall without supplementation. Table 8 shows the clinical features that are the sequelae of severe hypokalaemia in re-feeding syndrome.

HYPOMAGNESAEMIA

1. Magnesium is a major intracellular cation and is mandatory for optimal cell function.

Table 8 Clinical features that are the sequelae of severe hypokalaemia in re-feeding syndrome

Cardiac	Arrhythmias, hypotension, cardiac arrest, ECG changes (T wave flattening or inversion, U waves, St segment depression), increased digitalis sensitivity
Gastrointestinal	Nausea, vomiting constipation, paralytic ileus
Neuromuscular	Areflexia, hyporeflexia, paralysis, paresthesias, respiratory depression, rhabdomyolysis, weakness
Renal	Decreased urinary concentrating ability, polyuria and polydipsia, nephropathy with decreased glomerular filtration rate, myoglobinuria (secondary to rhabdomyolysis)
Metabolic	Metabolic acidosis, glucose intolerance

Table 9 Clinical features that are the sequelae of severe hypomagnesaemia

Cardiac	Arrhythmias, tachycardia, torsades de pointes, hypertension
Neuromuscular	Ataxia, confusion, fasciculations, hyporeflexia, irritability, muscle tremors, painful paresthesias, personality changes, positive Trousseau's sign, seizures, tetany, vertigo, weakness
Gastrointestinal	Abdominal pain, anorexia, diarrhoea, constipation, nausea, vomiting
Electrolyte	Hypokalaemia, hypocalcaemia

2. Magnesium is a co-factor for many enzymatic pathways.

There is intracellular movement of magnesium ions into cells with carbohydrate re-feeding and poor magnesium intake. Pre-existing poor magnesium status may exacerbate the degree of hypomagnesaemia. Hypomagnesaemia is often not clinically significant until severe (< 0.5 mmol/l). Table 9 demonstrates the clinical features that are the sequelae of severe hypomagnesaemia.

THIAMINE DEFICIENCY

Thiamine is an essential co-enzyme in intermediate carbohydrate metabolism. Thiamine deficiency can be measured biochemically but is rarely done in clinical practice as the risks of providing high doses of thiamine are small and the benefits potentially life-saving. Clinical manifestations of thiamine deficiency include Wernicke's encephalopathy (ataxia, ocular abnormalities, vestibular dysfunction, confusion and coma) and Korsakov's syndrome (short-term memory loss and confabulation).

CARDIAC DYSFUNCTION

Potentially fatal cardiopulmonary dysfunction can result from the electrolyte disturbances, vitamin deficiencies and body-fluid imbalances outlined above. There are, however, other factors that contribute to the cardiac dysfunction associated with starvation and re-feeding. Cardiac muscle mass is reduced in starvation. In patients with eating disorders, for example, the heart may be structurally atrophic secondary to long-standing hypovolaemia and they may have low cardiac outputs and demonstrate increased vascular resistance despite the presence of hypotension. Much of the mortality and morbidity in patients with eating disorders stems from cardiovascular complications such as arrhythmias, hypotension and bradycardia.[19]

WHEN DO THE CLINICAL FEATURES OF RE-FEEDING OCCUR?

Hypophosphataemia typically occurs within the first 2–3 days of nutrition support. Cardiac and neurological events are most likely to occur within the first weeks of re-feeding. Kohn *et al*.[20] described three adolescents admitted with anorexia nervosa who developed re-feeding syndrome and suffered acute cardiac complications – arrhythmias (bradycardia), pericardial effusion, hypotension and cardiac arrest. Two of the three developed hypophosphataemia; all had cardiac complications (arrhythmias) occurring within the first week of re-feeding and all had delirium during or after the second week of re-feeding.

MANAGEMENT/PREVENTION

There are no accepted comprehensive guidelines for the management of re-feeding syndrome in children. Afzal et al.[5] proposed evidence-based guidelines for the management of re-feeding syndrome with enteral nutrition in children and there is some information about re-feeding syndrome in the complications section of the recently published European Paediatric Parenteral Nutrition Guidelines.[21]

Being aware of the problem and recognising those patients who may be at risk of re-feeding syndrome is an important starting point. By involving hospital multidisciplinary nutrition support teams, who are experienced in the management of malnourished patients, potential complications associated with re-feeding may be avoided or dealt with in a safe and effective manner.

The key to the successful management and/or prevention of the re-feeding syndrome lies in a thorough nutritional assessment, continuous monitoring, cautious delivery of nutritional support and adequate supplementation of electrolytes and vitamins.

NUTRITIONAL ASSESSMENT

A detailed diet history is important. A thorough physical assessment is required to define nutritional status and may include the following measurements:

Body mass index (BMI)

$$BMI = Weight\ (kg)/Height\ squared\ (m^2) \qquad Eq.\ 1$$

BMI may not show the true significance of malnutrition if the child has stunted linear growth and should always be used with a BMI centile chart in paediatrics.

Percentage weight-for-height

Percentage weight (wt)-for-height (ht) can be used as an indicator to differentiate the stunted child from the wasted child.

$$\%\ Weight\text{-}for\text{-}ht = \frac{Actual\ wt}{Expected\ wt\text{-}for\text{-}ht\ age} \times 100 \qquad Eq.\ 2$$

where the expected weight-for-height age is the 50th centile weight for the age at which actual height is on the 50th centile.

Moderate wasting is defined as a weight-for-height ratio of 70–79%, severe wasting less than 70%. All children with percentage weight-for-height of < 80% should be deemed at risk for re-feeding syndrome.

Mid-arm circumference
This is an indicator of muscle growth.

Skin-fold thickness
This gives an estimate of body fatness.

MONITORING

Careful assessment of the following should be performed before initiating re-feeding and continued for at least the first week,

Hydration and nutritional state
Circulatory volume should be restored judiciously and fluid balance and overall clinical status monitored closely. Early weight gain may be secondary to fluid retention.

Cardiac status
Tachypnoea or tachycardia can be useful early signs of re-feeding syndrome after food intake has been re-started in a patient with nutritional deficiency.[22] Heart rate is a simple, non-invasive way to monitor fluid replacement and tachycardia has been reported to be a useful sign in detecting cardiac stress. ECG monitoring can be useful in detecting life-threatening arrhythmias and echocardiography may also be necessary to assess cardiac function.

Serum electrolytes
Daily measurements of serum phosphate, sodium, potassium, magnesium for at least the first 3–5 days of re-feeding and continue to monitor for the first week or longer if any evidence of abnormalities. Note that patients with initial normal levels of serum electrolytes can still be at high risk of developing re-feeding syndrome and even those with high base-line electrolyte levels may still have whole body depletion and, therefore, may need supplementation as re-feeding progresses. Plasma glucose and albumin should be measured and, if possible, urinary electrolytes.

ROUTE OF NUTRITION INTERVENTION

If possible, the gastrointestinal tract should be used for re-feeding. When the gastrointestinal tract is unable to absorb sufficient protein and energy to meet the individual's requirements then parenteral nutrition may be necessary.[23] Historically, re-feeding syndrome has most commonly been reported in patients who have received overzealous administration of total parenteral nutrition; however, it can occur in patients administered intravenous saline-dextrose, tube feeding or an oral diet. In enteral tube or parenteral feeding, re-feeding problems are precipitated because excessive feeding levels can be achieved easily. Problems of re-feeding are less likely to arise with oral feeding since starvation is usually accompanied by loss of appetite; however, care still needs to be taken in the prescription of oral nutrition.

ENERGY REQUIREMENTS

One approach is to estimate previous intake and begin by providing at least that amount.[15] Initial intake should be sufficient at least to prevent further weight loss. Keeping increases in calories modest during the first week, allows the body to re-establish a more anabolic milieu.

The National Collaborating Centre for Acute Care guidelines[13] in adults suggest starting nutrition support at a maximum of 10 kcal/kg/day and increasing levels slowly to meet or exceed full needs by 7–14 days. These guidelines suggests using only 5 kcal/kg/day in extreme cases, *e.g.* with a BMI less than 14 kg/m^2 or negligible intake of food for > 15 days.

The WHO guidelines for the management of malnourished children[6] advise the following age-specific regimen for energy intake: < 7 years old, 80–100 kcal/kg/day; 7–10 years, 75 kcal/kg/day; 11–14 years, 60 kcal/kg/day; and 15–18 years, 50 kcal/kg/day.

It should be noted that, in more severe cases, an initial starting volume of 75% of total daily requirements has been used. Also each requirement should be tailored to an individual's need and the above energy intake values may need to be adjusted by as much as 30%.

VOLUME

Frequent small feeds are recommended. When using liquid or milk-based diets, feeds should provide a minimum of 1 kcal/ml to minimise volume overload.

PROTEIN REQUIREMENTS

If a milk-based feed induces diarrhoea with positive faecal reducing substances, a hydrosylate-based feed may be used. An initial regimen for malnourished children suggests 0.6–1 g protein/kg/day.[23] The feed should be rich in essential amino acids and gradually increased as an intake of 1.2–1.5 g/kg/day is needed for anabolism to occur.[15]

Earlier literature reporting adults at risk of re-feeding syndrome suggested that all feeding should be withheld in those patients with low levels of potassium, magnesium or phosphate until their electrolyte abnormalities had been corrected. Current opinion is that prefeeding correction of plasma electrolyte levels is unlikely to change whole body electrolyte status significantly and does not reduce the risk of subsequent electrolyte disturbances. Current management strategies are based on the rationale that the vast majority of electrolyte deficits in these patients are intracellular and, therefore, cannot be corrected without low-level energy provision.

Although slow increments in feeding are usually advised, Flesher *et al.*[24] demonstrated that early feeding (*i.e.* reaching goal rate or calories within 48 h) even in patients assessed to be at-risk of re-feeding syndrome showed no observed negative clinical effects if a standardised enteral feeding protocol and electrolyte replacement protocol were implemented. They did, however, recommend that patients who are not haemodynamically stable, volume resuscitated or receiving norepinephrine should be fed cautiously.

SUPPLEMENTS

There are no randomised control trials for the treatment of re-feeding syndrome. The largest uncontrolled trial for the treatment of hypophosphataemia in adults with re-feeding syndrome is by Terlevich and Hearing.[25] Thirty patients with re-feeding syndrome, normal renal function and phosphate concentration less than 0.5 mmol/l were treated with a specified standard phosphate solution intravenously over 24 h. Out of the 30 patients, 28 achieved a serum phosphate concentration of 0.5 mmol/l or more after 4 days. Importantly, five patients required further phosphate as severe hypophosphataemia recurred after initial correction. None of the patients developed renal failure, although three developed mild transient hypophosphataemia and four developed asymptomatic hypocalcaemia.

One approach is to monitor serum phosphate levels and correct the deficit as needed. However, De Cock et al.[26] suggested an alternative approach by using a preventative schedule of phosphate administration. They proposed that, in the presence of normal kidney function, administering 2 x 10 mmol/day of oral phosphate or between 10–30 mmol intravenously may prevent the development of hypophosphataemia and, thereby, avoid serious complications such as sudden death. They demonstrated this regimen with two adult case reports. They recommend, however, that, in the presence of kidney malfunction, keeping to the corrective schedule is prudent.

The National Collaborating Centre for Acute Care guidelines[13] recommend the likely requirement of phosphate in adults at high risk of re-feeding is 0.3–0.6 mmol/kg/day orally or intravenously, potassium is 2–4 mmol/kg/day orally or intravenously, and magnesium is 0.2 mmol/kg/day intravenously or 0.4 mmol/kg/day orally unless prefeeding levels are high.

Oral thiamine (200–300 mg) is strongly recommended in adult practice immediately before and during the first 10 days of feeding. It can be given intravenously if necessary. A balanced multivitamin/trace element supplement is also recommended once a day.

There is less information on the use of supplements in children at risk of re-feeding syndrome. Oral supplements may not be tolerated because of an unpleasant taste, poor gut function or development of diarrhoea. Clinical judgement is, therefore, necessary to determine the most effective and safest route of administration. What is crucial is careful monitoring of the patient with serial electrolyte measurements to assess response to any treatments given and adjust dosing regimens or routes of administration accordingly.

In the proposed re-feeding syndrome guidelines by Afzal et al.,[5] the following supplement doses are recommended: sodium, 1 mmol/kg/day; potassium, 4 mmol/kg/day; magnesium, 0.6 mmol/kg/day; phosphate, up to 1 mmol/kg/day intravenously; and oral supplements, up to 100 mmol/day for children over 5 years. Hypocalcaemia may occur during phosphate supplementation.

Thiamine, folic acid, riboflavin, ascorbic acid, pyridoxine as well as fat-soluble vitamins A, D, E and K should be supplemented. Trace elements including selenium may also be deficient.

In my own clinical practice, I would usually administer supplements orally if tolerated and use the doses recommended in the British National Formulary for Children. The decision to give intravenous supplementation would depend on the clinical status of the patient, the severity of the underlying electrolyte abnormalities or if there was no improvement in electrolyte levels with oral supplements. Continuous assessment is mandatory.

Key points for clinical practice

- Re-feeding syndrome is a potentially lethal condition defined as severe electrolyte and fluid shifts with metabolic abnormalities in malnourished patients undergoing re-feeding orally, enterally or parenterally.

- Generally, any patient who has been chronically deprived of adequate nutrition is at risk of re-feeding syndrome. This includes any patient unfed in 7–10 days with evidence of stress and depletion, prolonged fasting and prolonged intravenous hydration.

- Patients especially at risk of developing the syndrome include, those with protein-energy malnutrition, anorexia nervosa and Crohn's disease.

- Clinical features may be life-threatening and are secondary to the effects of fluid intolerance, abnormal glucose metabolism, hypophosphataemia, hypokalaemia, hypomagnesaemia and thiamine deficiency on the cardiovascular, respiratory and neuromuscular systems.

- A multidisciplinary approach by expert nutrition teams who can recognise those patients at risk, co-ordinate their continuous assessment and provide appropriate and effective supplementation is the key to avoiding the dangers of re-feeding.

- Carefully monitor electrolytes, including phosphate, sodium, potassium, magnesium, glucose, at least daily over the first week of re-feeding.

- Start with small and frequent feeds and increase calorie delivery slowly.

- Look out for potential cardiovascular and neuromuscular complications in the first weeks of re-feeding.

- Start oral supplements if any indication of electrolyte abnormalities. Give replacement intravenously if not tolerated orally.

References

1. Crook MA, Hally V, Panteli JV. The importance of the refeeding syndrome. *Nutrition* 2001; **17**: 632–637.
2. Schnitker MA, Mattman PE, Bliss TL. A clinical study of malnutrition in Japanese prisoners of war. *Ann Intern Med* 1951; **35**: 69–96.
3. Keys A, Brozek J, Henschel A *et al. The Biology of Human Starvation*, vols 1,2. Minneapolis, MN: University of Minnesota Press, 1950.
4. Weinsier RL, Krumdieck CL. Death resulting from overzealous total parenteral nutrition: the refeeding syndrome revisited. *Am J Clin Nutr* 1980; **34**: 393–399.
5. Afzal NA, Addai S, Fagbemi A, Murch S, Thompson M, Heuschkel R. Refeeding syndrome with enteral nutrition in children: a case report, literature review and clinical guidelines. *Clin Nutr* 2002; **21**: 515–520.

6. World Health Organization. *Management of Severe Malnutrition: a manual for physicians and other senior health workers*. Geneva: WHO, 1999.

7. Manary MJ, Hart CA, Whyte MP. Severe hypophosphataemia in children with kwashiorkor is associated with increased mortality. *J Pediatr* 1998; **133**: 789–791.

8. Kellogg ND, Lukefahr JL. Criminally prosecuted cases of child starvation. *Pediatrics*, 2005; **116**: 1309–1316.

9. Melchoir JC. From malnutrition to refeeding during anorexia nervosa. *Curr Opin Clin Nutr Metab Care* 1998; **1**: 481–485.

10. Katzman DK. Medical complications in adolescents with anorexia nervosa: a review of the literature. *Int J Eat Disord* 2005; **37**: s52–s59.

11. Fung AT, Rimmer J. Hypophosphataemia secondary to oral refeeding syndrome in a patient with long-term alcohol misuse. *Med J Aust* 2005; **183**: 324–326.

12. Mason EE. Starvation injury after gastric reduction for obesity. *World J Surg* 1998; **22**: 1002–1007.

13. National Collaborating Centre for Acute Care. *Nutrition support in adults oral nutrition support, enteral tube feeding and parenteral nutrition*. London: NICE, 2006.

14. Palesty JA, Dudrick SJ. The Goldilocks paradigm of starvation and refeeding. *Nutr Clin Pract* 2006; **21**: 147–154.

15. Solomon SM, Kirby DF. The refeeding syndrome: a review. *J Parenteral Enteral Nutr* 1990; **14**: 90–97.

16. Worley G, Claerhout SJ, Combs SP. Hypophosphatemia in malnourished children during refeeding. *Clin Pediatr* 1998; **37**: 347–352.

17. Marinella MA. Refeeding syndrome and hypophosphataemia. *Intensive Care Med* 2005; **20**: 155–159.

18. Haglin L. Hypophosphataemia in anorexia nervosa. *Postgrad Med J* 2001; **77**: 305–311.

19. Casiero D, Frishman WH. Cardiovascular complications of eating disorders. *Cardiol Rev* 2006; **14**: 227–231.

20. Kohn MR, Golden NH, Shenker IR. Cardiac arrest and delirium: presentations of the refeeding syndrome in severely malnourished adolescents with anorexia nervosa. *J Adolesc Health* 1998; **22**: 239–243.

21. Koletzko B, Goulet O, Hunt J, Krohn K, Shamir R, Parenteral Nutrition Guidelines Working Group: European Society for Clinical Nutrition and Metabolism; European Society of Paediatric Gastroenterology, Hepatology and Nutrition (ESPGHAN): European Society of Paediatric Research (ESPR). Guidelines on paediatric parenteral nutrition of the European society of paediatric gastroenterology, Hepatology and nutrition (ESPGHAN) and the European Society for Clinical Nutrition and Metabolism (ESPEN), supported by the European Society of Paediatric Research (ESPR). *J Pediatr Gastroenterol Nutr* 2005; **41 (Suppl 2)**: S1–S87.

22. Mallet M. Refeeding syndrome. *Age Ageing* 2002; **31**: 65–66.

23. Goulet O. Nutritional support in malnourished paediatric patients. *Baillières Clin Gastroenterol* 1998; **12**: 843–876.

24. Flesher ME, Archer KA, Leslie BD, McCollum RA, Martinka GP. Assessing the metabolic and clinical consequences of early enteral feeding in the malnourished patient. *J Parenteral Enteral Nutr* 2005; **29**: 108–117.

25. Terlevich A, Hearing SD, Woltersdorf WW *et al*. Refeeding syndrome: effective and safe treatment with phosphates polyfusor. *Aliment Pharmacol Ther* 2003; **17**: 1325–1329.

26. De Cock A, Mana F, Velkeniers B, Urbain D. Hypophosphataemia and refeeding: a corrective or preventative attitude? *Acta Clin Belg* 2006; **61**: 134–137.

Michael L. Moritz

6

The evaluation and management of salt poisoning

Hypernatraemia in children in the out-patient setting is usually due to gastroenteritis or a renal concentrating defect and carries a favourable prognosis. When a patient presents in the out-patient setting with either unexplained severe hypernatraemia (serum sodium > 170 mEq/l), and either death or neurological impairment as a complication of hypernatraemia, then sodium poisoning must be considered. The diagnosis of sodium poisoning is not an easy one to make, as sodium is a naturally occurring substance in the body and there are a variety of rare conditions that can produce severe hypernatraemia (Table 1). It is tempting to assume that intentional sodium poisoning is the cause of hypernatraemia when there is no other obvious explanation. Intentional salt poisoning is a serious allegation with legal repercussions including the potential for criminal charges and the involvement of child protective services. In order to make a diagnosis of salt poisoning there must be both a scrupulous collection of forensic evidence and a sufficient understanding of body water homeostasis and of hypernatraemia in order to interpret the data properly. This report will discuss when to consider sodium poisoning, how to arrive at a proper diagnosis, and how to manage this condition when it occurs.

PATHOGENESIS OF HYPERNATRAEMIA

The body has two defences to protect against the development of hypernatraemia – the ability to produce a concentrated urine and a powerful thirst mechanism. Arginine vasopressin release (AVP) occurs when the plasma osmolality exceeds 275–280 mosmol/kg and results in a maximally concentrated urine when the plasma osmolality exceeds 290–295 mosmol/kg.

Michael L. Moritz MD
Associate Professor of Pediatrics, Division of Nephrology, University of Pittsburgh School of
Medicine, Department of Pediatrics, Children's Hospital of Pittsburgh, 3705 Fifth Ave, Pittsburgh, PA
15213-2538, USA.   E-mail: Michael.Moritz@chp.edu

89

Table 1 Causes of out-patient hypernatraemia in children

Decreased free-water intake
    Adypsia
    Restricted access to water
    Neurological impairment
    Infancy
    Gastrointestinal disease
        Gastro-oesophageal reflux, bowel obstruction, ileus, short gut
        syndrome, gastrostomy fed, pyloric stenosis
    Institutionalised
    Vomiting
    Reset osmostat
    Breast feeding

Urinary free-water losses
    Congenital nephrogenic diabetes insipidus
    Acquired nephrogenic diabetes insipidus
        Renal dysplasia/hypoplasia
        Obstructive uropathy
        Reflux nephropathy
        Sickle cell disease
    Central diabetes insipidus
        Pan hypopituitarism
        Head trauma
        Brain tumour
        Hypothalamic syndrome
    Loop diuretics
    Lithium
    Diabetes mellitus
    Solute diuresis
        High-protein feeds
        Improperly mixed infant formula

Gastrointestinal free-water losses
    Infectious diarrhoea
    Malabsorption
    Short gut syndrome
    Laxatives
        Lactulose
        Polyethylene glycol; electrolytes

High insensible free-water losses
    Fever
    High ambient temperature
        Desert climate
    Heat stroke
    Hyperthermia
    Burns
    Neuroleptic malignant syndrome
    Skin disorder
    Haemorrhagic shock and encephalopathy syndrome

Sodium ingestion
    Sodium chloride
        Table salt
        Rock salt
        Salt tablets
        Hypertonic saline solutions
        Sea water
        Food seasonings
        Salt as an emetic
    Sodium bicarbonate
        Baking soda
        Alka-seltzer
        Sodium bicarbonate tablets
        Sodium bicarbonate solutions
    Sodium citrate
        Bicitra (Scholl's solution)

Thirst is the body's second line of defence, but provides the ultimate protection against hypernatraemia. If the thirst mechanism is intact and there is unrestricted access to free water, it is rare for someone to develop sustained hypernatraemia from either excess sodium ingestion or a renal concentrating defect.[1]

CLINICAL MANIFESTATIONS

Hypernatraemia results in an efflux of fluid from the intracellular space to the extracellular space to maintain osmotic equilibrium. This leads to transient cerebral dehydration with cell shrinkage. Brain cell volume can decrease by as much as 10–15% acutely, but then quickly adapts.[2] Within one hour, the brain can significantly increase its intracellular content of sodium and potassium, amino acids and unmeasured organic substances called idiogenic osmoles. Within one week, the brain regains approximately 98% of its water content. If severe hypernatraemia develops acutely, the brain may not be able to increase its intracellular solute sufficiently to preserve its volume, and the resulting cellular shrinkage can cause structural changes. Cerebral dehydration from hypernatraemia can result in a physical separation of the brain from the meninges; the rupture of the delicate bridging veins leading to subdural and subarachnoid haemorrhages, intracranial or intracerebral haemorrhages[3,4] and retinal haemorrhages.[5] It can also result in venous sinus thrombosis and ischaemic infarctions.[6] Acute hypernatraemia has also been shown to cause cerebral demyelinating lesions in both animals and humans.[2,7] Patients with hepatic encephalopathy are at the highest risk for developing demyelinating lesions.

Children with hypernatraemia are usually agitated and irritable but can progress to lethargy, listlessness and coma.[8] On neurological examination they frequently have increased tone, nuchal rigidity and brisk reflexes. Myoclonus, asterixis and chorea can be present; tonic-clonic and absence seizures have been described. Hyperglycaemia is a particularly common consequence of hypernatraemia in children. Severe hypernatraemia can also result in rhabdomyolysis. While earlier reports showed that hypocalcaemia was associated with hypernatraemia, this has not been found in more recent literature.[9]

Hypernatraemia is associated with a mortality rate of 15% in children; this rate is estimated to be 15 times higher than the age-matched mortality in hospitalised children without hypernatraemia.[9] The high mortality is unexplained. Most of the deaths are not directly related to central nervous system pathology and appear to be independent of the severity of hypernatraemia. Recent studies have noted that patients who develop hypernatraemia following hospitalisation and patients with a delay in treatment have the highest mortality.[9,10] Approximately 40% of the deaths in children with hypernatraemia occurred while patients were still hypernatraemic.[9]

A subset of patients that have a particularly high morbidity and mortality in the out-patient setting includes infants with hypernatraemic dehydration and children with salt poisoning.[1] Most of the deaths or neurological damage directly attributable to hypernatraemia have been from brain injury, particularly vascular thrombosis and intracranial haemorrhage (Table 2).

Table 2 Neuropathological findings associated with salt poisoning

- Cerebral oedema
- Diabetes insipidus
- Diffuse capillary haemorrhages
- Subdural haemorrhages
- Dural membrane haemorrhages
- Subarachnoid haemorrhages
- Cerebral vessel thrombosis or sludging
- Dural sinus thrombosis
- Intracerebral haemorrhages
- Capillary and venous congestion
- Cerebral myelinolysis

REASONS TO SUSPECT SALT POISONING

Salt poisoning should be suspected (see Table 3) whenever the severity of hypernatraemia, neurological manifestations or hospital course does not correlate with the history of present illness. Reasons to suspect salt poisoning would be: (i) a child presenting violently ill, without any apparent preceding illness, and is then found to have hypernatraemia on laboratory evaluation; (ii) severe hypernatraemia, exceeding 170 mEq/l, without an apparent cause or with a preceding illness of short duration; (iii) death or serious neurological injury directly related to hypernatraemia: (iv) repeated episodes of out-patient hypernatraemia without apparent cause; or (v) a rising serum sodium or failure of the serum sodium to correct despite the administration of adequate amounts of free water. While these situations are suspicious for salt poisoning, they are also suspicious for a disorder in renal concentration or osmoregulation, and both of these conditions must be ruled out first.

COMMON CLINICAL SCENARIOS OF SUSPECTED SALT POISONING

Salt poisoning is not uncommon; in most cases it is mild and non-fatal and does not receive medical attention. According to the 2005 report of the American Association of Poison Control Centers, there were 3181 reports of sodium poisoning in 2005, with most classified as unintentional.[11] Only six cases were classified as severe, two with death. Severe salt poisoning is a rare condition that can occur in a variety of clinical situations. The literature on this condition is scant and, in most reports, details are lacking as to how the diagnosis was confirmed or how the hypernatraemia developed. The best documentation of salt

Table 3 Reasons to suspect salt poisoning

- Unexplained hypernatraemia
- Acute CNS injury from out-patient hypernatraemia
- Elevated serum sodium out of proportion to history
- Serum sodium rising following hospitalisation
- Repeated episodes of out-patient hypernatraemia

poisoning is that of accidental salt poisoning[12, 32-41] (Table 4). Accidental salt poisoning has primarily been described following the administration of hypertonic saline solution as an emetic, the improper preparation of infant formula by parents or by hospitals that substituted salt for sugar, or the improper preparation of oral rehydration solution by using excess amounts of sodium chloride or sodium bicarbonate. Salt poisoning may occur voluntarily by the child or intentionally as a form of child abuse. These two conditions can be difficult to differentiate, especially if the child dies. These conditions are the least well documented in the literature; many of the reports described as intentional salt poisoning may, in fact, represent voluntary salt ingestion by children with psychobehavioural problems and represent a form of pica. The least well understood form of severe hypernatraemia is that of thirsting as a form of child abuse. In these cases, children present to medical attention with severe hypernatraemia, presumably due to water deprivation by caregivers. Each form of salt poisoning is summarised below.

ACCIDENTAL SALT POISONING

Salt water emetic
A once-common reason for accidental salt poisoning was the use of a salt water solution as an emetic after a possible poisoning.[32-36] Salt water was administered to children either by their parents to induce vomiting or as a

Table 4 Reports of accidental salt poisoning

Reference	n	Cause	Age (yrs)	Peak serum Na (mmol/l)	Outcome
Casavant et al. (2003)[32]	1	Salt water as an emetic	14	195	Death
Carter et al. (1971)[33]	2	Salt water as an emetic	2	N/A	Death
			2	176	Death
Barer et al. (1973)[34]	1	Salt water as an emetic	3	188	Death
DeGenaro et al. (1971)[35]	1	Salt water as an emetic	2	189	Death
Streat (1982)[36]	1	Salt water as an emetic	2	204	Death
Krige et al. (2002)[37]	1	Peritoneal irrigation with hypertonic saline	7	170	Death
Habbick et al. (1984)[38]	1	Hospital error in infant formula	0.5	182	Recovery
Miller et al. (1960)[39]	1	Parental error in oral rehydration solution	0.33	200	Recovery
Saunders et al. (1976)[40]	1	Parental error in oral rehydration solution	0.17	212	Recovery
Finberg et al. (1963)[12]	14	Hospital error in infant formula	≤ 0.25	160–274	6 deaths, 8 recovery
Paut et al. (1999)[41]	1	Parental error in infant formula	0.1	211	Recovery
Sanchez et al. (2000)[42]	2	Salt added to yoghurt	1.7	195	Death
		Parental error in oral rehydration solution	0.6	178	Death

gastric lavage prescribed by physicians.[37] This was common in the 1950s and 1960s; however, by the 1970s, multiple reports had called attention to the dangers of this practice, and the incidence decreased. This form of salt poisoning is associated with the highest mortality, presumably because it is the most acute form of hypernatraemia. Children typically become violently ill soon after the lavage, presenting comatose with fever and tachycardia. They usually die within 1–2 days of presentation with wide-spread neuro-pathological findings on autopsy.

Errors in infant formula or rehydration solution preparation

Reports of accidental salt poisoning from errors in infant formula or rehydration solution preparation do exist.[12,39–42] Most of these reports are from the time period preceding the advent of commercially available infant formulas and rehydration solutions. In most cases, hypernatraemia resulted from adding salt instead of sugar. Remarkably, the infants remained quite hungry and readily took the hypertonic formula, many times without inducing emesis. These children also did not appear quite as ill as those from salt poisoning from hypertonic saline as an emetic. This may be due to the fact that hypernatraemia from an error in infant formula preparation is not generally as acute as that from hypertonic saline as an emetic. Most of these infants presented with seizures or coma. The outcome for this disorder is surprisingly good if therapy is instituted early. Much of what we know about this condition is from a report of mass accidental salt poisoning occurring over a 5-day period at Binghamton General Hospital in 1962.[12] The hospital kitchen staff inadvertently used salt instead of sugar when preparing infant formula. Fourteen infants were identified with clinical manifestations of salt poisoning. The first five infants died prior to the identification of the problem and sodium values were not checked in these. There was only one death in the other nine. The death occurred in a child whose serum sodium was corrected from 244 mmol/l to 195 mmol/l with the use of peritoneal dialysis. The child had severe aspiration pneumonia which likely played a major impact on mortality. One child with a serum sodium of 274 mmol/l survived without apparent neurological sequelae despite the lowering of serum sodium by 120 mmol/l in less than 24 h via the use of peritoneal dialysis. It is not clear why these infants fared so well.

SEVERE HYPERNATRAEMIA FROM VOLUNTARY SODIUM INGESTION, THIRSTING, AND INTENTIONAL SALT POISONING

The exact mechanism of hypernatraemia could not be determined in all cases of salt poisoning in the literature[14–22, 43] (Table 5). The cases are similar in that many of these children were either adopted or in foster care, had psychological problems, or had parents with mental illness. The cases appear to represent severe psychopathology on the part of either the child or the parent, regardless of the exact cause. These three conditions will be classified as best as the literature permits, understanding that the distinction is not always clear.

Voluntary sodium ingestion

A poorly understood, but well-documented, condition is that of severe hypernatraemia from voluntary sodium ingestion. Many of these cases, unfortunately, may have been misclassified in the literature as child abuse

Table 5 Publications on severe hypernatraemia from voluntary sodium ingestion, thirsting, and intentional salt poisoning

Reference	n	Cause	Age (yrs)	Peak serum Na (mmol/l)	Outcome
Calvin et al. (1964)[14]	2	1.5 lb of table salt placed in crib as a toy	1.2 1.2	182 179	Recovery Recovery
Chesney et al. (1981)[18]	1	Unclear	1.75	206	Recovery
Dockery (1992)[17]	1	Table salt ingestion	5	220	Death
Zumwalt et al. (1980)[16]	1	Voluntarily ate overly salted food	6	176	Death
Kupiec et al. (2004)[15]	1	Voluntarily ate rock salt	6	234	Recovery
Pickel et al. (1970)[19]	3	Water deprivation Water deprivation Water deprivation	2.5 3.75 7	195 201 194	Recovery Recovery Recovery
Zumwalt et al. (1980)[16]	1	Water deprivation	2	177	Death
Baugh et al. (1983)[20]	1	Force fed salt for enuresis	5	184	Recovery
Rogers et al. (1976)[43]	1	Salt added to child's feeds	1	200	Death
Meadow (1977)[21]	1	Unclear	1	175	Death
Meadow (1993)[22]	12	Usually parental administration of table salt	0.1–3.5	150–228	11 recovery, 1 death

when they likely were not. Fatal voluntary salt poisoning is well described in adults, primarily in patients with psychiatric or developmental conditions.[13] The first well-described case of voluntary salt poisoning was by Calvin et al.[14] in 1964 where they reported on twin 14-month-old girls who presumably ate the better part of a 1.5-lb box of salt that was somehow placed in their crib to play with. The children presented to medical care because they would not drink or eat. They looked well on examination with the exception of slight dehydration and made an uneventful recovery.

They are four other reports of salt poisoning in the literature where it is not clear whether salt poisoning was voluntary or was the result of intentional abuse. In all cases there was overt psychopathology in the children. Presumed voluntary salt poisoning occurred in a 6-year-old boy in foster care who had a history of physical and sexual abuse, post traumatic stress disorder, attention deficit disorder, and pica for glass.[15] He presented to medical attention with a sodium of 234 mmol and made an uneventful recovery. He was suspected to have overdosed on rock salt secondary to his pica. A similar report appeared of a 6-year-old boy in foster care who had behavioural problems and craved salt.[16] His foster father intentionally heavily salted the child's food to 'teach him the taste of salt'. Remarkably, the child voluntarily ate the food and soon thereafter had a convulsion and died prior to arrival at the hospital. His serum sodium was 176 mmol/l. Fatal hypernatraemia has also been reported in a 5-year-old girl who was adopted at 2 years of age. The child had unusual eating habits and apparently voluntarily ingested salt 2 h prior to admission.[17] She presented to medical attention with a serum sodium of 189 mmol/l and a large sodium chloride concretion in her abdomen. Her serum sodium rose as high as

220 mmol/l prior to death. Finally, there is a report of 21-month-old girl who appeared to have been neglected by her parents and developed psychosocial dwarfism.[18] She had a history of eating rabbit food and faeces and drinking water out of the toilet bowl and bird bath. She presented emaciated with serum sodium of 206 mmol/l and a dilute urine, specific gravity 1.004, suspicious for a renal concentrating defect. In all these cases, the exact mechanism of salt poisoning could not be conclusively determined, but there was no evidence of forced salt feeding, physical abuse or trauma.

Thirsting

Severe hypernatraemia from water deprivation is an extreme form of child abuse which is not well described in the literature. The details provided in the reports are so scant that the true aetiology can not be determined. It is possible that some form of parental water restriction played a role in these cases as hypernatraemia can not practically occur in the absence of restricted access to free water. Fluid restriction alone is unlikely to cause severe hypernatraemia, so there may have been other factors that contributed to hypernatraemia that were not discovered by the investigating physicians.

Pickel et al.[19] described three children with severe hypernatraemia where parental fluid restriction was believed to be the main contributing factor. One of the three was adopted; another had a peculiar salt craving and was known to eat salt from a salt shaker. It is possible that voluntary salt poisoning or intentional salt poisoning also played a role. In a separate case, a 2-year-old girl with sickle cell disease was beaten by her mother's boyfriend then bound by her hands and feet and left alone in a vacant room.[16] Thirteen hours later, she was found dead with a vitreous sodium of 177 mmol. Intravascular sickling was a contributing factor to her death.

Intentional salt poisoning

Intentional salt poisoning, as a form of child abuse, is a potentially lethal condition that is not well documented in the medical literature. There have been multiple criminal investigations for alleged salt poisoning; however, most of these have never been published in the medical literature, so the forensic data to make this diagnosis are not well described. The force feeding of salts should not be difficult to achieve when added to infant formula or via a gastrostomy tube. More difficult to achieve would be the force feeding of salt to an older child, who would resist and would likely spit out or vomit the salt. In order for forced salt ingestion to prove lethal there would have to be an added component of fluid restriction, as copious intake of water would readily correct the hypernatraemia. There is only one documented report of forced salt poisoning to an older child in the literature, a 5-year-old who admitted that he was fed salt by the spoonful for enuresis.[20] All other reports are in infants.

Meadow's reports

Most recorded incidents of intentional salt poisoning have occurred in the UK and have been reported by Professor Sir Roy Meadow, a prominent paediatrician who was one of the first to describe the Munchausen syndrome by proxy. In 1977, Meadow first reported a case of intentional salt poisoning involving a child with recurrent hypernatraemia since 6 weeks of age.[21]

Endocrine and renal disorders were apparently ruled out, but details were not given as to what tests were done. Meadow's investigations of the child included the administration of a salt load of 20 g of sodium chloride (344 mmol, or 3 teaspoons of salt) which resulted in a serum sodium of 147 mmol/l. The child eventually died with severe hypernatraemia, but the serum sodium was not provided nor were details of the postmortem, other than the discovery of gastric erosions.

In 1993, Meadow published a case series of 12 children with non-accidental salt poisoning.[22] These children were almost all young infants, with a median age of 2.5 months. This in itself is problematic as errors in infant formula reconstitution can produce severe hypernatraemia from the high solute content. This innocent error may be confused with salt poisoning.[23] Meadow also outlined four criteria for the diagnosis of salt poisoning, one of which is clearly incorrect: 'Illness associated with high serum sodium concentration and even higher urine sodium concentrations'. A spot urine sodium in the absence of a spot urine creatinine is not diagnostic of excess sodium excretion as a low fractional excretion of sodium can be achieved with a high urine sodium concentration. Further, an elevated urine sodium would not be unexpected if collected after the child was volume resuscitated. There was also no data provided to confirm that diabetes insipidus had been ruled out. Another error in Meadow's report is that his calculations grossly underestimated how much sodium would be needed to produce hypernatraemia. Meadow's calculations were based on the volume of distribution of extracellular water rather than total body water. The most convincing evidence that Meadow presents in the manuscript for salt poisoning is that in seven cases the mothers actually confessed to salt poisoning and in nine of the cases there was evidence that the child was poisoned while resident in the hospital. Unfortunately, insufficient details were provided to generalise about salt poisoning and, because these cases were in young infants, it is difficult to apply these data to the older child with suspected salt poisoning. In all likelihood some of these children did suffer salt poisoning as five had serum sodium concentrations between 190–228 mmol/l and there was one death with a serum sodium of 200 mmol/l.

HOW MUCH SODIUM IS TOXIC?

There is no good data as to how much sodium is toxic. The dose is largely dependent on how acutely it is administered and whether or not there is access to water. A review of the literature suggests than acute elevation in serum sodium of about 30 mmol/l or a rise in serum sodium to 170 mmol/l is needed to generate significant hypernatraemic encephalopathy. One mmol/kg of sodium, in general, will raise the serum sodium by 2 mmol/l; therefore, a dose of at least 15 mmol/kg of sodium or 1 g/kg of sodium chloride would be necessary to poison. As little as 3 teaspoons of salt (375 mmol sodium; see Table 6) acutely administered to a 5-year-old child weighing 20 kg could be dangerous. Doses in excess of this could be lethal. The probability of a lethal ingestion is much reduced if there is unrestricted access to water in an otherwise healthy individual. The kidneys can excrete sodium at a concentration as high as 400 mmol/l. Therefore, in 3 litres of urine produced in a 24-h period, as much as 1200 mmol of

Table 6 Doses of sodium and sodium chloride

	Measure	Quantity of sodium (mmol)
Sodium (Na; MW 23)	1 g	43
Sodium chloride (NaCl; MW 58)	1 g	17
Table salt	1 teaspoon (7.25 g NaCl)	125
Table salt	1 tablespoon (21.75 g NaCl)	375
MW = molecular weight		

sodium, or 10 teaspoons of salt, could be excreted. Hypertonic sodium chloride is a gastric irritant, and its ingestion could prevent free water intake.

EVALUATION OF SODIUM POISONING

The most convincing evidence of salt poisoning is a history, confession, or witness account describing the type and quantity of sodium ingested. In the absence of this, sodium poisoning is difficult to prove in a court of law unless critical forensic evidence is obtained. Simple tests can be done that can conclusively prove salt poisoning. Below are the most important data that must be obtained to confirm a suspicion of salt poisoning (see also Table 7).

GASTRIC CONTENTS

There is good reason to suspect salt poisoning when a child appears violently ill with unexplained, severe hypernatraemia. If salt poisoning did occur, it likely happened acutely in the preceding 4–12 h and there is a good chance that some of the ingested sodium could be recovered from the gastric contents. A gastric sodium concentration exceeding that of the plasma sodium is virtually diagnostic of recent sodium ingestion, as the gastric sodium concentration is always lower then the plasma sodium due to the presence of other cations such as potassium and protons. The gastrointestinal absorption of sodium is rapid, so it is unlikely that a gastric aspirate will be diagnostic of salt poisoning if obtained more than 12 h after ingestion. The stoichiometric ratio between gastric sodium and chloride is also important as the gastric chloride concentration normally exceeds the gastric sodium concentration. When the gastric sodium and chloride are of similar concentration, this is suggestive of sodium chloride ingestion. When the gastric sodium exceeds the chloride concentration, this is suggestive of sodium bicarbonate ingestion.

CLOTHING AND VOMITUS

If evidence of salt poisoning is not determined by a gastric aspirate, it is still possible to collect evidence of salt poisoning from residues of gastric contents that may be found on clothing, bedding and linen, or even a car seat. Hypertonic saline solutions are gastric irritants and can induce vomiting. Sodium administered orally might be forcefully spat out or might be purged through emesis in an older child who was intentionally salt poisoned; evidence of this should be sought. In order to determine the aetiology of a stain, it is

Table 7 Evaluation of suspected salt poisoning

Immediate hospital evaluation

Accurate vitals

Weight, temperature, pulse, blood pressure

Physical examination

Assessment of volume status: quality of pulses, capillary refill time, skin turgor, peripheral oedema, sunken eyes or fontanelle, cardiac gallop, pulmonary congestions

Physical evidence of abuse: oral lacerations, bruising, petichiae, scratches, abrasions, retinal haemorrhages

Gastric aspirate

Sodium, potassium, chloride, pH

Serum samples

Biochemical assays: sodium, potassium, chloride, blood urea nitrogen, glucose, anion gap, calcium, magnesium, phosphorous, uric acid, total protein, albumin, liver function tests, creatinine kinase, lactate dehydrogenase, osmolality, arginine vasopressin level

Complete blood count

Blood cultures and coagulation profile as clinically indicated

Urine samples

Spot urine: urinalysis, sodium, potassium, chloride, creatinine, osmolality

Begin a *timed urine collection* for volume and further biochemical analyses

Stool

Cultures and chemical analysis in cases of diarrhoea or as clinically indicated

Forensic evaluation

History

Vomiting

Diarrhoea

Fever

Polyuria

Polydypsia

Adypsia

Pica

Behavioural/emotional problems

Salt cravings

Collect samples for evidence of sodium poisoning

Clothes

Linen, blankets

Medications

Feeds

Vomitus

Vomit stains on mattress, car seat, rugs, upholstery

Infant formula

Submit forensic material for analysis of sodium, potassium, chloride and creatinine, possibly protein

Radiography

Abdominal X-ray to rule out salt bezoar

Skeletal survey to rule out fractures

Neuro-imaging to rule out subdural or intracranial haemorrhages, infarcts, thrombosis, cerebral oedema

Renal sonogram (if renal failure or renal concentrating defect suspected)

Record composition and quantity of all intake

Collect all urine

Calculate sodium balance from intake and output if possible

critical to measure the serum sodium, potassium, chloride and protein content. The source of a stain as being either a naturally occurring gastric content or that of ingested sodium chloride or bicarbonate can be determined by assessing the stoichiometric relationship of these components.

URINE CHEMISTRY AND TIMED URINE SAMPLE

A spot urine analysis for electrolytes, creatinine and osmolality should be obtained as soon as salt poisoning in suspected. These tests can be added on to urine that was previously sent for a toxicology screen or urinalysis. A renal concentrating defect or diabetes insipidus must be ruled out as either can contribute to the development of severe hypernatraemia, even if evidence for excess sodium ingestion or extra-renal free water losses exists. Hypernatraemia is a stimulus for vasopressin production and should produce a maximally concentrated urine. A urine osmolality less than, or equal to, the plasma is suspicious for a renal concentrating defect.

The fractional excretion of sodium (FENa) should be calculated on the very first urine sample obtained. A FENa of < 1% is suggestive of dehydration or other states of effective circulation volume depletion and a FENa of > 2% is suggestive of sodium excess. Many clinical situations can affect the FENa and interfere with the diagnosis of salt poisoning. A FENa could be low in salt poisoning if there is shock, circulatory collapse, capillary leak or hypotension. A FENa could be elevated in the absence of salt poisoning if there is tubular injury, underlying chronic renal insufficiency, or adrenal insufficiency, or if the urine sample was collected following volume expansion with saline.

A timed urine collection is the most useful test in the diagnosis of salt poisoning. In salt poisoning, the patient should be in negative sodium balance during rehydration unless there is shock, capillary leak, or acute renal failure. A 24-h urine collection should be performed, and urine electrolyte excretion should be compared to intake over the same time period. A negative electrolyte excretion is highly suggestive of sodium poisoning as the cause of hypernatraemia.

PITFALLS IN THE DIAGNOSIS OF SALT POISONING

Certain misconceptions in the evaluation of hypernatraemia have led to the false assumption of salt poisoning by physicians. First and foremost is that severe hypernatraemia in the absence of severe clinical signs of volume depletion rules out hypernatraemic dehydration. This is incorrect. The extracellular volume is relatively well preserved in hypernatraemic dehydration from free water loss, and clinically signs of volume depletion are significantly reduced. Supposing a patient had a serum sodium of 200 mmol/l from pure free-water loss, this would require a staggering loss of 24% of body weight, but only one-third of this loss (8% body weight) would be from the extracellular space, as the water loss is evenly distributed from the intracellular and extracellular space. In cases of diabetes insipidus, hypernatraemia is usually due to a combination of free-water loss and sodium retention, so clinical signs of extracellular volume depletion could be mild. It is also a false assumption that there will be biochemical parameters of dehydration including pre-renal azotemia and acute renal failure. Renal failure is less commonly seen when volume depletion is due to polyuric state, such a diabetic ketoacidosis or diabetes insipidus, rather than extrarenal losses. Polyuria seem to have some renoprotective affect to developing acute renal failure. Lastly, a high FENa does not necessary rule out hypernatraemic dehydration as, in most cases of suspected salt poisoning, urine is not collected until the patient has been massively rehydrated with isotonic fluid and made euvolaemic and hypernatraemic. High urine sodium excretion could be an expected finding following massive fluid resuscitation in a patient with severe hypernatraemia from dehydration.

DISTINGUISHING SALT POISONING FROM A DISORDER IN OSMOREGULATION?

Disorders in osmoregulation that produce severe hypernatraemia have been referred to by the names adipsic hypernatraemia, hypodipsic hypernatraemia and essential hypernatraemia, or resetting of the osmostats.[24] These conditions can be difficult to diagnose and are usually made by evaluating the thirst and arginine vasopressin response to treatment. In these conditions, there is a disorder in the thirst mechanism with or without a defect in arginine vasopressin secretion. These children can present with severe hypernatraemia, serum sodium exceeding 190 mEq/l, without overt signs of volume depletion. The hypernatraemia is chronic in nature, developing at least over many days if not weeks or months. Most children have presented with irritability, anorexia, abnormal behaviour, lethargy, or volume depletion. Some have presented obtunded. Structural lesions involving the hypothalamus may or may not be found. In some cases, there appears to be a true 'resetting' of the osmostats, where the serum osmolality cannot be returned to normal despite parenteral hydration.[25] In other cases, arginine vasopressin production cannot be suppressed with volume expansion and lowering of the serum osmolality below normal.[26] In essence, these patients manifest features of the syndrome of inappropriate diuretic hormone secretion when hydrated. This can potentially make the condition difficult to distinguish from salt poisoning as fractional excretion of sodium will be high following volume expansion. One would anticipate that children with a disorder of osmoregulation would present for medical attention with less severe symptoms than those with salt poisoning, since this is a chronic rather than an acute hypernatraemia. An exception would be during an acute illness or under extreme environmental conditions where increased insensible or urinary losses would be poorly tolerated and acute on chronic hypernatraemia could develop. The main distinguishing features at presentation between a disorder in osmoregulation and salt poisoning are the history of absent thirst and the absence of signs of cerebral dehydration on neuroradiological examination. It is not clear whether a disorder in osmoregulation can result in a fatal hypernatraemia as there are no reports in the literature of death. One could argue that this is because a diagnosis could not be made if a child with this condition died prior to evaluation.

MANAGEMENT OF SALT POISONING

Patients with acute salt poisoning can present critically ill with poor vascular tone, circulatory collapse and renal failure. The initial step in management should be re-establishing good circulatory perfusion and urine output. Boluses of 0.9% sodium chloride should be administered until this is achieved. Once circulatory perfusion has been established, hydration to correct the hypernatraemia can be initiated. Hydration with hypotonic fluids should be sufficient to correct the hypernatraemia if there is normal renal function. The optimal rate of correction of hypernatraemia is unclear and is largely dependent on how acutely hypernatraemia developed and on its severity. Rapid correction of hypernatraemia can lead to cerebral oedema due to the relative inability of the brain to extrude unmeasured organic substances called idiogenic osmoles. Surprisingly, there are few reports of death or serious neurological morbidity in humans resulting from rapid correction of hypernatraemia. In the case of mass accidental salt poisoning, there are reports of infants with serum sodium greater than 200 mmol/l/h who were corrected by as much as 120 mmol/l in 24 h without adverse neurological sequelae.[12] While there are no definitive studies that document the optimal rate of correction that can be undertaken without developing cerebral oedema, empirical data have shown that unless symptoms of hypernatraemic encephalopathy are present, a rate of correction not exceeding 1 mmol/l/h or 15 mmol/l/24-h is reasonable.[1] In acute salt poisoning, the generation of idiogenic osmoles is likely to be incomplete and a relatively rapid initial rate of correction can probably be safely tolerated. In severe hypernatraemia where there are signs of encephalopathy, a more rapid rate of initial correction is likely to be beneficial. Once the serum sodium has decreased to below 170 mmol/l, an average rate of correction of 0.5–1 mmol/l/h should be sufficient. In cases of severe hypernatraemia (> 170 mEq/l), once the serum sodium is 150–160 mEq/l, correction should proceed more slowly and the patient should be kept mildly hyperosmolar in the first 48–72 h.[27] Seizures occurring during the correction of hypernatraemia are not uncommon in children, and may be a sign of cerebral oedema.[28-30] They can usually be managed by slowing the rate of correction or by giving hypertonic saline to increase the serum sodium a few milliequivalents. Seizures are usually self-limited and not a sign of long-term neurological sequelae.[27,31] Patients with acute hypernatraemia, corrected by the oral route, can tolerate a more rapid rate of correction with a much lower incidence of seizures.[28] Patients with severe hypernatraemia can develop ischaemic brain injury with cerebral oedema. If there is evidence of increased intracranial pressure, then the serum sodium cannot be safely lowered and hypernatraemia will have to be tolerated in order to avoid cytotoxic cerebral oedema and potential herniation.

Multiple approaches can been taken in the management of salt poisoning. One reasonable approach would be to administer 0.22% NaCl in 2.5% dextrose at a rate of two times maintenance, or 3200 cc/M²/day. In general, 4 ml/kg of free water will decrease the serum sodium by 1 mmol/l, so about this much free water should be provided on an hourly basis to begin with. Frusemide can be added if there are signs of fluid overload or inadequate urine output. The serum sodium should be checked every 2 h and urine electrolytes monitored to see if there is a natriuresis. The serum sodium may fall more rapidly than anticipated if there is a large natriuresis, in which case the intravenous fluid rate may need to be decreased and/or the sodium composition increased. Hyperglycaemia is a frequent complication of severe hypernatraemia so a reduced dextrose concentration of intravenous fluids is advisable.

Dialysis has been used for the treatment of salt poisoning but, in general, this is not indicated unless there is oliguric acute renal failure, chronic renal insufficiency, or signs of fluid overload such as pulmonary oedema. Peritoneal dialysis has been used in previous reports of salt poisoning; however, in most cases, it was questionable whether it was indicated or of any benefit. Continuous haemo-diafiltration would be the preferred dialytic for the treatment of salt poisoning as there is better control over the amount of fluid and sodium removal.

Key points for clinical practice

- Salt poisoning should be suspected when there is: (i) unexplained severe hypernatraemia; (ii) death or a severe CNS injury from out-patient hypernatraemia; (iii) repeated episodes of out-patient hypernatraemia; or (iv) a rise in serum sodium following the initiation of therapy.

- The body's primary defences against the development of hypernatraemia are: (i) the ability to produce a concentrated urine; and (ii) an intact thirst mechanism. Hypernatraemia should not develop if there is an intact thirst mechanism and unrestricted access to water.

- Disorders in renal concentration, osmoregulation and thirst can present in a similar fashion to salt poisoning.

- The primary neurological sequelae of hypernatraemia are from cerebral dehydration which can lead to intracranial haemorrhages and thrombosis.

- The highest mortality directly related to hypernatraemia in children is in infants with hypernatraemic dehydration and from acute salt poisoning.

- Salt poisoning is not uncommon; the vast majority of incidents are mild and non-fatal and do not receive medical attention.

- Fatal salt poisoning is usually due to a hyperacute sodium ingestion producing a serum sodium that exceeds 170 mmol/l.

- Salt poisoning can be: (i) accidental; (ii) voluntary on the part of the patient; or (iii) intentional as a form of child abuse.

- Accidental salt poisoning is usually from the use of hypertonic saline as an emetic or substituting salt for sugar in the preparation of infant formula.

- Fatal voluntary sodium ingestion has been reported in children with psychobehavioural problems and pica.

- Intentional salt poisoning has primarily been reported in infants where salt was added to the feeds.

- Fatal intentional salt poisoning is rare in the older child with only one well documented case in the literature.

(Continued on next page)

Key points for clnical practice *(Continued)*

- Salt poisoning is unlikely to be fatal if there is unrestricted access to fluids without vomiting.

- Salt poisoning can be difficult to prove in court in the absence of a confession or a witness account. A scrupulous collection of forensic data is necessary to confirm a diagnosis.

- The most convincing forensic evidence of salt poisoning is: (i) a gastric sodium concentration that exceeds the plasma concentration; (ii) evidence of sodium on clothing or bedding; or (iii) negative sodium balance based on a timed urine collection.

- A fractional excretion of sodium (FENa) is usually elevated in salt poisoning and low in hypernatraemic dehydration, but there are exceptions.

- The FENa can be low in salt poisoning if there is decreased renal perfusion from shock, hypotension, third spacing, or other forms of effective circulating volume depletion.

- The FENa may be elevated in hypernatraemic dehydration if it is collected following massive fluid resuscitation or if there is renal failure or tubular dysfunction.

- Rapid correction of hypernatraemia can lead to cerebral oedema due to the brain's relative inability to extrude unmeasured organic substances called idiogenic osmoles. In acute salt poisoning, the generation of idiogenic osmoles is likely to be incomplete and a more rapid initial rate of correction can probably be safely tolerated..

- If increased intracranial pressure develops in a patient with salt poisoning, then the serum sodium cannot be safely lowered and hypernatraemia will have to be tolerated in order to avoid cytotoxic cerebral oedema and potential herniation.

References

1. Moritz ML, Ayus JC. Preventing neurological complications from dysnatremias in children. *Pediatr Nephrol* 2005; **20**: 1687–1700.
2. Ayus JC, Armstrong DL, Arieff AI. Effects of hypernatraemia in the central nervous system and its therapy in rats and rabbits. *J Physiol* 1996; **492**: 243–255.
3. Finberg L, Luttrell CN, Redd H. Pathogenesis of lesions in the nervous system in hypernatremic states. II. Experimental studies of gross anatomic changes and alterations of chemical composition of the tissues. *Pediatrics* 1959; **23**: 46–53.
4. Luttrell CN, Finberg L. Hemorrhagic encephalopathy induced by hypernatraemia. I. Clinical, laboratory, and pathological observations. *AMA Arch Neurol Psychiatry* 1959; **81**: 424–432.
5. Fenton S, Murray D, Thornton P, Kennedy S, O'Keefe M. Bilateral massive retinal hemorrhages in a 6-month-old infant: a diagnostic dilemma. *Arch Ophthalmol* 1999; **117**: 1432–1434.
6. Grant PJ, Tate GM, Hughes JR, Davies JA, Prentice CR. Does hypernatraemia promote thrombosis? *Thromb Res* 1985; **40**: 393–399.

7. Brown WD, Caruso JM. Extrapontine myelinolysis with involvement of the hippocampus in three children with severe hypernatraemia. *J Child Neurol* 1999; **14**: 428–433.
8. Finberg L. Pathogenesis of lesions in the nervous system in hypernatremic states. I. Clinical observations of infants. *Pediatrics* 1959; **23**: 40–45.
9. Moritz ML, Ayus JC. The changing pattern of hypernatraemia in hospitalized children. *Pediatrics* 1999; **104**: 435–439.
10. Moritz ML. Hypernatraemia in hospitalized patients. *Ann Intern Med* 1996; **125**: 860.
11. Lai MW, Klein-Schwartz W, Rodgers GC *et al.* 2005 Annual Report of the American Association of Poison Control Centers' national poisoning and exposure database. *Clin Toxicol* 2006; **44**: 803–932.
12. Finberg L, Kiley J, Luttrell CN. Mass accidental salt poisoning in infancy. A study of a hospital disaster. *JAMA* 1963; **184**: 187–190.
13. Ofran Y, Lavi D, Opher D, Weiss TA, Elinav E. Fatal voluntary salt intake resulting in the highest ever documented sodium plasma level in adults (255 mmol L^{-1}): a disorder linked to female gender and psychiatric disorders. *J Intern Med* 2004; **256**: 525–528.
14. Calvin ME, Knepper R, Robertson WO. Hazards to health. Salt poisoning. *N Engl J Med* 1964; **270**: 625–626.
15. Kupiec TC, Goldenring JM, Raj V. A non-fatal case of sodium toxicity. *J Anal Toxicol* 2004; **28**: 526–528.
16. Zumwalt RE, Hirsch CS. Subtle fatal child abuse. *Human Pathology* 1980; **11**: 167–174.
17. Dockery WK. Fatal intentional salt poisoning associated with a radiopaque mass. *Pediatrics* 1992; **89**: 964–965.
18. Chesney RW, Brusilow S. Extreme hypernatraemia as a presenting sign of child abuse and psychosocial dwarfism. *Johns Hopkins Med J* 1981; **148**: 11–13.
19. Pickel S, Anderson C, Holliday MA. Thirsting and hypernatremic dehydration – a form of child abuse. *Pediatrics* 1970; **45**: 54–59.
20. Baugh JR, Krug EF, Weir MR. Punishment by salt poisoning. *South Med J* 1983; **76**: 540–541.
21. Meadow R. Munchausen syndrome by proxy. The hinterland of child abuse. *Lancet* 1977; **2**: 343–345.
22. Meadow R. Non-accidental salt poisoning. *Arch Dis Child* 1993; **68**: 448–452.
23. Moritz ML. Errors in diagnosing salt poisoning in children. *Pediatr Emerg Care* 2007; **23**: 280.
24. Robertson GL, Aycinena P, Zerbe RL. Neurogenic disorders of osmoregulation. *Am J Med* 1982; **72**: 339–353.
25. Gossain VV, Kinzel T, Strand CV, Rovner DR. Essential hypernatraemia. *Am J Med Sci* 1978; **275**: 353–358.
26. Conley SB, Brocklebank JT, Taylor IT, Robson AM. Recurrent hypernatraemia; a proposed mechanism in a patient with absence of thirst and abnormal excretion of water. *J Pediatr* 1976; **89**: 898–903.
27. Rosenfeld W, deRomana GL, Kleinman R, Finberg L. Improving the clinical management of hypernatremic dehydration. Observations from a study of 67 infants with this disorder. *Clin Pediatr (Phila)* 1977; **16**: 411–417.
28. Hogan GR, Pickering LK, Dodge PR, Shepard JB, Master S. Incidence of seizures that follow rehydration of hypernatremic rabbits with intravenous glucose or fructose solutions. *Exp Neurol* 1985; **87**: 249–259.
29. Hogan GR, Dodge PR, Gill SR, Pickering LK, Master S. The incidence of seizures after rehydration of hypernatremic rabbits with intravenous or *ad libitum* oral fluids. *Pediatr Res* 1984; **18**: 340–345.
30. Hogan GR, Dodge PR, Gill SR, Master S, Sotos JF. Pathogenesis of seizures occurring during restoration of plasma tonicity to normal in animals previously chronically hypernatremic. *Pediatrics* 1969; **43**: 54–64.
31. Banister A, Matin-Siddiqi SA, Hatcher GW. Treatment of hypernatraemic dehydration in infancy. *Arch Dis Child* 1975; **50**: 179–186.
32. Casavant MJ, Fitch JA. Fatal hypernatraemia from saltwater used as an emetic. *J Toxicol Clin Toxicol* 2003; **41**: 861–863.
33. Carter RF, Fotheringham FJ. Fatal salt poisoning due to gastric lavage with hypertonic

saline. *Med J Aust* 1971; **1**: 539–541.

34. Barer J, Hill LL, Hill RM, Martinez WM. Fatal poisoning from salt used as an emetic. *Am J Dis Child* 1973; **125**: 889–890.

35. DeGenaro F, Nyhan WL. Salt – a dangerous 'antidote'. *J Pediatr* 1971; **78**: 1048–1049.

36. Streat S. Fatal salt poisoning in a child. *NZ Med J* 1982; **95**: 285–286.

37. Krige JE, Millar AJ, Rode H, Knobel D. Fatal hypernatraemia after hypertonic saline irrigation of hepatic hydatid cysts. *Pediatr Surg Int* 2002; **18**: 64–65.

38. Habbick BF, Hill A, Tchang SP. Computed tomography in an infant with salt poisoning: relationship of hypodense areas in basal ganglia to serum sodium concentration. *Pediatrics* 1984; **74**: 1123–1125.

39. Miller NL, Finberg L. Peritoneal dialysis for salt poisoning. Report of a case. *N Engl J Med* 1960; **263**: 1347–1350.

40. Saunders N, Balfe JW, Laski B. Severe salt poisoning in an infant. *J Pediatr* 1976; **88**: 258–261.

41. Paut O, Andre N, Fabre P *et al.* The management of extreme hypernatraemia secondary to salt poisoning in an infant. *Paediatr Anaesth* 1999; **9**: 171–174.

42. Martos Sanchez I, Ros Perez P, Otheo de Tejada E, Vazquez Martinez JL, Perez-Caballero C, Fernandez Pineda L. [Fatal hypernatraemia due to accidental administration of table salt]. *Anales espanoles de pediatria* 2000; **53**: 495–498.

43. Rogers D, Tripp J, Bentovim A, Robinson A, Berry D, Goulding R. Papers and originals. *BMJ* 1976; **1**: 793–796.

Carson R. Harris Matthew Morgan

7

Dangerous drug and poison ingestion

Based on US Poison Center data compiled by the American Association of Poison Control Centers (AAPCC), approximately 51% of the 2.4 million human-exposure calls involved children younger than age 6 years.[1] Of the total cases, 38% involved children under the age of 3 years. According to the National Poisons Information Service (Birmingham Centre), 35% of all enquiries were related to children less than age 5 years, 4% between the ages of 5–9 years, and 12% aged 10–19 years.[2] The majority of cases called to poison centres originates from the home and tend to be minor; however, there are several ingestions where minimal exposure may lead to severe toxicity or even death. It is, therefore, paramount that healthcare providers be familiar with presenting signs and symptoms, emergent management, and thoughtful disposition of the potential deadly paediatric ingestions.

GENERAL MANAGEMENT

Given that the majority of dangerous ingestions by children are of adult dose medications, it is easy to see how a child's smaller size can have an impact. Other differences in assessing and treating the poisoned child include those that are size-dependent (*e.g.* inability to use effective gastric lavage in a toddler) and those that are age-dependent (*e.g.* drug absorption and metabolism).[3]

Carson R. Harris MD FACEP FAAEM (for correspondence)
Director, Clinical Toxicology Service and Associate Professor, Department of Emergency Medicine, University of Minnesota Medical School, Minneapolis, Minnesota, USA; Senior Staff Emergency Medicine Department, and Director, Clinical Toxicology Service, Emergency Medicine Department, 640 Jackson Street, Regions Hospital, Saint Paul, MN 55101, USA.
E-mail: harri037@umn.edu

Matthew Morgan MD
Medical Toxicology Fellow, HealthPartners Institute of Medical Education, Regions Hospital, Saint Paul, Minnesota and Hennepin Regional Poison Center, Minneapolis, Minnesota, USA

GENERAL CONSIDERATIONS

It is important to remember that children less than 6 years of age rarely, if ever, ingest something to harm themselves deliberately.[4] This combined with the fact that children are pleasure seekers and most medicines are generally not to their liking, young children are inclined to ingest only small amounts. This does not necessarily translate to small import.

The initial approach to triage and management begins with stabilisation of the vital signs and assessment of mental status. Important historical features include the amount and substance the child was exposed to, time of ingestion, and whether emesis occurred. A minimal toxicological examination includes assessment of vital signs, mental status, pupils, skin, and lungs. Following stabilisation, consider decontamination and the need for an antidote.

Inducing emesis with ipecac and gastric lavage are techniques that enjoy little support among the European and American toxicology community except under the narrowest of circumstances.[5] More recently, the administration of charcoal (either in a single dose or in multiple doses) appears to be the mainstay of gut decontamination.

ACTIVATED CHARCOAL

Activated charcoal should be considered in potentially toxic ingestions that have occurred within the last hour and if airway protection is assured. It is not effective and can be potentially harmful in ingestions of heavy metals, hydrocarbons, toxic alcohols, or corrosives. When given as a single dose, the recommendation is to administer 1 g/kg unless the amount of toxin is known in which case it should be given in a 10:1 ratio by weight. Adding chocolate milk and cola may improve the palatability. With the knowledge that charcoal has never been established to make a clinical difference, the authors rarely use a nasogastric tube to instil charcoal in paediatric patients.

MULTIPLE-DOSE ACTIVATED CHARCOAL

Use of multiple doses of activated charcoal has been suggested as possibly beneficial in an overdose involving carbamazepine, theophylline, phenytoin, dapsone, and quinine.[6] Additionally, there is reason to suspect it is helpful in salicylate overdose when bezoar formation is suspected. Multiple-dose charcoal can be given at a 1 g/kg dose initially, then every 2–3 h. Only the first dose of activated charcoal should be given with sorbitol to avoid issues of electrolyte imbalance.

WHOLE BOWEL IRRIGATION

Whole bowel irrigation will most often be used in the paediatric setting of iron ingestions. Other possible uses include removal of ingested metals such as lead, packets of illicit drugs (older children more often), and button batteries. The dose in children is 500 ml/h for ages 9 months to 6 years, and 1000 ml/h in ages 7–12 years, until the effluent is clear, which should occur in most cases within 6 h. Whole bowel irrigation is best accomplished by placing a nasogastric tube due to the amount of fluid that must be instilled.

Table 1 Common antidotes

Poison	Antidote
Acetaminophen	N-acetylcysteine
Cholinesterase inhibitors	Atropine
Iron	Desferoxamine
Cardio-active steroids	Digi-FAB
Opiates	Naloxone
Methemoglobinaemia	Methylene blue
Isoniazid	Pyridoxine
Anticholinergic syndrome	Physostigmine
Lead	Di-mercapto-succunic acid (Succimer, DMSA)
Sulphonylureas	Octreotide
β-Blockers	High-dose insulin
Ethylene glycol/methanol	Fomepazole

ANTIDOTES

Most treatment for poisoning is supportive; however, there is a limited number of effective antidotes available for various possible ingestions. Some of the more common antidotes and the overdoses they treat are given in Table 1.

SULPHONYLUREAS

GENERAL OVERVIEW

Toxic exposure to oral hypoglycaemics continues to increase at a steady rate. Over 190 million people world-wide are affected by type-2 diabetes, and sulphonylurea agents are considered to be one of the primary treatments. This disease transcends all community, cultural, racial, and gender boundaries; thus, the acquisition of sulphonylurea agents represents a clear and present danger to all paediatric populations.

The second generation sulphonylureas (glimepiride, glipizide, and glyburide) exert their action by binding to specific membrane receptors within pancreatic β-islet cells, with subsequent release of preformed insulin into the systemic circulation.[7] Sulphonylureas also suppress endogenous glycogenolysis, creating further potential for symptomatic and life-threatening hypoglycaemia.[8] Case reports indicate that one or two tablets of a sulphonylurea have the potential to cause permanent neurological disability or death.[9]

CLINICAL PRESENTATION

Many of the signs and symptoms of this ingestion are related to hypoglycaemia. The child may be profusely diaphoretic, tremulous, anxious and typically tachycardic. Although the child may initially be asymptomatic, he or she can progress to overt coma and imminent death if treatment is delayed. Dizziness, lethargy, anorexia, and seizure have all been associated with significant sulphonylurea ingestion.[9,10] A wide pulse pressure with elevated systolic pressure and a decreased diastolic pressure is common. In general, the child will have hypothermia. Symptomatic hypoglycaemia may occur some hours after the ingestion.

LABORATORY FINDINGS

Blood glucose levels begin to decline early after the ingestion or can be delayed up to 48 h after ingestion. A recurrence of hypoglycaemia may persist for up to 96 h.[11] Rapid glucose testing is essential. Baseline electrolytes may be beneficial in some patients especially if the history is suspect. Other tests that may be helpful when the history is uncertain include an electrocardiogram, CT scan of the head, and chest radiography.

MANAGEMENT

Rapid stabilisation of the patient's airway, breathing, and circulation is crucial. During the initial evaluation, bedside glucose testing is done (early intervention is likely to improve mental status quickly), along with any deficiencies encountered during the primary survey. Treatment of hypoglycaemia should be weight-based administration of dextrose bolus (25% dextrose, 2–4 ml/kg in children aged 1–24 months and 50% dextrose, 1–2 ml/kg in children > 24 months). We do not recommend administering glucose prophylactically when there is no evidence of hypoglycaemia. Removal of the toxin from the patient may be partially facilitated with the use of activated charcoal (1 g/kg); however, benefits exceeding 1 h post ingestion are questionable.[12]

Glucose supplementation

The blood glucose level should be above 60 mg/dl in order to optimise ample glucose reserves. It is important to remember that continuous glucose infusion may potentiate further insulin release thereby resulting in breakthrough hypoglycaemic episodes.[8] Careful blood glucose monitoring, every 1–2 h, and frequent neurological evaluation may indicate the need for supplemental intravenous dextrose.

Octreotide

Octreotide has been studied and used as an adjunct to treatment for sulphonylurea-induced hypoglycaemia and is currently recommended for serious sulphonylurea toxicity or refractory hypoglycaemia.[13] Octreotide is a somatostatin analogue that directly inhibits insulin secretion. Its utility has been suggested through multiple case studies and reviews; however, evaluation within the paediatric population has been limited. One case report indicates the successful management with octreotide in a 5-year-old child presenting with profound hypoglycaemia and status epilepticus after a glipizide overdose.[14] Octreotide should be considered in cases of symptomatic hypoglycaemia or in cases of hypoglycaemia refractory to initial intravenous infusions or boluses of dextrose. Published dosing recommendations include 4–5 mcg/kg/day of subcutaneous octreotide given in divided doses every 6 h to a maximum dose of 50 mcg every 6 h.[9]

Glucagon

When oral glucose replacement is contra-indicated and peripheral intravenous access has proven difficult, intramuscular glucagon is a viable option. Glucagon is an endogenous catabolic hormone produced and released from pancreatic α-cells in the islets of Langerhans. It raises the glucose level by stimulating hepatic glycogenolysis and the induction of gluconeogenesis. In children, administer 0.025–0.1 mg/kg subcutaneously or intramuscularly and repeat dosing every 20 min as required. Vomiting and aspiration are risks since glucagon is well known to cause emesis. Glucagon is only a temporary modality in the emergent treatment of sulphonylurea-induced hypoglycaemia.

Observation

Considerable controversy exists regarding the exact length of observation for the asymptomatic child with suspected sulphonylurea overdose. Based on personal experience, we advocate a 24-h observation period to allow safe disposition to home with planned follow-up. However, others advocate earlier disposition if the serum glucose remains above 60 mg/dl (3.33 mmol/l) for 8 h.[9] Any documented hypoglycaemic episodes or neurological deterioration would warrant an obvious extension of observation time. In the absence of documented hypoglycaemia or mental status deterioration, feeding the child is encouraged.

CALCIUM-CHANNEL ANTAGONISTS

GENERAL OVERVIEW

Calcium-channel antagonists (Table 2) are widely used in the management of a variety of medical conditions, such as hypertension, angina pectoris, supraventricular dysrrhythmias, subarachnoid haemorrhage, and migraine prophylaxis. In many parts of the world, calcium-channel antagonists are used as an initial therapy for tocolysis in threatened preterm labour, and there is some data to support their use in bipolar disorders[15] and persistent hyperinsulinaemia hypoglycaemia of infancy.[16] The wide-spread use and

Table 2 Calcium channel antagonists

Class	Agent	Trade name
Dihydropyridines	Amlodipine	Norvasc, Istin
	Felodipine	Cardioplen, Plendil, Keloc, Vascalpha
	Nicardipine	Cardene
	Isradipine	Prescal
	Nifedipine	Adalat, Nifedipress, Slofedipine, Coracten
	Nimodipine	Nimotop
	Nisoldipine	Sular, Syscor
Phenylalkylamine	Verapamil	Verelan, Verapress, Ethimil, Securon, Univer, Cordilox
Benzothiazepine	Diltiazem	Adizem, Calcicard, Dilzem, Tildiem, Dilcardia

availability of these drugs increase the potential for a child to have access to, and accidentally ingest, one or several of the pills.

CLINICAL PRESENTATION

Calcium antagonists block the entry of calcium through voltage-sensitive, L-type, cellular membrane, calcium channels resulting in arterial smooth muscle relaxation and hypotension. In cardiac cells, these agents slow depolarisation in sino-atrial and atrioventricular nodes, leading to depressed contractility and bradycardia. Insulin release from pancreatic islet cells is inhibited by calcium antagonists and, consequently, leads to hyperglycaemia.[17] Lactic acidosis is a common finding, likely due to tissue hypoperfusion.

The classic presentation of this overdose is bradycardia with hypotension. Children can become symptomatic or could possibly die from the ingestion of one or two tablets, especially in the toddler age group.[18,19] The onset of symptoms usually occurs within 1–2 h of ingestion but may be delayed up to 24 h with extended-release preparations. Other dysrrhythmias that may occur include junctional escape rhythms, idioventricular rhythms, AV conduction abnormalities, and complete AV block. With dihydropyridine (nifedipine and others) ingestion, the child may present with hypotension and reflex tachycardia due to lack of significant SA node effect. Tachycardia may occur alone after nifedipine overdose. Typically, conduction abnormalities are rare with dihydropyridines due to absent AV node blockade.[17]

The child may present with symptoms that include unsteady gait or dizziness, obtunded, coma, and seizure activity due to cerebral hypoperfusion. Gastrointestinal symptoms may include nausea and vomiting secondary to diminished gastric motility. Bowel hypoperfusion may cause mesenteric ischaemia.[20] Ileus and small bowel obstruction have also been described and may prolong drug absorption and make decontamination efforts challenging. Metabolic features include hyperglycaemia and lactic acidosis. Finally, pulmonary oedema may result from poor myocardial function, but non-cardiogenic pulmonary oedema has been described as well.[21]

LABORATORY EVALUATION

Electrolytes, glucose, blood urea nitrogen, and creatinine should be analysed. Also consider a basic haemogram, chest radiograph and cardiac monitoring for patients in extremis. One of the primary concerns is hypoglycaemia.

MANAGEMENT

Children with suspected calcium-channel antagonist ingestions of any amount should be evaluated in a healthcare facility and monitored closely for signs of delayed toxicity. Whenever a child presents with depressed blood pressure or heart rate, the carers should be closely questioned to determine if anyone in the household is taking blood pressure or heart medicine.

Supportive care

Treatment of severe hypotension, bradycardia should begin with intravenous crystalloid, atropine, and calcium chloride. Additional pressors such as epinephrine, dopamine, and norepinephrine may be required. Atropine is notorious for being ineffective or at least inconsistently effective.

Hyperinsulinaemia euglycaemia

More recently, the addition of insulin and glucose, known as hyperinsulinaemia euglycaemic treatment, has gained acceptance as an early intervention in the treatment of toxin-induced shock states.[22] Although the ideal starting regimen for this treatment has not been established, a continuous infusion of insulin at a rate of 0.5–1 IU/kg/h has been used to reverse cardiovascular collapse due to calcium-channel antagonist overdose (anecdotally, we have successfully used doses as high as 6 IU/kg/h]. Even with this high-dose insulin therapy, some patients may not require supplemental glucose.[23] Potassium should be assessed frequently (at least every hour at the initiation of treatment) and glucose monitored closely. It has been suggested that hyperinsulinaemia euglycaemic therapy may be considered as a first-line therapy in calcium-channel antagonist intoxication. Of course, more human data are needed before this treatment modality can be recommended as first-line treatment.

Glucagon

Glucagon has been used as adjunct therapy to improve inotropic, chronotropic, and dromotropic effects of calcium antagonist overdose. However, review of animal models of calcium antagonist poisoning treated with glucagon indicates that it does not improve survival.[24]

TRICYCLIC ANTIDEPRESSANTS

GENERAL OVERVIEW

Tricyclic antidepressants have been replaced in recent years in the treatment of depression by safer alternatives. However, in Germany, tricyclic antidepressants still constitute a large percentage of the medicinal therapy for depression.[25] These agents are used for insomnia and chronic pain syndromes and, thus, maintain their availability and potential access for accidental ingestion by children. They can be extremely dangerous to children in relatively small doses due to the narrow therapeutic window. Tricyclics have effects as antimuscarinics, antihistamines, bioamine uptake inhibitors, sodium and potassium channel blockers, α-blockers, and as antiGABA agents. From these activities, their toxic manifestations can be gleaned.

In therapeutic doses, tricyclic antidepressants reach peak absorption in 2–8 h. Antimuscarinic effects in overdose can delay absorption and may be a reason to give charcoal later than current recommendations (perhaps up to 2 h).[26]

CLINICAL PRESENTATION

Common presentations after ingestion of tricyclic antidepressants include the anticholinergic toxidrome, central nervous system effects such as somnolence, agitation, or seizure, and conduction abnormalities. The anticholinergic toxidrome is characterised by flushing, fever, dry mucous membranes and skin, mydriasis and psychosis. The most severely affected patients will show signs of intoxication within 2 h; almost all patients will show signs of intoxication within 6 h.

LABORATORY EVALUATION

Workup consists of an ECG, blood chemistry and, in the case of a suicidal ingestion, a paracetamol level should be obtained to rule out concomitant ingestion. ECG findings that would be consistent with toxicity at a level that requires treatment include R'> 3 mm in aVR, or an R/S ratio greater than 0.7. Both are indicators of rightward shift of the terminal 40 ms of the QRS. The paediatric ECG, unfortunately, may have a rightward shift normally making this distinction more difficult.[27] A QRS of greater than 100 ms in someone without previously known conduction delay would also be concerning. QT interval prolongation can also be seen. A wide complex tachycardia would be the ultimate cardiac manifestation. Those with QRS durations of greater than 100 ms have been found to have greater likelihood of seizure.

MANAGEMENT

Management of tricyclic antidepressant intoxication includes decontamination with charcoal – keeping in mind that precipitous deterioration is possible and that airway protection must be taken into account. Cardiac monitoring is necessary, as is adequate intravenous access such that resuscitation can commence should it be necessary.

Sodium bicarbonate
A wide complex rhythm or the above indicators should prompt administration of sodium bicarbonate to overcome sodium channel blockade. In addition, displacement of the drug from the receptor site may be enhanced due to the increased alkalinity of the blood. Blood pH should be maintained between 7.5 and 7.55. The initial dose is 1–2 mEq/kg and repeated every 3–5 min until the desired result of narrowing of the QRS interval is attained. An infusion or repeated bolus of sodium bicarbonate can then be administered to maintain the effect. Beware of hypernatraemia if multiple doses are needed.

Hypertonic saline
If the pH becomes a limiting factor before correction of ECG abnormalities, hypertonic saline can be infused. In this circumstance, we generally recommend 3–4 ml/kg of 7.5% saline solution by intravenous push.

Other treatments
Wide complex tachyarrhythmias that persist despite the above measures should be treated with lidocaine (lignocaine). Seizures should be treated with benzodiazepines followed by barbiturates. Acidosis attributable to seizures will exacerbate tricyclic antidepressant toxicity. Hypotension, unresponsive to intravenous crystalloid, will need vasopressor therapy. There is theoretical reason to believe that norepinephrine may be preferable as it is a direct vasopressor. The toxic effects of tricyclic antidepressants can be persistent and

monitoring should continue 24 h beyond the disappearance of ECG abnormality.

TOXIC ALCOHOLS

GENERAL OVERVIEW

Unlike the other poisons discussed in this review, the toxic alcohols (ethanol, methanol, isopropanol, and ethylene glycol) are not therapeutics (with the exception of ethanol). They are included, though, as they are easily available to curious toddlers and melancholy adolescents and can cause great harm in relatively small doses.

Methanol is commonly found in windshield wiper fluid and 'wood' alcohol. The toxic metabolite of methanol is formate, which is eventually metabolised to carbon dioxide and water, with the help of folate. Ethylene glycol is a common component of antifreeze and some brake fluids. Isopropanol is most commonly encountered as rubbing alcohol. All of the mentioned alcohols are absorbed quickly and efficiently through the stomach. Isopropanol is known to be approximately twice as intoxicating as ethanol or ethylene glycol. Its metabolite, acetone, has a half-life of 22 h making the duration of intoxication longer. All of the above alcohols will cause an elevation in osmolar gap proportional to their molecular weights. Only the metabolites of methanol and ethylene glycol traditionally cause an elevation in the anion gap.

CLINICAL PRESENTATION

Ethanol

Ethanol's acute effects are well known to the general public. It often has a disinhibitory effect followed by central nervous system depression. Central nervous system depression can be profound, potentially conveying risk of aspiration. Mild hypotension may be seen due to peripheral vasodilation. In children, especially younger children, there is risk of hypoglycaemia and seizure. Workup, in general, can be minimal including blood sugar analysis. In cases where there is question of an adolescent wanting to harm themselves, a blood chemistry, paracetamol level, and ECG may be useful to rule out other ingestants such as those causing an anion gap, paracetamol co-ingestion, and those causing interval prolongation, respectively.

Isopropanol

In terms of presentation, there is little difference between isopropanol and ethanol. The child may appear intoxicated and an odour of acetone (the metabolite of isopropanol) present on the child's breath. With a significant ingestion, the child is also at risk of developing haemorrhagic gastritis, respiratory depression, hypotension and coma. Effects otherwise are essentially the same as with ethanol.

Methanol

Methanol is known for its toxic effects on the retina. In addition to blindness, methanol can cause a profound metabolic acidosis and the organ dysfunction that follows. It is notorious for causing a delayed syndrome of obtundation, acidosis, visual disturbance, and death. Granted, the visual effects will be difficult to assess in the toddler, but attempts should be made to examine the retina and assess visual acuity. Methanol is oxidised to formaldehyde and then formate which is responsible for its toxicity.

Ethylene glycol

Ethylene glycol produces a profound metabolic acidosis. The metabolites that likely cause most problems in ethylene glycol poisoning include glycolate and oxalic acid. Note that glycolate is responsible for most of the acidosis and that oxalate is responsible for renal and other organ dysfunction. Toxic manifestations are usually divided into three stages. The first stage involves central nervous system ranging from intoxication to coma. The second stage involves cardiovascular and pulmonary dysfunction and is thought to begin at 12 h and end at 24 h post-ingestion. Metabolic acidosis can become profound during this period. Cardiopulmonary dysfunction often includes hypertension initially, tachycardia, tachypnoea, heart failure and acute respiratory distress syndrome. This is the stage during which most deaths occur due to progressive cardiovascular collapse.[28] Organ dysfunction results from the altered metabolic milieu as well as deposition of calcium oxalate crystals in the viscera. The third stage begins thereafter (24–72 h) and involves renal dysfunction. Deposition of calcium oxalate crystals in the renal tubules is likely the reason for this dysfunction. Provided diagnosis is made early in the patient's course and support of renal function commences, renal compromise is often reversible.

LABORATORY STUDIES

The initial investigation of the child suspected of a toxic alcohol ingestion is to obtain basic blood chemistry, urea, creatinine, glucose, and ionised calcium levels. In addition, lactate level and ECG may be beneficial. Levels of the suspected alcohols should be ordered. Since some products contain fluorescein, the child's urine may fluoresce; however, this not a reliable indication of ingestion or non-ingestion. Oxalate crystals may be present in the urine after ethylene glycol ingestion. Chest radiograph is warranted if aspiration or pulmonary oedema is suspected.

MANAGEMENT

The treatment of isopropanol and ethanol ingestions is generally supportive care. Airway and blood pressure should be managed appropriately. Hypoglycaemia can be treated with glucose boluses and seizures managed initially with benzodiazepines.

The metabolism of ethylene glycol proceeds through successive oxidation steps that begin through the enzyme alcohol dehydrogenase. This enzyme is also the first step in the metabolism of ethylene glycol and methanol. Metabolic pathways that circumvent oxalate production may be encouraged by administration of the co-factors thiamine and pyridoxine. Treatment includes inhibition of the first step of the metabolism by a substance with a higher affinity for the enzyme.

Fomepizole (4-methylpyrazole)

Most often, when it is available, fomepizole is used to inhibit alcohol dehydrogenase. It is administered as a loading dose of 15 mg/kg followed by 10 mg/kg every 12 h for 4 doses; then the dose is increased to 15 mg/kg every 12 h because of auto-induction of metabolism. Treatment should continue until the level of methanol or ethylene glycol is less than 20 mg/dl (3222 μmol/l).

Ethanol (10%)

When fomepizole is not available, ethanol can be used for inhibition of alcohol dehydrogenase. Ethanol is administered initially at 600 mg/kg and then ethanol levels maintained at 100–150 mg/dl (21.7–32.6 mmol/l). The maintenance rate is typically 0.8–0.9 ml/kg/h. Obviously, intensive care monitoring will be necessary.

Haemodialysis

The volumes of distribution are less than 1 l/kg making the alcohols dialysable. If metabolism has already occurred to the degree that there is uncorrectable acidosis or there is significant renal dysfunction (creatinine > 3.0 mg/dl or 265 μmol/l) in the case of ethylene glycol or visual disturbance in the case of methanol poisoning, haemodialysis should be performed. Currently, haemodialysis is indicated if the methanol or ethylene glycol levels are greater than 50 mg/dl (15.6 mmol/l methanol, 8.05 mmol/l for ethylene glycol).

Other management

Other supportive care might include treatment of acidosis with sodium bicarbonate to achieve a pH of 7.30, intravenous crystalloid and pressors for hypotension, administration of metabolic cofactors – folate (or folinic acid) in methanol toxicity, and pyridoxine and thiamine in ethylene glycol poisoning.[29]

CLONIDINE

GENERAL OVERVIEW

Clonidine is a centrally acting α-adrenoreceptor agonist and is widely prescribed as a treatment for hypertension, attention deficit hyperactivity disorder, and Tourette's syndrome. It has also been used to treat opiate withdrawal syndrome.[30] Due to its wide-spread use within all age populations, clonidine remains a common paediatric ingestion. The toxic effects on the CNS and cardiovascular systems primarily contribute to the lethality of the ingestion. Death may occur with doses as small as 10 mcg/kg. The typical scenario is the child visiting grandparents and medications have been left unattended and poorly secured, making easy access for the child.

CLINICAL PRESENTATION

Clonidine toxicity chiefly resembles an opioid toxidrome due to a functional overlap of the α_2-receptors affected by clonidine and the μ-receptors affected by opioids. Symptoms include altered mental status ranging from somnolence to coma, miosis, respiratory depression, bradycardia, and hypotension. Transiently, the child may present with hypertension. Dose-related responses have been documented with cardiovascular effects seen with ingestions between 10–20 mcg/kg and respiratory depression and apnoea occur with ingestions greater that 20 mcg/kg. Most children will have signs or symptoms of toxicity within 30–90 min.[31] If attention to the child is not expeditious, cardiopulmonary arrest may ensue. Convulsions are rare but may occur with significant overdoses.

LABORATORY STUDIES

Obtaining a chemistry panel may be prudent since occasionally these patient will develop hypoglycaemia. Continuous ECG monitoring is paramount in the evaluation of these patients.

MANAGEMENT

The management of clonidine overdose remains largely supportive. Careful attention must be focused on the establishment and maintenance of a patent airway. Due to risks of bradycardia, heart block, and hypotension, continuous cardiac monitoring and a 12-lead ECG should be utilised. Activated charcoal should be administered if the patient presents within 1 h of ingestion. If a clonidine patch is ingested, whole bowel irrigation may be of benefit.

Naloxone

Due to opioid receptor overlap as described above, naloxone has been used with variable success to reverse both cardiovascular and respiratory depression. The suggested naloxone dose is 0.1 mg/kg up to a maximum of 10 mg.[32] Although this treatment is only weakly supported in the literature through case reports, it is a relatively benign modality to attempt.

Supportive care

Refractory cases of bradycardia will usually respond to atropine. Hypotension should be managed with aggressive fluid resuscitation. Dopamine is a good starting vasopressor, initially at 5 mcg/kg/min and increasing in 5 mcg/kg/min increments as needed. Norepinephrine can be added once the maximum infusion dose of dopamine is attained (more than 20 mcg/kg/min). At moderate doses, dopamine may provide sufficient blood pressure support while its chronotropic properties may assuage clonidine-induced bradycardia.[31]

Disposition

Admission to a paediatric intensive care unit is recommended for patients with altered mental status, respiratory depression, or cardiac abnormality. Those without evidence of toxicity within 6–8 h post-ingestion can be safely discharge following an observation period of 6–8 h.[32]

SALICYLATES

GENERAL OVERVIEW

Salicylates are used less frequently for paediatric patients since the awareness of its controversial association with Reye's syndrome.[33] There are the adult formulations and other forms of salicylates can be found in high concentration in several products commonly used in the home and accessible to children; most notably, oil of wintergreen (methyl salicylate) which is contained in liniments or rubefacients. One millilitre of a 98% concentration of oil of wintergreen is equivalent to 1400 mg of salicylate. The toxic dose of salicylate is reported as 200 mg/kg; thus, an ingestion of less than 5 ml of this product is potentially lethal to the curious toddler. Liquid preparations undergo rapid absorption, typically within 1 h, and are converted quickly to salicylate. It should be remembered that Chinese herbal medications or Chinese medicated oils may also contain salicylates. At toxic doses in children, the elimination half-life of salicylates increases from 2 h to 4 h (at therapeutic levels) to 15–29 h.[34]

MECHANISMS OF TOXICITY

The pathophysiological mechanisms of salicylates include: (i) stimulation of the respiratory centre in the brainstem causes hyperventilation; and (ii) uncoupling of oxidative phosphorylation resulting in increased oxygen consumption, further respiratory stimulation, metabolic acidosis and compensatory response by the kidney to excrete bicarbonate, potassium and sodium. Toxic doses can lead to an increase in pulmonary vascular permeability and an increase in leukotrienes resulting in pulmonary oedema. Glucose consumption is increased, gluconeogenesis is inhibited, and insulin secretion is enhanced.[35] These toxic actions can lead to significant hypoglycaemia, particularly in children.

Solid or pill preparations are absorbed more slowly through the stomach. Pylorospasms, which result from salicylate may contribute to delayed absorption and can lead to bezoar formation. Bezoar formation is associated with continued and erratic absorption causing a prolonged and fluctuating clinical course.

CLINICAL PRESENTATION

The characteristic presentation of salicylate toxicity include gastrointestinal distress, hyperventilation, tinnitus and metabolic acidosis. Initial presentation also includes nausea and vomiting. Hyperventilation results from respiratory centre stimulation and, later, a response to the progressive metabolic acidosis. Children under the age of 2 years generally present with metabolic acidosis, whereas, older children may present with respiratory alkalosis. Classically, vital signs are increased and the patient will present with tachypnoea, tachycardia, fever, and occasionally hypertension. Diaphoresis is also a classic finding. The uncoupling of oxidative phosphorylation results in inefficient energy production and hyperthermia. A lactic acidosis is the result of less efficient anaerobic metabolism. Salicylates are also known to cause hypoglycaemia in children as a result of additional inhibition of gluconeogenesis and increased insulin secretion.

Patients may complain of hearing disturbances. Mental status can range from normal to comatose. Dehydration will occur from gastrointestinal losses, tachypnoea, and fever. Ultimately, pulmonary oedema, cerebral oedema, coma and subsequent multi-organ failure are the characteristics of end-stage poisoning.

LABORATORY FINDINGS

Laboratory findings include an anion gap acidosis, hypokalaemia, hypoglycaemia, and an indication of pre-renal insufficiency. Imaging may reveal pulmonary or cerebral oedema. The basic chemistry panel will give valuable information. Salicylate levels should be obtained and followed, but do not totally rely on levels; the clinical condition of the child will ultimately dictate management.

MANAGEMENT

Management begins with resuscitation. The combination of altered mental status and vomiting may necessitate airway protection. Care should be taken if the child is tracheally intubated. Ventilator settings must be adjusted appropriately. Patients who were previously compensating for the metabolic acidosis can suddenly deteriorate in the situation of a forced decrease in minute ventilation. The same applies to over-sedation of the agitated, salicylate-poisoned patient. Severely poisoned patients will be hypovolaemic and will need volume resuscitation. Charcoal should be administered if there is a secure airway. Crystalloid fluids with sodium bicarbonate should be given in severely poisoned children or children with levels over 30 mg/dl (0.22 mmol/l) 150 mEq of bicarbonate in 850 ml of D5W at a rate twice that of maintenance should be given. This creates a nearly isotonic solution; however, the patient should be monitored for fluid overloading. Alternatively, in a child, you may administer sodium bicarbonate 25–50 mmol (25 ml of an 8.4% solution) intravenously over 1 h and give additional boluses intravenously to maintain urine pH in the range 7.5–8.5. This will trap the ionised form of salicylates in the renal tubule and increase excretion of the salicylic acid. Serial salicylate levels should be followed until two successive decreasing non-toxic levels are obtained. We generally recommend levels every 2–3 h. The end-point of alkalinisation is when the salicylate level is less than 25 mg/dl.[36] Those with altered mental status, fluid overload, or uncorrectable metabolic acidaemia should be haemodialysed.

PARACETAMOL (ACETAMINOPHEN)

GENERAL OVERVIEW

Paracetamol is widely used in over-the-counter and prescription preparations and is, therefore, one of the most common toxic ingestions in children. The dilemma associated with paracetamol toxicity is an asymptomatic period which is longer than the threshold time for administering a completely effective antidote. Children seem to be somewhat protected from toxicity due, in part, to better conjugation of paracetamol. Before age 9–12 years, children are known to metabolise paracetamol predominantly with sulphation; this being relatively more important that glucuronidation which is the predominant conjugation pathway in adolescents and adults. In the case of paracetamol, this appears to contribute to lesser hepatotoxicity in children. Hepatotoxicity can develop in this younger age group, but at a lesser rate than in adults with similar levels. Glutathione helps to detoxify N-acetyl-pbenzoquinoneimine, the toxic metabolite of paracetamol, and children may have a greater production of glutathione than adults.[37]

CLINICAL PRESENTATION

The initial period after a toxic ingestion of paracetamol, anytime between 0–24 h, can be asymptomatic or can lead to gastric irritation, nausea and vomiting. At 24–48 h, the patient can again be asymptomatic or appear to improve. They may develop some right, upper-quadrant, abdominal pain and tenderness. During this period, transaminases will begin to rise. At 48 h, overt signs of hepatotoxicity may develop such as jaundice, bleeding diatheses, altered mental status and so on. From days 3–5, patients will show signs of recovery or deterioration towards death.

LABORATORY STUDIES

A paracetamol level should be drawn 4-h post-ingestion or immediately if the child presents after 4 h. In a single acute ingestion, this level is placed on the Rumack–Matthew nomogram to assess potential toxicity. The basic chemistry panel, hepatic function tests, coagulation studies, glucose, and urea with creatinine should be obtained and followed at least daily or as clinically indicated. Other tests that may be helpful are lactate and phosphorus levels.

MANAGEMENT

If the ingestion has occurred within 1 h of the child's arrival, activated charcoal should be administered. The Rumack–Matthew nomogram is available for determining the toxicity of the obtained level. A 4-h level above 200 mcg/ml (1325 μmol/l) is considered toxic and necessitates treatment with the antidote. The antidote, N-acetylcysteine, is nearly 100% effective if given within 8 h.[39] If a paracetamol level cannot be obtained before this time, the antidote should be administered empirically based on the history of a potentially toxic ingestion and can be stopped if the level is non-toxic. The antidote most often can be given according to the Prescott protocol which is administered over 20 h. A loading dose of 150 mg/kg is followed by 50 mg/kg over 4 h and then 100 mg/kg over 16 h. Prior to stopping N-acetylcysteine therapy, aspartate transaminase and paracetamol levels should be determined. If the aspartate transaminase is declining and less than 1000 IU/l and paracetamol level less than 10 μg/ml (66.2 μmol/l), the infusion can safely be discontinued. Otherwise, a repeat of the 16-h infusion can be administered. In children weighing less than 20 kg, carefully monitor the amount of fluids given.

Other management issues

Criteria for liver transplant considerations consist of the following: blood pH < 7.3 after adequate fluid resuscitation; or prothrombin time 100 s or INR 6.5, and creatinine > 3.4 mg/dl (301 mmol/l) plus grade III or IV encephalopathy; lactate > 3 mmol/L after fluid resuscitation. Any intentional ingestion should be evaluated in light of the unreliability of the history and for psychiatric or social conditions placing the child at risk.

OPIOIDS

GENERAL OVERVIEW

Opioids are extremely popular for controlling moderate-to-severe pain. In addition to their therapeutic use, they are one of the most abused categories of drugs. Because of their wide-spread use in modern medicine and as an illicit drug, they have become easily accessible to children in the home setting. Methadone and oxycodone are frequently incriminated as a cause of paediatric deaths due to accidental overdose. The minimal lethal paediatric dose is not known; a small child who ingests even residual amounts of methadone suspension left in a bottle can progress from drowsiness to coma within 30 min.[40] With their increased mobility after infancy, curiosity, and oral fixation, toddlers are at high risk of ingesting illicit narcotics that are left unattended by adults.

CLINICAL PRESENTATION

Opioids bind to three main receptors (mu, kappa, and delta) located throughout the CNS and peripheral nervous systems and in the gastrointestinal tract. Activation of these receptors by the opioids results in a variety of life-threatening complications.[41] The classic triad of CNS depression, respiratory depression and miosis should signal the clinician to probable opioid ingestion. Additionally, dizziness, euphoria or dysphoria, depressed reflexes, altered sensory perception, lethargy and coma are typically seen. The child may ignore painful stimuli, or present with coma, bradycardia, and quickly progress to non-cardiogenic pulmonary oedema, apnoea, circulatory collapse, and cardiac arrest. If a child presents with suspicion of narcotic ingestion, it is vitally important to quiz the adult caretaker regarding the possibility of access to narcotics.

MANAGEMENT

If the child presents within 1 h of ingesting a delayed-absorption product such as diphenoxylate-atropine (Lomotil) or sustained release morphine or oxycodone, 1 g/kg of activated charcoal should be administered paying close attention to the mental status and respiratory depression. Activated charcoal should be given either orally or by naso- or orogastric tube.

Naloxone

The usual initial dose of naloxone for patients with CNS depression without respiratory depression is 0.1–0.4 mg intravenously for both adults and children. If there is partial or absent response, then naloxone 2 mg should be administered as an intravenous bolus and repeated every 3 min up to a total dose of 10–20 mg. When there is respiratory depression, initial higher doses of naloxone should be given, starting with 1–2 mg. The effective dose may have to be repeated every 20–60 min, depending on the half-life of the opioid ingested and patient's response. A continuous infusion may be appropriate, titrated to patient's respiratory status and level of conscious if long-acting narcotics, such as methadone, are ingested. The infusion rate may be started at two-thirds the amount needed to reverse the child's respiratory depression per hour.[42]

Naloxone can be given by almost any route, including intranasally and nebulised. Although the intranasal route is not as effective as intramuscular, it is still effective in reversing opiate-induced respiratory depression.[43]

Nalmefene

The long-acting narcotic antagonist, nalmefene, is an option in children that are non-opioid-dependent and not at risk of withdrawal. Although there is limited literature on this treatment in children, it appears to be safe and effective in opioid toxicity.

Disposition

Children who have ingested long-acting or delayed absorption opioids, have recurrent respiratory depression after treatment with naloxone, or have signs of pulmonary oedema should be admitted. Consider the home environment and safety of the child when deciding to release versus admit the child.

QUININE AND QUINIDINE

GENERAL OVERVIEW

Both quinine and quinidine are well known for their narrow therapeutic windows. Quinine remains the drug of choice for severe *Plasmodium falciparum* malaria and *Babesia microti* infection. The intravenous formulation is recommended in severe cases of malaria in the UK.[5] Quinine was, until recently, routinely prescribed for the restless leg syndrome. Although the amount of quinine readily available to the general population of children is less and declining, it is one of the more concerning overdoses due to its high potential for toxicity. Quinidine, the optical isomer of quinine, has been prescribed for its anti-dysrrhythmic properties (both are class IA anti-dysrrhythmics). It is used much less now as there are safer alternatives. Both medicines are highly protein bound but less so in children under age 2 years, which may predispose them to more serious toxicity. Both medicines are quickly and efficiently absorbed from the small intestine.

CLINICAL PRESENTATION

Manifestations of toxicity can be seen as early as 30 min and peak serum levels are seen 1–4 h after ingestion. The major morbidity and mortality are due to the neurological and cardiovascular manifestations. Typically, cardiovascular effects precede the neurological effects. Sodium and potassium channels are antagonised leading to prolongation of the QRS and QT intervals and, eventually, to ventricular dysrrhythmias and asystole. Decreases in contractility of the myocardium can also be seen with higher doses of quinine and quinidine. Neurological manifestations of the drugs include seizure, coma, visual and hearing abnormalities. Hearing and visual disturbances are part of a largely reversible syndrome termed cinchonism, so named for the cinchona tree from which both drugs are derived. Other manifestations of the syndrome include gastrointestinal symptoms such as abdominal pain, vomiting, and diarrhoea, skin flushing, and nervous system disturbances. Visual disturbances, which are seen predominately with quinine, can include progressive visual loss that can result in permanent blindness. Direct toxicity to the retina is the aetiology of visual loss.

There are two cases of toxicity resulting in death, one each for quinine and quinidine, resulting from ingestion of just two tablets.[44] For this reason, any ingestion of these compounds in a child that is more than a therapeutic dose should prompt an evaluation in emergency department.

MANAGEMENT

Asymptomatic children should be watched for 6 h for regular preparations and 12 h for extended-release preparations. Symptomatic patients will need admission and monitoring for a period extending until disappearance of manifestations and normalisation of the ECG for 24 h. Treatment will depend on the manifestations. Strong consideration should be given to administering activated charcoal in ingestions that have occurred within the previous hour. Precipitous deterioration can occur and should be taken into account, as should current level of consciousness.

Cardiac abnormalities
Lengthening of the QRS interval should prompt treatment of the sodium channel blockade with sodium bicarbonate. Dosing is outlined in the section on tricyclic antidepressants. Prolongation of the QT interval, evidence of potassium channel blockade, can be managed by ensuring adequate potassium and magnesium levels. Torsade de Pointes, the feared evolution of a prolonged QT interval is managed in the usual way. Ventricular tachycardia and fibrillation should be treated with the class 1B antidysrrhythmic lidocaine provided the patient has been given sodium bicarbonate and this has been ineffective.

Seizure management
Seizures should be treated with benzodiazepines followed by barbiturates. Propofol is also a useful anti-seizure medication in the case of intubated patients. Care is otherwise supportive with vasopressors given to those whose blood pressure does not respond to fluids.

Key points for clinical practice

- Level of development needs to be considered in the evaluation of a poisoned child. A child over the age of 6 years should at least have motive considered and appropriately dealt with.

- Most of the care for a poisoned patient is supportive; however, in each patient, decontamination, specific antidotal therapy, and ruling out of co-ingestion should be undertaken when appropriate.

Key points for clinical practice *(continued)*

- Quinine and quinidine are known for cardiovascular and neurological toxicity manifest by arrhythmia and seizure. These drug are associated with cinchonism, symptom complex associated with quinine (or cinchona bark) ingestion.

- Of the toxic alcohols, ethylene glycol and methanol produce the most profound metabolic effects and are thus life-threatening.

- Isopropanol produces a state of drunkenness more profound than ethanol but is otherwise a less severe toxic alcohol poisoning.

- Early consideration of bicarbonate and awareness of the potential need for dialysis are essential to the management of salicylate toxicity.

- Care should be taken in taking away respiratory drive in the salicylate poisoned patient as with any patient with a severe metabolic acidosis.

- Priority should be given to administering *N*-acetylcysteine within 8 h to those with toxic ingestion of paracetamol.

- Life-threatening tricyclic antidepressant poisoning often manifests within 2 h of ingestion. Toxic manifestations should definitely be seen within 6 h if they are going to occur.

- Infusion of sodium bicarbonate therapy is the mainstay of treatment for wide-complex rhythms in tricyclic antidepressant toxicity. The purpose is to alkalinise the blood not the urine as in salicylate poisoning.

- The presentation of clonidine poisoning is similar to narcotic overdose. Naloxone may be attempted to reverse the symptoms. The child may present initially with hypertension.

- Death from clonidine ingestion may occur with doses as small as 10 mcg/kg.

- In sulphonylurea ingestion, octreotide should be considered in cases of symptomatic or refractory hypoglycaemia.

- After sulphonylurea ingestion, an observation period of 12–24 h is recommended to allow safe disposition to home.

- Methadone and oxycodone are frequent causes of paediatric deaths due to accidental overdose.

- Naloxone can be administered by almost any route, including intranasal and nebulised.

- High-dose insulin infusion while maintaining euglycaemia has gained acceptance as an early intervention in the treatment of calcium-channel blocker overdose.

References

1. Lai M, Klein-Schwartz W, Rodgers GC *et al*. 2005 Annual Report of the American Association of Poison Control Centers' National Poisoning and Exposure Database. *Clin Toxicol* 2005; **22**: 335–404.
2. Annual Report 2003. NPIS (Birmingham Center). <http://www.npis.org/NPIS/Annual%20report%202003.pdf> [Accessed 22 February 2007].
3. Gussow L, Bizovi K. Acetaminophen. In: Erickson TB, Ahrens WR, Aks SE, Boom CR, Ling LJ. (eds) *Pediatric Toxicology*, 1st edn. New York: McGraw Hill, 2005; 212–218.
4. Fine JS. Pediatric principles. In: Flomenbaum NE, Howland MA, Goldfrank LR, Lewin NA, Hoffman RS, Nelson LS. (eds) *Goldfrank's Toxicologic Emergencies*, 8th edn. New York: McGraw Hill, 2006; 487—500.
5. Vale JA. Position statement: Gastric lavage. American Academy of Clinical Toxicology; European Association of Poison Centres and Clinical Toxicologists. *J Toxicol Clin Toxicol* 2004; **42**: 933–943.
6. Krenzelak EP, Vale JA, Barceloux DG. Multiple-dose activated charcoal. In: Brent J, Wallace KL, Bunjhart KK, Phillips SD, Donovan JW. (eds) *Critical Care Toxicology*, 1st edn. St Louis, MO: Mosby, 2005; 61–65.
7. Buse JB, Polonsky KS, Burant CF. Type 2 diabetes mellitus. In: Larsen PR, Kronenberg HM, Melmed S, Hardin R,. Polonsky KS. (eds) *Williams' Textbook of Endocrinology*, 10th edn. Philadelphia, PA: WB Saunders, 2003; 1427–1468.
8. Wolf LR, Smeeks F, Policastro M. Oral hypoglycemic agents. In: Ford MD, Delaney KA, Ling LJ, Erickson T. (eds) *Clinical Toxicology*, 1st edn. Philadelphia, PA: WB Saunders, 2001; 423–432.
9. Little G, Boniface K. Are one or two dangerous? Sulfonylurea exposure in toddlers. *J Emerg Med* 2005; **28**: 305–310.
10. Spiller HA. Prospective multicenter study of sulfonylurea ingestion in children. *J Pediatr* 1997; **131**: 68–78.
11. Koken L, Dart RC. Oral hypoglycemics: ACMTnet concurs. *Clin Toxicol* 1996; **34**: 271–272.
12. Krenzelok EP, Vale JA. Single-dose activated charcoal. *Clin Toxicol* 2005; **43**: 61–87.
13. McLaughlin SA, Crandall CS, McKinney PE. Octreotide: an antidote for sulfonylurea-induced hypoglycemia. *Ann Emerg Med* 2000; **36**: 133–138.
14. Mordel A, Sivilotti MLA, Old AC, Ferm RP. Octreotide for pediatric sulfonylurea poisoning [Abstract]. *J Toxicol Clin Toxicol* 1998; **36**: 437.
15. Levy NA, Janicak PG. Calcium channel antagonists for the treatment of bipolar disorder. *Bipolar Disorder* 2000; **2**: 108–119.
16. Eichmann D, Hufnagel M, Quick P *et al*. Treatment of hyperinsulinemic hypoglycemia with nifedipine. *Eur J Pediatr* 1999; **158**: 204–206.
17. Anderson AC. Calcium channel blockers overdose. *Clin Pediatr Emerg Med* 2005; **6**: 109–115.
18. Spiller HA, Romoska EA. Isradipine ingestion in a two-year-old child. *Vet Hum Toxicol* 1993; **35**: 233.
19. Bar-Oz B, Levichek Z, Koren G. Medications that can be fatal for a toddler with one tablet or teaspoonful: a 2004 update. *Paediatr Drugs* 2004; **6**: 123–126.
20. Wax PM. Intestinal infarction due to nifedipine overdose. *J Toxicol Clin Toxicol* 1995; **33**: 725–728.
21. Rasmussen L, Husted SE, Johnsen SP. Severe intoxication after an intentional overdose of amlodipine. *Acta Anaesthesiol Scand* 2003; **47**: 1038–1040.
22. Boyer EW, Shannon M. Treatment of calcium channel blocker intoxication with insulin infusion. *N Engl J Med* 2001; **344**: 1721–1722.
23. Yuan TH, Kerns II WP, Toamszewski CA, Ford MD, Kline JA. Insulin-glucose adjunctive therapy for severe calcium channel antagonist poisoning. *J Toxicol Clin Toxicol* 1999; **37**: 463–474.
24. Bailey B. Glucagon in beta-blocker and calcium channel blocker overdoses: a systematic review. *J Toxicol Clin Toxicol* 2003; **41**: 595–602.
25. Fegert JM, Kolch M, Zito JM, Glaeske G, Jahnsen K. Antidepressant use in children and adolescents in Germany. *J Child Adolesc Psychopharmacol* 2006; **16**: 197–206.
26. Rosenbaum J, Kau M. Are one or two dangerous? Tricyclic antidepressant exposure in toddlers. *J Emerg Med* 2005; **28**: 169–174.

27. Harrigan RA. Tricyclic antidepressants. In: Chan TC, Brady WJ, Harrigan RA, Ornato JP, Rosen P. (eds) *ECG in Emergency Medicine and Acute Care*, 1st edn. New York: Elsevier, 2005; 272–274.

28. White ML, Liebelt E: Update on antidotes for pediatric poisoning. *Pediatr Emerg Care* 2006; **22**: 740–746.

29. Harris CR, Henry K. Deadly ingestions. *Pediatr Clin North Am* 2006; **53**: 293–315.

30. Wallen MC, Lorman WJ, Gosciniak JL. Combined buprenorphine and clonidine for short-term opiate detoxification: patient perspectives. *J Addict Dis* 2006; **25**: 23–31.

31. Henretig FM. Clonidine and central-acting antihypertensives. In: Ford MD, Delaney KA, Ling LJ, Erickson T. (eds) *Clinical Toxicology*, 1st edn. Philadelphia, PA: WB Saunders, 2001; 391–396.

32. Tenenbein M. Naloxone in clonidine toxicity. *Am J Dis Child* 1984; **138**: 1084.

33. Bzduch V, Behulova D, Lohnert W *et al*. Metabolic cause of Reye-like syndrome. *Bratisl Lek Listy* 2001; **102**: 427–429.

34. Levy G. Pharmacokinetics of salicylate elimination in man. *J Pharm Sci* 1965; **54**: 959–967.

35. Donovan JW, Akhtar J. Salicylates. In: Ford MD, Delaney KA, Ling LJ, Erickson T. (eds) *Clinical Toxicology*, 1st edn. Philadelphia, PA: WB Saunders, 2001; 275–280.

36. Proudfoot AT, Krenzelok EP, Vale JA. Position paper on urine alkalinization. *J Toxicol Clin Toxicol* 2004; **42**: 1–26.

37. Gussow L, Bizovi K. Acetaminophen. In: Erickson TB, Ahrens WR, Aks SE, Boom CR, Ling LJ. (eds) *Pediatric Toxicology*, 1st edn. New York: McGraw-Hill, 2005; 212–218.

38. Kearns GL. Acetaminophen poisoning in children. Treat early and long enough. *J Pediatr* 2002; **140**: 495–498.

39. Smilkstein MJ, Knapp GL, Kulig KW, Rumack BH. Efficacy of oral *N*-acetylcysteine in the treatment of acetaminophen overdose. Analysis of the national multicenter study (1976 to 1985). *N Engl J Med* 1988; **319**: 1557–1562.

40. Blatman S. Narcotic poisoning of children through accidental ingestion of methadone and *in utero*. *Pediatrics* 1974; **54**: 329–332.

41. Kleinschmidt KC, Wainscott M, Ford MD. Opioids. In: Ford MD, Delaney KA, Ling LJ, Erickson T. (eds) *Clinical Toxicology*, 1st edn. Philadelphia, PA: WB Saunders, 2001; 627–639.

42. Erickson TB. Opioids. In: Erickson TB, Aherns WR, Aks SE, Baum CR, Ling LJ. (eds) *Pediatric Toxicology: Diagnosis and Management of the Poisoned Child*. New York: McGraw-Hill, 2005; 409–415.

43. Kelly AM, Kerr D, Dietze P, Patrick I, Walker T, Koutsogiannis Z. Randomised trial of intranasal versus intramuscular naloxone in prehospital treatment for suspected opioid overdose. *Med J Aust* 2005; **182**: 24–27.

44. Huston M, Levinson M. Are one or two dangerous? Quinine and quinidine exposure in toddlers. *J Emerg Med* 2006; **31**: 395–401.

Peter S. Blair Peter Fleming

8

Co-sleeping and infant death

Co-sleeping is a normal infant-care behaviour in many different cultures and is commonly practiced in Western society. In England, almost half of all neonates bed-share at some time with their parents: a fifth of infants are brought into the parental bed on a regular basis over the first year of life.[1] Similar or higher rates of bed-sharing at 3 months of age have recently been reported in other European countries, including Ireland (21%), Germany (23%), Italy (24%), Scotland (25%), Austria (30%), Denmark (39%) and Sweden (65%).[2] Even in countries where bed-sharing is uncommon, such as The Netherlands, Norway and the US, all have reported an increase in the prevalence of bed-sharing in the last decade.[3–5] Proposed physiological benefits of close contact between infants and care-givers include improved cardiorespiratory stability and oxygenation, fewer crying episodes, better thermoregulation, an increased prevalence and duration of breast-feeding, and enhanced milk production.[6,7] The postulated benefits of breast-feeding are increasingly being recognised and actively promoted by the World Health Organization, United Nations Children's Fund and the UK National Health Service. Co-sleeping can facilitate breast-feeding and the promotion of one practice can lead to the promotion of the other. However, the parental bed, particularly in Western societies, is not designed with infant safety in mind and co-sleeping has been implicated in rare accidental infant deaths due to entrapment and parental overlaying.[8] More recently, epidemiological studies investigating sudden infant death syndrome (SIDS) have shown a proportional increase of these deaths in the co-sleeping environment,[9–12] which

Peter S. Blair MSc PhD (for correspondence)
Senior Research Fellow, Institute of Child Life and Health, University of Bristol, UK and FSID
Research Unit, Level D, St Michael's Hospital, Southwell Street, Bristol BS2 8EG, UK
E-mail: p.s.blair@bris.ac.uk

Peter Fleming PhD MB ChB FRCP FRCP(C) FRCPCH
Professor of Infant Health and Developmental Physiology, Institute of Child Life and Health,
University of Bristol, UK

has led some authorities, including the American Academy of Pediatrics,[13] to recommend against bed-sharing. The unusual level of criticism and hostility[14–17] generated by this recommendation is a testament to the current polarised debate both within and beyond the field of SIDS of the potential risk and perceived benefits of parents and infants sharing the same bed. In the UK, the current advice is to place the sleeping infant in a cot beside the parental bed for the first 6 months of life but falls short of advising indiscriminately against bed-sharing. This is a review of the evidence surrounding the debate on whether infants should share the parental bed to sleep with particular reference to the field of SIDS research.

Explained accidental deaths in the infant sleeping environment

Explained accidental infant deaths are rare in the sleeping environment and much less common than SIDS deaths, which, by definition, are unexplained. The cause usually attributed to accidental death is mechanical asphyxia and occurs unobserved in both the solitary and co-sleeping environments, though evidence for asphyxia is often only circumstantial. Infants found wedged between a mattress and wall, piece of furniture or cot frame is the most usual scenario and is primarily a pattern amongst the 3–6-month-old infants[18] who have begun to develop several motor skills including moving from side to side, pushing themselves up and being able to roll over. Thus, they have the capability to move around the bed or cot but not necessarily the muscle development, particularly in the neck, to extricate the head (which is 15–20% of the total body weight) from a wedged position. Accidental asphyxia may also occur when the infants are found face down with the mouth and nose obstructed by non-permeable materials, found suspended usually involving head entrapment or caught clothing, entangled round the neck or found smothered or compressed under the weight of an object including parental overlaying. The carotid arteries in the soft tissues of the infant neck are relatively unprotected and vulnerable to compression; as little as 2 kg of pressure exerted on the neck can result in vascular occlusion.[19] Particular hazards within the infant sleeping environment include ill-fitting cot mattresses, faulty furniture, small gaps between the adult mattress and wall, headboard or adjacent furniture, filled plastic bags, railed bunk-beds, waterbeds and trailing cords (curtain, telephone, dummy, *etc.*). Pressure on the carotid sinus leads to a profound fall in heart rate, particularly in infants; this, in the presence of defective vasomotor control, could lead to lethal circulatory failure, suggesting another possible mechanism than asphyxia for the pathogenesis of lethal entrapment.[20]

Less than 10% of all accidental deaths in the infant sleeping environment are attributed to parental overlaying.[18] Statistics are not routinely available although the tenth revision of the *International Classification of Diseases* does list the much wider category of 'accidental suffocation and strangulation in bed' as a specific code. Between 2001 and 2004, on average 17 infants a year were assigned this code in England and Wales, suggesting a rate of 0.024 deaths per 1000 live-births,[21,22] compared to more than 300 deaths a year diagnosed as SIDS in the same population over the same time period. Infants found overlaid are often very young; reports from a large US study of 121 such deaths over a

7-year period suggest that around 60% were less than one month old.[19] When an infant is overlain, the infant's airway may be obstructed, the thorax or abdomen may be compressed, or the neck circulation impaired but a conclusive diagnosis is sometimes difficult. Post mortem findings are often negative and the prevalence of bruising, contusions and petechiae are not clear.[23] The lividity pattern may support the position of the infant as well as show blanching due to the pressure; however, pressure marks from the co-sleeper, the bedding or from the compressing object can occur after the death so are not conclusive evidence in themselves. The lividity that develops within 30–60 min after death in an infant is indicative of the position in which the infant has been lying; if the infant has been lying in that position for less than 3–4 h after death (which is almost always the case), then the pattern of lividity will change over the next few hours, to that of the position (almost always supine) in which the infant has been placed after death has been confirmed. Thus, unless careful observations of the presence and distribution of lividity are made by those who see the infant shortly after the death is discovered, the observations made hours or days later by the pathologist will be potentially misleading in terms of infant position. The majority of post-neonatal infant deaths are unexplained (*i.e.* SIDS), occur unobserved during infant and parental sleep and a proportion are expected to occur in the parental bed. It is, therefore, entirely possible that overlaying may also occur in some instances after this unexplained final event.

Historical perspective of bed-sharing and unexplained SIDS death

The diagnosis of SIDS is unique in that it is derived by exclusion, by failing to demonstrate an adequate cause of death after reviewing the clinical history of the infant, investigating the death scene and conducting a thorough post mortem examination. It is an admission that we do not know why the baby died. The acceptance of SIDS as an international classification was only agreed in 1969 but unexpected and unexplained infant deaths have occurred throughout history. Prior to the 20th century, most infants slept in bed with their parents. The majority of unexpected infant deaths thus occurred in bed with an adult and were attributed to overlaying of the infant by one or both parents. The prevalence of overlaying was not recorded but the prevention was a matter of great concern for many scientific academies. In 1732, the Royal Society in London was presented with the *arcuccio*, a cradle often used in Florence, with iron arches above the sleeping place, to prevent overlaying.[24] By implication, the assumption of overlaying meant that the death of the infant was considered an accident and, therefore, did not need to be investigated; parents were dealt with by the ecclesiastical rather than the secular courts. The *Births and Deaths Registration Act* of 1836 required the certification of the medical cause of every death in England and Wales, yet the evidence for overlaying was mainly circumstantial. Coroners such as Wakely of Middlesex, editor of *The Lancet*, dismissed, except very rarely, the assumption of death from overlaying and called for thorough investigation by uniform post mortem examinations.[24] Cots became widely used in the 20th century, yet unexpected infant deaths continued to occur in this solitary environment leading to the term 'cot death' more precisely now described as SIDS. In the

1960s, parents were encouraged not only to take the infant out of the parental bed, but also the cot out of the parental bedroom to facilitate infant independence.[25] The wisdom of such advice has since been questioned whilst more recent findings from SIDS studies suggest that sharing the parental bedroom, if not the bed, affords protection to the infant.[26,27] The evidence associated with bed-sharing prior to the fall in SIDS rates in the 1990s was mixed – two studies reported a risk[28,29] whilst one suggested a possible protective effect.[30]

The proportional increase of SIDS victims found in the parental bed

The 'Back to Sleep' intervention campaign encouraging parents to place their infant in the supine position to sleep was initiated in 1991 and has led to a 75% fall in SIDS deaths in England & Wales over the last 15 years (Fig. 1).

In Avon, we have a unique longitudinal cohort of 300 consecutive SIDS deaths from 1984 to 2003 and, for many of these (96%), we have accurately recorded the sleeping environment in which they were discovered. The majority (74.3%) were found sleeping alone in a cot or sleeping place designed specifically for the infant (Moses basket, carry cot, pram, *etc.*), 19.4% were found co-sleeping in the parental bed, 3.8% co-sleeping with a parent on a sofa and 2.4% elsewhere (found dead in a baby seat, in the parental bed alone, in the parents arms, *etc.*). These proportions, however, dramatically change over time confirming reports from recent studies[9–12] of a proportional increase in co-sleeping deaths amongst SIDS infants (Fig. 2). The proportion of SIDS infants found in a solitary sleeping environment in Avon has halved over the 20-year period from 88% to 42%, whilst the proportion found co-sleeping in the parental bed or sofa has increased from 12% to 50%.

However, if we look at the numbers rather than the relative proportions, a different picture emerges (Fig. 3). The dominating feature is the fall in those SIDS infants who died in a cot. Prior to the UK 'Back to Sleep' campaign in November 1991, around 22 SIDS infants a year in Avon were discovered dead sleeping alone in a cot, compared to just 3 deaths a year after this campaign – a 7-fold difference. Amongst those SIDS infants found in the parental bed, around 4 deaths a year occurred in Avon prior to the campaign compared to 2

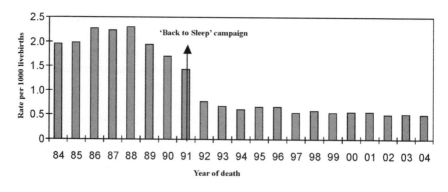

Fig. 1 SIDS rate in England and Wales, 1984–2004. Source: Office for National Statistics (ONS) and Foundation for the Study of Infant Deaths (FSID).

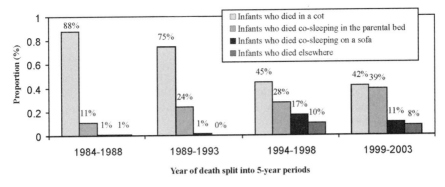

Fig. 2 Proportion of SIDS deaths in Avon by sleeping environment. Source: Avon Longitudinal Study (*n* = 288 SIDS deaths).

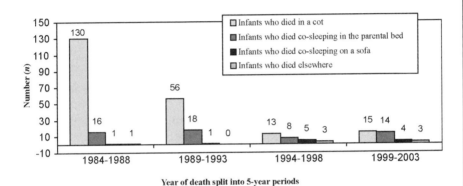

Fig. 3 Number of SIDS deaths in Avon by sleeping environment. Source: Avon Longitudinal Study (*n* = 288 SIDS deaths).

deaths a year subsequently. Thus, although the proportion of SIDS deaths in the parental bed may have dramatically risen, the actual number of deaths in this environment has halved. The number of co-sleeping SIDS deaths occurring on a sofa are smaller but a worrying observation is that only 2 deaths occurred in this environment in the 10 years between 1984 and 1993 but 9 such deaths occurred in the subsequent 10 years.

The dramatic reduction in the number of SIDS deaths found sleeping alone in a cot has largely been brought about by closely scrutinising the solitary sleeping environment in which they were found. A similar approach to co-sleeping deaths, which is essentially a different sleeping environment, may bring similar rewards.

Co-sleeping on a sofa

In Avon, both the prevalence and number of SIDS infants found co-sleeping with a parent on a sofa has increased. Despite the possibility of overlaying in such circumstances (particularly when the infant was found between the adult and the back of the sofa), the evidence, even with careful scene investigation, was usually not sufficient to identify overlaying confidently, although the possibility is never entirely ruled out. Thus, most such deaths are labelled as SIDS. In our population-based case control study conducted between 1993 and 1996, we reported 20 (6%) such SIDS deaths; more recent studies from Scotland[9] and Northern Ireland[31] suggest an increasing prevalence of co-sleeping SIDS deaths on sofas and chairs of 13% and 24% of the total SIDS, respectively. Regardless of whether these deaths are SIDS or accidental suffocation, clearly the infants are co-sleeping in an inappropriate environment.

The interaction between bed-sharing and common characteristics of SIDS

SIDS deaths occurring in the parental bed have, therefore, fallen but not at the same rate as SIDS deaths of infants found in the cot. One potential reason for this may be a consequence of the intervention campaign itself. Prior to the 'Back to Sleep' campaign, the Avon data showed that, of those SIDS infants found sleeping alone in the cot, 91% were discovered in the prone sleeping position; however, amongst those SIDS infants found in the parental bed only 55% were found prone.[32] A speculative explanation for this differece might be that co-sleeping mothers who breast-feed tend to place the infant in a more amenable position, often placing infants on their side or back to feed before sleep. Thus, any campaign aimed at changing sleeping position was going to have a reduced effect for those infants sleeping with someone than those infants sleeping alone.

As well as finding solitary sleeping SIDS victims in the prone position, another common observation is finding the face or head of these infants covered with bedclothes. It is not clear whether this is a result of the agonal struggle or part of some causal mechanism. What is clear is that this is an observation more often reported amongst SIDS infants found in a cot than those co-sleeping in a parental bed. Head covering occurs in over a quarter of SIDS victims but two recent studies in Scotland[9] and England[27] both suggest only 7% of co-sleeping SIDS victims were found with their head covered. Home studies of healthy infants in New Zealand with overnight video and physiological recordings showed that head covering was more common during sleep amongst bed-sharing infants than those sleeping alone in a cot but also that parents tended to adjust the infant covering during sleep.[33]

Another unique characteristic of SIDS infants is the age at death. Few deaths occur in the first month of life or after 6 months with a large peak at 3–4 months of age. However, recent studies have shown that co-sleeping SIDS infants die at a younger age, with a peak at 8 weeks compared to 16 weeks amongst solitary sleeping infants.[12,27] The increased vulnerability of younger infants may suggest that these co-sleeping SIDS deaths are being misdiagnosed and perhaps point to accidental death, although the peak age of deaths identified as being from overlaying is, according to Nakamura et al.,[19] in the first 4 weeks of life when infants are at their most vulnerable rather than at 8 weeks.

These differences may be important in trying to understand causal mechanisms. They also have implications in terms of how we interpret multivariate findings in SIDS studies if major risk factors such as sleeping position, head covering and age appear to have a different emphasis depending on the environment in which the infant sleeps. There is no reason to suppose there is just one mode of death amongst SIDS victims and future studies may need to analyse co-sleeping deaths separately from solitary sleeping deaths to understand the association of potential risk factors.

Bed-sharing as a risk-factor for SIDS

Several recent studies have investigated the role of bed-sharing amongst SIDS victims and reported a significant multivariate risk.[9-12,34,35] How bed-sharing was defined and whether sufficient adjustment was made for potential confounding in these studies is questionable. In most studies, no differentiation was made between sleeping on a sofa or sleeping in the parental bed and, in some studies, victims were labelled as co-sleeping deaths even though the infants were put back and subsequently died in the cot. Factors potentially associated with unsafe co-sleeping environments, related both to the co-sleeping parents (*e.g.* recent alcohol or drug consumption) and to the bed (*e.g.* softness of the adult mattress and composition of the bedding) were not routinely collected. Nevertheless, there is general agreement amongst researchers that SIDS now occurs more often in the parental bed than expected. Bed-sharing is perceived to be, and treated as, a risk factor in the field of SIDS epidemiology; dealt with in this rudimentary way, there is ample evidence to advise against such a practice. On closer inspection, however, there are several aspects to be considered. Studies have also reported a significant interaction between maternal smoking and bed-sharing,[34,35] making it difficult to generalise findings when the majority of bed-sharing SIDS mothers smoke whilst the majority of bed-sharing mothers in the population do not. In a large European study, the risk of bed-sharing was 10-fold greater amongst mothers who smoked.[12] The magnitude of any increase in risk for non-smoking, breast-feeding mothers who are bed-sharing on a firm flat surface, and who have not taken alcohol or other drugs, is unclear, but certainly small.[12,36-38] From our own work, adjusting for potential confounders specifically associated with the adult co-sleeping environment (such as recent alcohol consumption, sleep deprivation, overcrowded conditions and adult-sized duvets) rendered bed-sharing as a non-significant risk factor suggesting it is not bed-sharing itself but the particular circumstances in which bed-sharing occurs that puts an infant at risk.[27] Similar findings were reported in Ireland by McGarvey *et al.*,[11] although neither study collected adequate information on other potential confounding factors in the bed-sharing environment, such as the recent consumption of other sleep-inducing drugs, both legal and illegal, the size and composition of the adults nor the softness of the adult mattress. Further analysis has also shown an increase in the risk of SIDS amongst pre-term and low birth-weight infants co-sleeping in the first few weeks of life.[39]

Prevalence of bed-sharing and SIDS in different cultures

In certain cultures, bed-sharing is the common infant care practice and the SIDS prevalence is high. These include the black populations in the US and the Maori and Aboriginal populations in the Southern hemisphere. Intriguingly, however, there are other cultures where bed-sharing is also the common practice but the SIDS rates quite low, including Japan and Hong Kong, the Bangladeshi and Asian communities in the UK, and Pacific Islander communities in New Zealand. It is not bed-sharing that distinguishes these cultures but there are other mediating factors such as maternal smoking which is particularly low in Japan and Hong Kong[40] and parental alcohol consumption which is higher amongst the Maori and Aboriginal populations[41,42] that may combine with co-sleeping and play a role in SIDS deaths. Another mediating factor might be the sleeping environment itself – the Japanese futon for instance, a firm thin mattress placed on the floor is intrinsically different from the elevated often softer mattresses used in Western societies.

The potential benefits of co-sleeping

Co-sleeping begins in infancy and often continues through to childhood as part of early nurturing practices. In evolutionary terms, the human infant is the most neurologically immature primate at birth and develops the most slowly; thus, intense and prolonged mother–infant contact acts as a protective mechanism against physiological difficulties and environmental assaults. Studies of pre-term and newborn infants have reported beneficial physiological effects of mother–infant contact using skin-to-skin care or the kangaroo method of baby care, which increase infant skin temperature, stabilise heart rates, reduce crying and increases milk production.[6,7] Cross-over studies of post neonatal infants and mothers in sleep laboratories have shown that the average breast-feeding intervals follow the duration of the adult sleep cycle (approximately 1.5 h) when co-sleeping, an interval half that observed when the mother and infant are sleeping apart. Thus, breast-feeding occurs more frequently when co-sleeping, although the duration of episodes is often shorter.[43] Breast-feeding mothers also tend to sleep for longer when co-sleeping with their infant than when sleeping apart.[44] Polysomnographic recordings of mother–infant pairs show that infants follow maternal cues in terms of breathing and sleep stages whilst infra-red videos reveal that infants initiate arousals and interactions with a relatively high response on the part of the mother. This heightened sensitivity might increase the chances that mothers could more quickly detect and intervene against a life-threatening event that night-time separation from the baby precludes. Over-night recordings in the home setting show the infant usually sleeps beside the mother, separated from fathers and siblings if present, facing the mother, with the head at the mother's breast level, touching or with the mother cradling the infant,[45] whilst longer term sleep diaries in this setting suggest co-sleeping helps prolong the duration of breast-feeding.[46]

Far fewer epidemiological studies have investigated potential benefits associated with infant-care practices than have investigated practices possibly linked with infant morbidity and mortality. Studies have shown that breast-feeding mothers are much more likely to bed-share than bottle-feeding mothers,[1,3,47] although it is difficult to untangle whether co-sleeping encourages breast-feeding or the other way round. Studies have also shown possible psychological and emotional benefits associated with co-sleeping, with higher self-esteem in later life, less psychiatric problems and improved cognitive performance.[41,48] The importance of breast-feeding should not be underestimated in terms of its nutritional, immunological and developmental benefits to both the mother and infant. The demonstration by Chen and Rogan,[49] in a multivariate analysis, that the post neonatal infant mortality rate in the US was 26% higher for bottle-fed than breast-fed infants raises the possibility that any action leading to reduced rates or duration of breast-feeding may increase infant mortality. While many factors potentially contributed to this difference, it is likely that breast-feeding itself has an important contributory effect, and thus any fall in breast-feeding rates may lead to a significant increase in post neonatal infant mortality, even in Western societies. There is, therefore, a need for a careful assessment of potential adverse consequences before any public pronouncement on the desirability or otherwise of practices such as bed sharing that may affect breast-feeding rates.

CONCLUSIONS

There has been little in the way of direct observational data until recently, but it is becoming clear that bed-sharing both for infants and mothers results in complex interactions which are completely different to isolated sleeping and which need to be understood in detail before applying crude labels such as 'safe' or 'unsafe'. The scientific rigor with which data are gathered is not easily applied to the dissemination of the results, and formulating advice can be a subjective exercise of weighing up the available evidence and constrained by attempts to simplify the message. Simply advising parents to avoid co-sleeping may conceivably reduce the SIDS rates even further, but not necessarily infant mortality in general. To give such a message based on current evidence not only precludes specific advice on how one can co-sleep safely but also reduces the options of where mothers can feed their infants during night-time sleep. If bed-sharing is actively discouraged, breast-feeding mothers may choose to feed at night on a chair or sofa and some will inevitably fall asleep in the process; yet this environment appears to be by far the most unsafe and the only environment in which the number of unexplained SIDS deaths are actually increasing. Current advice in the UK does not advise against bed-sharing but describes particular circumstances when bed-sharing should be avoided including if either parent smokes, has recently taken alcohol or a sleep-inducing drug, or is excessively tired. Parents are also advised not to bed-share with pre-term or low birth-weight infants or when infants have a high temperature. Co-sleeping with an infant on a sofa should always be avoided.

Key points for clinical practice

- Infants co-sleeping with parents is the normal infant-care practice in many cultures and common in Western society.
- Co-sleeping facilitates breast-feeding and studies suggest an association with enhanced milk production, longer maternal sleep and prolonged duration of breast-feeding.

Key points for clinical practice *(continued)*

- Parental overlaying is probably rare, but difficult to identify with certainty, even with careful scene evaluation and post mortem examination.

- Unexplained sudden infant death syndrome (SIDS) deaths are more common, over 300 a year occurring in England and Wales. Recent studies suggest an increasing proportion of these deaths are occurring in the parental bed. This has led to authorities such as the American Academy of Pediatrics to advise against bed-sharing.

- A closer inspection of longitudinal data in Avon suggests the number of co-sleeping SIDS deaths in the parental bed has fallen (halved) but not to the same degree of solitary SIDS deaths occurring in the infant cot, which have fallen 7-fold.

- Both the proportion and number of co-sleeping SIDS deaths on a sofa have increased.

- Parental smoking and recent alcohol consumption have both been implicated in co-sleeping SIDS deaths.

- The safest place for an infant to sleep is in the cot by the parental bed for the first 6 months of life.

- If the parents smoke, they should be encouraged to stop smoking if they intend to co-sleep with the infant; otherwise, they should be discouraged from co-sleeping.

- Current policy in the UK does not advise against bed-sharing but describes particular circumstances when bed-sharing should be avoided – if parents have recently consumed alcohol or a sleep-inducing drug, are excessively tired, if the infant is pre-term or low birth-weight or when infants have a high temperature.

- Parents should be advised never to place themselves and infants in a situation where they may fall asleep in an unsafe or inappropriate environment such as on a chair, sofa or waterbed.

- Parents should also be advised never to leave infants to sleep unattended on adult beds, bunk beds or any environment that was not designed with infant safety in mind.

References

1. Blair PS, Ball HL. The prevalence and characteristics associated with parent-infant bed-sharing in England. *Arch Dis Child* 2004; **89**: 1106–1110.
2. Nelson EAS, Taylor BJ. International child care practices study: infant sleeping environment. *Early Hum Dev* 2001; **62**: 43–55.
3. Willinger M, Ko CW, Hoffman HJ, Kessler RC, Corwin MJ. National Infant Sleep Position Study. Trends in infant bed sharing in the United States, 1993–2000. *Arch Pediatr Adolesc Med* 2003; **157**: 43–49.
4. Arnestad M, Andersen M, Vege A, Rognum TO. Changes in the epidemiological pattern of sudden infant death syndrome in southeast Norway, 1984–1998: implications for

future prevention and research. *Arch Dis Child* 2001; **85**: 108–115.

5. De Jonge GA, Hoogenboezem J. Epidemiology of 25 years of crib death (sudden infant death syndrome) in The Netherlands; incidence of crib death and prevalence of risk factors in 1980–2004. *Ned Tijdschr Geneeskd* 2005; **149**: 1273–1278.

6. Anderson GC. Current knowledge about skin-to-skin (kangaroo) care for preterm infants. *J Perinatol* 1991; **11**: 216–226.

7. Ludington-Hoe SM, Hadeed AJ, Anderson GC. Physiological responses to skin-to-skin contact in hospitalised premature infants. *J Perinatol* 1991; **11**: 19–24.

8. Kemp JS, Unger B, Wilkins D *et al*. Unsafe sleep practices and an analysis of bedsharing among infants dying suddenly and unexpectedly: results of a four-year, population-based, death-scene investigation study of sudden infant death syndrome and related deaths. *Pediatrics* 2000; **106**: e41.

9. Tappin D, Brooke H, Ecob R, Gibson A. Used infant mattresses and sudden infant death syndrome in Scotland: case-control study. *BMJ* 2002; **325**: 1007.

10. Hauck FR, Herman SM, Donovan M *et al*. Sleep environment and the risk of sudden infant death syndrome in an urban population: the Chicago Infant Mortality Study. *Pediatrics* 2003; **111**: 1207–1214.

11. McGarvey C, McDonnell M, Chong A, O'Regan M, Matthews T. Factors relating to the infant's last sleep environment in sudden infant death syndrome in the Republic of Ireland. *Arch Dis Child* 2003; **88**: 1058–1064.

12. Carpenter PR, Irgens PL, Blair PS *et al*. Sudden unexplained infant death in 20 regions in Europe: case control study. *Lancet* 2004; **363**: 185–191.

13. American Academy of Pediatrics. The changing concept of sudden infant death syndrome: diagnostic coding shifts, controversies regarding the sleeping environment, and new variables to consider reducing the risk. *Pediatrics* 2005; **116**: 1245–1255.

14. Gessner BD, Porter TJ. Bed sharing with unimpaired parents is not an important risk factor for sudden infant death syndrome. *Pediatrics* 2006; **117**: 990–991.

15. Eidelman AI, Gartner LM. Bed sharing with unimpaired parents is not an important risk factor for sudden infant death syndrome. *Pediatrics* 2006; **117**: 991–992.

16. Bartick M. Bed sharing with unimpaired parents is not an important risk factor for sudden infant death syndrome. *Pediatrics* 2006; **117**: 992–993.

17. Pelayo R, Owens J, Mindell J, Sheldon S. Bed sharing with unimpaired parents is not an important risk factor for sudden infant death syndrome. *Pediatrics* 2006; **117**: 993.

18. Drago DA, Dannenberg AL. Infant mechanical suffocation deaths in the United States, 1980–1997. *Pediatrics* 1999; **103**: e59.

19. Nakamura S, Wind M, Danello MA. Review of hazards associated with children placed in adult beds. *Arch Pediatr Adolesc Med* 1999; **153**: 1019–1023.

20. Ledwidge M, Fox G, Matthews T. Neurocardiogenic syncope: a model for SIDS. *Arch Dis Child* 1998; **78**: 481–483.

21. Office for National Statistics. *Series DH2. Mortality statistics—by cause*. London: Office for National Statistics, 2006.

22. Office for National Statistics. *Series DH3 Mortality statistics—childhood, infant and perinatal*. London: Office for National Statistics, 2006.

23. Collins KA. Death by overlaying and wedging: a 15-year retrospective study. *Am J Forensic Med Pathol* 2001; **22**: 155–159.

24. Limerick SR. Sudden infant death in historical perspective. *J Clin Pathol* 1992; **45 (Suppl)**: 3–6.

25. Spock B. The striving for autonomy and regressive object relationships. *Psychoanal Study Child* 1963; **18**: 361–364.

26. Scragg RK, Mitchell EA, Stewart AW *et al*. Infant room-sharing and prone sleep position in sudden infant death syndrome. New Zealand Cot Death Study Group. *Lancet* 1996; **347**: 7–12.

27. Blair PS, Fleming PJ, Smith IJ *et al*. and the CESDI SUDI research group. Babies sleeping with parents: case-control study of factors influencing the risk of sudden infant death syndrome. *BMJ* 1999; **319**: 1457–1462.

28. Carpenter RG. Sudden and unexpected deaths in infancy (cot death). In: Camps FE, Carpenter RG. (eds) *Sudden and unexpected deaths in infancy (cot death)*. Bristol: J Wright, 1972; 7–15.

29. Luke JL. Sleeping arrangements of sudden infant death syndrome victims in the District of Columbia – a preliminary report *J Forensic Sci* 1978; **23**: 379–383.
30. Lee NNY, Chan YF, Davis DP, Lau E, Yip DCP. Sudden infant death syndrome in Hong Kong: confirmation of a low incidence. *BMJ* 1989; **298**: 721–722.
31. Glasgow JF, Thompson AJ, Ingram PJ. Sudden unexpected death in infancy: place and time of death. *Ulster Med J* 2006; **75**: 65–71.
32. Blair PS, Ward Platt MP, Smith I, Fleming PJ. Major changes in the epidemiology of sudden infant death syndrome: a 20 year population based study of all unexpected deaths in infancy. *Lancet* 2006; **367**: 314–319.
33. Baddock SA, Galland BC, Bolton DPG, Williams SM, Taylor BJ. Differences in infant and parent behaviours during routine bed sharing compared with cot sleeping in the home setting. *Pediatrics* 2006; **117**: 1599–1607.
34. Fleming PJ, Blair PS, Bacon C *et al.* Environment of infants during sleep and risk of the sudden infant death syndrome: results from 1993–5 case-control study for confidential inquiry into stillbirths and deaths in infancy. *BMJ* 1996; **313**: 191–195.
35. Mitchell EA, Tuohy PG, Brunt JM *et al.* Risk factors for sudden infant death syndrome following the prevention campaign in New Zealand: a prospective study. *Pediatrics* 1997; **100**: 835–840.
36. Wailoo M, Ball H, Fleming PJ, Ward-Platt M. Infants bedsharing with mothers: helpful, harmful or don't know? *Arch Dis Child* 2004; **89**: 1082–1083.
37. Fleming PJ, Blair PS, McKenna JJ. New knowledge, new insights and new recommendations. *Arch Dis Child* 2006; **91**: 799–801.
38. McGarvey C, McDonnell M, O'Regan M, Matthews T. An eight year study of risk factors for SIDS: bedsharing vs non bedsharing. *Arch Dis Child* 2006; **91**: 318–323.
39. Blair PS, Ward Platt MP, Smith IJ, Fleming PJ. Sudden infant death syndrome and sleeping position in pre-term and low birthweight infants: an opportunity for targeted intervention. *Arch Dis Child* 2006; **91**: 101–106.
40. Nelson EAS, Taylor BJ. International child care practices study: infant sleep position and parental smoking. *Early Hum Dev* 2001; **64**: 7–20.
41. Chikritzhs T, Brady M. Fact or fiction? A critique of the National Aboriginal and Torres Strait Islander Social Survey 2002. *Drug Alcohol Rev* 2006; **25**: 277–287.
42. Scragg R, Mitchell EA, Taylor BJ *et al.* Bed sharing, smoking, and alcohol in the sudden infant death syndrome. New Zealand Cot Death Study Group. *BMJ* 1993; **307**: 1312–1318.
43. Quillin SI, Glenn LL. Interaction between feeding method and co-sleeping on maternal–newborn sleep. *J Obstet Gynecol Neonat Nurs* 2004; **33**: 580–588.
44. McKenna JJ, Mcdade T. Why babies should never sleep alone: a review of the co-sleeping controversy in relation to SIDS, bedsharing and breast feeding. *Paediatr Respir Rev* 2005; **6**: 134–152.
45. Ball H. Breastfeeding, bed-sharing, and infant sleep. *Birth* 2003; **30**: 181–188.
46. Baddock SA, Galland BC, Taylor BJ, Bolton DPG. Sleep arrangements and behaviour of bed-sharing families in the home setting. *Pediatrics* 2007; **119**: 200–207.
47. McCoy RC, Hunt CE, Lesko SM *et al.* Frequency of bed sharing and its relationship to breastfeeding. *Dev Behav Pediatr* 2004; **25**: 141–149.
48. Forbes F, Weiss DS, Folen RA. The cosleeping habits of military children. *Military Med* 1992; **157**: 196–200.
49. Chen A, Rogan WJ. Breastfeeding and the risk of postneonatal death in the United States. *Pediatrics* 2004; **113**: 435–439.

Richard Morton

9

Botulinum for cerebral palsy

In 1994, a group of paediatric orthopaedic surgeons working in Northern Ireland were amongst the first to publicise the benefits of botulinum toxin in cerebral palsy, demonstrating an improvement in walking when injected into the lower limbs.[1] At the same time, they reported that a single injection to infant mice with hereditary spasticity produced 30% more growth in the calf muscle.[2] It was presumed this was because muscle needs to be stretched to grow, and this was facilitated by botulinum toxin A. They predicted it could be used routinely to improve function in cerebral palsy and, in the longer term, prevent contracture formation. While the lead author, Cosgrove, stayed in Ireland to promote these ideas, the senior partner Graham, moved to Australia to form another research team which has continued to make a major contribution to the field, notably with physiotherapist Rosalind Boyd. Almost 15 years later, has this treatment been the success anticipated? Undoubtedly, it has been used to good effect as a 'concomitant' treatment with physiotherapy and splinting in the lower and upper limbs. However, evidence remains scarce that it has any other than short-term benefit, and significantly prevents deformity in the clinical setting.

EVIDENCE OF EFFICACY

There have been numerous studies into the effectiveness of botulinum toxin A in the lower limbs, which have been classified according to Sackett criteria[3] by Boyd and Hayes.[4] These studies consisted of six randomised, controlled trials all involving the calf muscle; four compared botulinum toxin A with saline placebo[5–8] and two with casting.[9,10] All used the Physicians' Rating Scale[11] to score gait according to kinematics (joint angles) at different stages of walking and a meta-analysis of the first and the second group of studies was

Richard Morton BA BM BCh FRCHP
Consultant Paediatrician, Derbyshire Children's Hospital, Uttoxeter Road, Derby DE22 3NE, UK
E-mail: richard.morton@derbyhospitals.nhs.uk

performed. A difference of two points for the botulinum toxin A subjects on the Physicians' Rating Scale was taken as a mark of success. This was achieved by around 25% for each group, a significant, albeit modest, result.

There have only been two randomised, controlled trials evaluating botulinum toxin A in the upper limb. One showed improvement in some active movements compared to placebo,[12] and the other demonstrated better function compared to untreated controls in terms of the QUEST and some aspects of the PEDI.[13]

The effect of a disability can be assessed in terms of pathophysiology, impairment, functional loss and participation in society. The latter two aspects are the most important, reflecting real improvement in quality of life appreciated by the child and their carers. These outcomes are notoriously lacking for most interventions in cerebral palsy, at any level of evidence. The evaluation of botulinum toxin A is no exception and this provides an important research challenge for the future.

BASIC SCIENCE

There are seven major forms of botulinum toxin (types A–G), of which type A is used mainly clinically, and all consist of a heavy and a light chain, linked by a disulphide bond. The heavy chain has two major functions (Fig. 1). First, it attaches the complex specifically to a protein ganglioside receptor on the pre-synaptic membrane of cholinergic nerve terminals, following which an endosome is incorporated into the cell. Second, the heavy chain forms a channel to extrude the light chain into the cytosol by the process of translocation. The light chain is an endopeptidase acting on the snare proteins necessary for the release of acetyl choline from the vesicle into the post synaptic space by the process of exocytosis. Botulinum toxin A lyses Snap-25 and is effective within 48 h. While the synapse is inactive, sprouting of new nerve terminals occurs but these are resorbed once normal activity is resumed after around 4 months. This is longer than for other forms of botulinum toxin, possibly because of a slower breakdown of the light chain.[14] When injected into muscle, botulinum toxin A affects nerve transmission at the neuro-

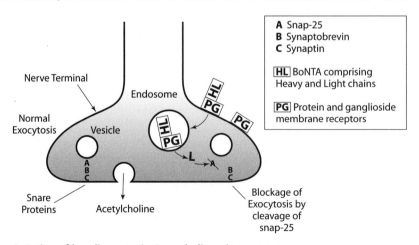

Fig. 1 Action of botulinum toxin A on cholinergic nerve synapse.

muscular junction, but it can also act at other cholinergic parasympathetic and preganglionic sympathetic synapses.

COMMERCIAL BOTULINUM TOXIN

There are two types of botulinum toxin A commercially available which are very different – Botox (Allergan) and Dysport (Ipsen). Dose–response curves for each are not linear, but logarithmic, so equivalence between the two varies with dose. They are conveniently compared in practice using the amount required for half-maximal paralysis of muscle, which gives an equivalence ratio of Botox 1 unit to Dysport 3 units.[15] The commercial rivalry between the two is healthy and ensures that, in practice, they are of equal cost relative to their effectiveness. It does appear from clinical studies that Botox diffuses from the injected muscle less than Dysport, which is attributed to it being a larger molecule.[16] However, attempts to replicate this directly in animals have been contradictory. In rats, diffusion from the injected muscle to local muscle was about the same for both preparations,[15] whereas in mice, Dysport was associated with a significantly greater amount of local and systemic spread.[16] Any such differences are not relevant in the treatment of cerebral palsy at conventional dosages, but may be important with high-dose, multilevel treatment.

In the US, a commercial preparation of botulinum toxin B is available (Nevrobloc, Solstice Neuroscience) but this is effective for a relatively short time and is only indicated in the rare situation when immune resistance has developed to botulinum toxin A.

PRINCIPLES OF INJECTION

Botulinum toxin A is dissolved in normal saline and injected into muscle where it binds avidly to the local motor end plates. Some diffuses across fascial boundaries to local muscle, and small amounts escape further into the systemic circulation. Side effects take the form of excessive weakness of the injected muscle, local spread to antagonists which reduces the effect on the target muscle, and systemic effects of mild botulism. The latter are uncommon at conventional dosage, and consist of generalised tiredness and weakness, constipation and incontinence. Accepted recommendations are up to 30 U/kg Dysport or 1000 U in total,[17] or 12 U/kg, 300 U total Botox.[18] These levels can be exceeded if divided between several muscles in multilevel treatment in bilateral cerebral palsy.[19] However, care must be taken in gradually increasing the dosage as the response is idiosyncratic and some individuals tolerate botulinum toxin A much less than others.[20]

IDENTIFICATION OF MUSCLE

The muscle to be injected can often be identified in the lower limb using simple surface anatomical markers.[21] It is useful to manipulate the joint gently with the needle in place to prove the needle is correctly situated and not resting in overlying connective tissue. This should be sufficient for muscles such as hamstrings, hip adductors, calves and the elbow flexors. If the muscle is small or hidden under others, a simple electrical stimulator can be used together with an insulated or 'Pole' needle, to produce the characteristic muscle twitch required. This technique is applicable to all the muscles in the forearm and the tibialis posterior in the lower limb. Psoas injections are perhaps most challenging and best performed with ultrasound guidance.[22] Ultrasound can be used instead of a stimulator on other muscles which are difficult to locate; some recommend this technique for all muscles to confirm accurate injection.[23] EMG will identify both the muscle and the sites of maximal concentration of motor end plates.[24] However, it has limited application as it requires the services of a neurophysiologist and many children are unable to co-operate sufficiently in moving their limbs in the right direction for the recording.

INJECTION TECHNIQUE

Increasing the amount of botulinum toxin A injected into a muscle improves the peak and duration of effect to a certain point after which the response deteriorates, probably due to diffusion to local antagonists.[25,26] Dysport (10–15 U/kg) or Botox (3–5 U/kg) is recommended to muscles in the lower limbs, with about a quarter of these amounts to smaller muscles in the upper limbs. One usually has to make do with only one or two injections into the main muscle belly when injecting under local anaesthetic. A larger volume of injection has been shown to be more effective in rabbits,[27] although this may promote local escape of the toxin.[28] Therefore, it may be advisable to use lower concentrations in big muscle and higher in smaller muscle.

Motor end plates are situated in different configurations, according to the type of muscle. In fusiform muscle, they are spread around the mid-belly, and in pennate muscle throughout its length (Fig. 2). Since the objective of injection is to target as many motor end-plates as possible without wastage, multiple small injections would be beneficial, especially in pennate muscles. This has been shown in animal models,[29] and is the best approach when toxin needs to be used most efficiently, such as in multilevel treatment in cerebral palsy. For this treatment approach, a general anaesthetic would be needed.

Many centres nowadays administer botulinum toxin A to children mainly under local anaesthetic, as a simple out-patient procedure. Local anaesthetic

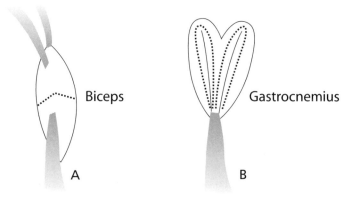

Fig. 2 Distribution of motor end plates in: (A) fusiform muscle (*e.g.* biceps) and (B) pennate muscle (*e.g.* gastrocnemius). Adapted from[38]

ointments are used together with oral midazolam for relaxation. A recent audit of our botulinum clinic[30] showed that significant pain and upset was still occurring in some children, who already have much extra stress in their lives. Following this, we now also use a strong analgesic (*e.g.* Diclofenac) and nitrous oxide for those able to take it (about 5 year mental age). For the younger child, we are now more inclined to return to the use of general anaesthesia, particularly if they have more than half a dozen injections.

TREATMENT PROGRAMMES

Therapy colleagues are essential to help in determining the specific goals for treatment, which can be categorised as active functioning, aiding nursing care or simple cosmesis. They identify the overactive muscles needing injection and monitor response for a couple of months afterwards, ideally using a video or an objective scale such as the Physicians' Rating Scale for the lower limbs[11] and its equivalent for the upper limbs.[18] Gait analysis is particularly helpful in identifying problems in the lower limb in a complex hemi- or diplegic. Injections should be combined with physiotherapy or occupational therapy to encourage better movement, sometimes also with splints to help prevent further contracture. In the future, it is hoped that therapists themselves may give the injections, fully integrated with the rest of their treatment programme for the child.

Immunological resistance to botulinum toxin A may be a problem if injections are repeated less than 4 months apart.[31] If given at the recommended 6-month intervals, there is still often a gradual reduction in efficacy but this is usually due to contracture formation. The best evidence to date that botulinum toxin A can actually help prevent contractures is provided by Koman *et al.*,[32] who found that equinus surgery could be put off by 3–4 years on average, although unlikely to be cancelled completely. Most centres plan blocks of 4–6 treatments, and concentrate on the younger child who is more responsive; however, some children have been treated for many years with continuing good results. Long-term treatment can, therefore, be given if it remains effective, and with the chance that orthopaedic surgery will be delayed. There must, however, remain some caution as concerns have been expressed about inducing long-term weakness in spastic muscle, especially in the lower limbs of a mobile diplegic.[33]

INDIVIDUAL MUSCLE INJECTIONS

Calf
This is the most commonly injected muscle (Fig. 3). Treatment has been shown to improve all aspects of gait according to standard criteria.[34] These are: (i) there is better foot clearance because of increased ankle dorsiflexion during foot swing; and (ii) improved foot placement by means of improved ankle contact, leading to greater stride length and a flatter foot and, therefore, greater stability in stance.

In addition, ankle–foot orthoses are easier to put on and better tolerated. If the foot has limited dorsiflexion with the knee bent, soleus is tight and will need to be injected. If dorsiflexion is further reduced by extending the knee,

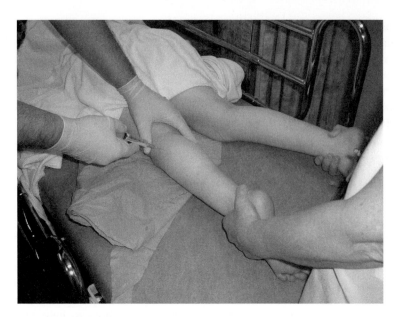

Fig. 3 Botulinum injections to the calf under local anaesthesia.

thus stretching gastrocnemius, then this muscle will also need treatment. Care must be taken with diplegics, however, who usually need good soleus tone to control the ankle; if this muscle is over weakened, they could collapse with excessive dorsiflexion. For this reason, surgeons often prefer elongation of only the gastrocnemius rather than the whole tendo-Achilles. Additional serial below-knee casting can be helpful to reduce existing calf contracture. This is disliked by many children, however, and should only be necessary if passive ankle dorsiflexion is restricted to 10° below neutral. Once dorsiflexion has deteriorated beyond this point, a heel rise may be helpful; however, this only delays inevitable tendon surgery.

Hamstrings

Diplegics often have a squat gait due to overactive hamstrings causing excessive knee bend; this can be effectively treated with botulinum toxin A. Care must be taken to distinguish this from squat gait due to hamstrings which have normal function but are stretched over an anteverted pelvis – so-called 'hamstring shift'. Some children also have a squat gait because of excessive ankle dorsiflexion or plantarflexion. Gait analysis may be needed in difficult and mixed cases. By contrast, few mistakes can be made with hamstring injections in the quadriplegic sitting uncomfortably on the sacrum. The difficulty here is in preventing contractures in these immobile children, and injections must be supplemented with use of a standing frame, muscle stretches and, possibly, night splints.

Hip adductors

Diplegics benefit from adductor treatment for scissor gait, although this is often exacerbated by accompanying femoral anteversion.

Quadriplegics will benefit from regular adductor injections to reduce subluxation of the hips, as part of a 24-h programme of therapy and positioning. This also helps prevent scoliosis and includes correct seating (possibly using a hip spica) and a night abduction bed. When severe adductor tone is present from a young age, such management will need to be started in the first year.[35] From around 30 months, hip X-rays can reliably indicate the degree of subluxation according to the 'hip migration percentage',[36] and repeated to guide intervention. This approach also includes the aggressive use of soft-tissue hip surgery if the hip migration exceeds 35%. By means of these procedures, it is hoped that hip dislocation can be avoided in many cases. If this does occur, it is frequently painful but the child now can be generally too frail for bony surgery. In these circumstances, botulinum toxin A injections to the hip adductors and sometimes psoas can be extremely helpful.[37]

Psoas
This muscle is injected in diplegics with hip flexion contractures, which upsets posture and limits stride length. It is difficult to treat and the best way is aided by ultrasound, with injection above the inguinal ligament.[22]

Tibialis posterior
Overactivity of this muscle in hemi- or diplegics causes the mid-foot to invert. It lies just deep to the tibia and is located with a muscle stimulator.

Elbow flexors (biceps, brachialis and brachioradialis)
Treatment of these three muscles can help function considerably by extending the reach, especially if the hand is functional. If not, the limbs tend to lie motionless and the aim is to help dressing or appearance. Botulinum toxin A in such situations must be reinforced by elbow splinting during the day or night for at least 6 h to avoid further contracture.

Wrist flexors (flexor carpi ulnaris and radialis)
Both muscles are identified using the nerve stimulator. Treatment of the over-flexed wrist improves grasp. Additional wrist splintage can be used either functionally or to reduce contractures.

Finger flexors (flexor digitorum superficialis and profundus)
Using a stimulator, these muscles can be very successfully injected if the hand is functional but grasp-release is poor. It should also be considered for the young child with persistent grasp, in which a cognitive neglect is reinforced by a sensory absence in the hand. After opening the sensitive palm in this way, the child has greater awareness of the hand which stimulates its function.

Wrist pronators
Although limited supination is a major problem in many hemiplegics, this muscle is difficult to treat as it rapidly becomes fibrous and is annoyingly difficult to find with the muscle stimulator.

Thumb flexors (opponens pollicis and short thumb flexor)
Easily injected with tiny amounts of botulinum toxin A, this a very effective treatment for thumb-in-palm deformity to help grasp.

Key points for clinical practice

- Interventions for disability should be assessed in terms of their effect on pathophysiology, impairment, functional loss and participation in society.

- There are seven forms of botulinum toxin, all having a heavy chain which binds to the receptor membrane, and a light chain interrupting chemical export from the cell. There is considerable potential for the treatment of conditions other than the peripheral nervous system.

- Two forms of botulinum toxin A are commercially available, Dysport and Botox, with approximate relative equivalence of 3:1.

- Side-effects of botulinum toxin are over-weakness of the injected muscle, escape to neighbouring muscle and systemic spread causing mild botulism.

- Needle placement for injection is guided by surface markers, electrical stimulation, EMG and many now prefer ultrasonography.

- Increased volume and multiple injections have been shown to be beneficial in animals and adults, but there is no evidence of this yet in cerebral palsy.

- Adequate preparation for injection includes local anaesthetic creams, and either midazolam and Diclofenac, or inhaled nitrous oxide.

- Clear objectives should be set for treatment with carers and the child's therapists. These can be assessed 2 months after injection by video or the Physicians' Rating Scale for the lower or upper limbs.

- Contracture formation is the main factor inhibiting the effect of botulinum toxin. Younger children, therefore, benefit most from this treatment.

- Hip subluxation is common in children with bilateral cerebral palsy, and can lead to dislocation . This can be detected by hip X-rays from 30 months.

- Botulinum toxin A injection to the hip adductors can help prevent hip subluxation, in combination with a 24-h programme of postural management.

- Diplegics benefit from multilevel injections to psoas, hamstrings and calves. Hemiplegics are usually injected in the calves and tibialis posterior and quadriplegics in the hip adductors and hamstrings.

References

1. Cosgrove AP, Corry IS, Graham HK. Botulinum toxin in the management of the lower limb in cerebral palsy. *Dev Med Child Neurol* 1994; **36**: 386–396.
2. Cosgrove AP, Graham HK. Botulinum toxin A prevents the development of contractures in the hereditary spastic mouse. *Dev Med Child Neurol* 1994; **36**: 379–385.

3. Sackett D. Rules of evidence and clinical recommendations on the use of antithrombotic agents. *Chest* 1989; **39 (Suppl 2)**: 25–35.

4. Boyd RN, Hayes RM. Current evidence for the use of botulinum toxin type A in the management of children with cerebral palsy; a systematic review. *Eur J Neurol* 2001; **8 (Suppl 5)**: 1–2.

5. Koman LA, Mooney JF, Smith BP *et al.* Management of cerebral palsy with botulinum toxin A: preliminary investigation. *J Pediatr Orthop* 1993; **13**: 489–495.

6. Sutherland DH, Kauffmann KR, Wyatt MP *et al.* Double-blind study of botulinum A toxin injections into the gastrocnemius muscle in patients with cerebral palsy. *Gait Posture* 1999; **10**: 10–19.

7. Koman LA, Mooney JF, Smith BP *et al.* Botulinum toxin A neuromuscular blockade in the treatment of lower limb spasticity in cerebral palsy: a randomised double-blind placebo controlled trial. *J Pediatr Orthop* 2000; **20**: 108–115.

8. Ubbhi T, Bhakta BB, Ives HL *et al.* Randomised double-blind placebo controlled trial of the effect of botulinum toxin on walking in cerebral palsy. *Arch Dis Child* 2000; **83**: 481–487.

9. Corry IS, Cosgrove AP, Duffy CM *et al.* Botulinum toxin A compared with stretching casts in the treatment of spastic equines: a randomised prospective trial. *J Pediatr Orthop* 1998; **18**: 304–311.

10. Flett PJ, Stern LM, Waddy H *et al.* Botulinum toxin versus fixed cast stretching for dynamic calf tightness in cerebral palsy. *J Paediatr Child Health* 1999; **35**: 71–77.

11. Mackay AH, Lobb GL, Walt SE *et al.* The reliability and validity of the observational gait scale in children with spastic diplegia. *Dev Med Child Neurol* 2003; **45**: 4–11.

12. Corry IS, Cosgrove AOP, Walsh EG *et al.* Botulinum toxin A in the hemiplegic upper limb: a double blind trial. *Dev Med Child Neurol* 1997; **39**: 186–193.

13. Fehlings D, Rang M, Glazier J *et al.* An evaluation of botulinum-A toxin injections to improve upper extremity function in children with hemiplegic cerebral palsy. *J Pediatr* 2000; **8 (Suppl 5)**: 145–149.

14. Dolly JO, Lisk G, Foran PG *et al.* Insights into the extended duration of neuroparalysis by botulinum neurotoxin A serotypes: differences between motor end terminals and cultured neurons. In: Brin MR, Hallett M, Jancovic J. (eds) *Scientific and therapeutic aspects of botulinum toxin. London:* Lippincott Williams and Wilkins, 2002; 91–102.

15. Rosales RL, Bigalke H, Dressler D. Pharmacology of botulinum toxin; differences between type A preparations. *Eur J Neurol* 2006; **13 (Suppl 1)**: 2–10.

16. Foster KA, Bigalke H, Aoki R. Botulinum neurotoxin – from laboratory to bedside. *Neurotoxic Res* 2006; **9**: 133–140.

17. Bakheit AMO, Severa S, Cosgrove A *et al.* Safety profile and efficacy of botulinum toxin A (Dysport) in children with muscle spasticity. *Dev Med Child Neurol* 2001; **43**: 234–238.

18. Graham HK, Aoki KR, Autti-Romo I *et al.* Recommendations for the use of botulinum toxin type A in the management of cerebral palsy. *Gait Posture* 2000; **11**: 67–79.

19. Molenaers G, Desloovere K, Eyssen M *et al.* Botulinum toxin type A treatment of cerebral palsy; an integrated approach. *Eur J Neurol* 1999; **Suppl 40**: S51–S57.

20. Morton RE, Campbell V, Watson L. High dose botulinum treatment in cerebral palsy and the measurement of cardiac variability to predict systemic side effects. 2007; In press.

21. Morton RE, Murray-Leslie CF. The role of botulinum in the management of cerebral palsy. *Curr Paediatr* 2001; **11**: 235–239.

22. Westhoff B, Seller K, Wild A *et al.* Ultrasound guided botulinum toxin injection techniques for the ileopsoas muscle. *Dev Med Child Neurol* 2003; **45**: 829–832

23. Chin TY, Nattrass P, Selber P, Graham HK. Accuracy of intramuscular injections of botulinum toxin A in juvenile cerebral palsy; a comparison between manual needle placement and placement guided by electrical stimulation. *J Paediatr Orthop* 2005; **25**: 286–291.

24. Comella CL, Buchman AS, Tanner CM, Brown-Toms NC Goetz CG. Botulinum toxin injection for spasmodic torticollis; increased magnitude of benefit with electromyographic assistance. *Neurology* 1992; **42**: 878–882.

25. Polak F, Morton RE, Ward C *et al.* Double blind comparison study of two doses of botulinum toxin A injected into calf muscles in children with hemiplegic cerebral palsy. *Dev Med Child Neurol* 2002; **44**: 551–555.

26. Baker R, Jasinski M, Maciag-Tymecka I *et al.* Botulinum toxin treatment of spasticity in diplegic cerebral palsy; a randomised double-blind placebo controlled dose ranging study. *Dev Med Child Neurol* 2002; **44**: 666–675.

27. Kim HS, Hwang Yeong ST, Lee YT *et al.* Effect of muscle activity and botulinum toxin dilution and volume on muscle paresis. *Dev Med Child Neurol* 2003; **45**: 200–205.

28. Blackie JD, Lees AJ. Botulinum toxin in spasmodic torticollis, *J Neurosurg Psychiatry* 1990; **53**: 640–643.

29. Shaari CM, Sanders I. Quantifying how location and dose of botulinum toxin affects paralysis. *Muscle Nerve* 1993; **16**: 964–969.

30. Vater M. Personal communication.

31. Jancovic J, Swartz K. Response and immunoresistance to botulinum toxin injections. *Neurology* 1995; **45**: 1743–1746.

32. Koman LA, Smith BP, Tingey CT, Mooney JF, Slone S, Naughton MJ. The effect of botulinum type A injections on the natural history of equines foot deformity in paediatric cerebral palsy patients. *Eur J Neurol* 1999; **6 (Suppl 4)**: S19–S22.

33. Gough M, Fairhurst C, Shortland AP. Botulinum toxin and cerebral palsy; time for reflection. *Dev Med Child Neurol* 2005; **47**: 709–713.

34. Gage JR. *Gait analysis in cerebral palsy*. London MacKeith, 1991.

35. Gericke T. Postural management for children with cerebral palsy; consensus statement. *Dev Med Child Neurol* 2006; **48**: 244.

36. Scrutton D, Smeeton N. Hip dysplasia in bilateral cerebral palsy; incidence and natural history in children age 18 months to 5 years. *Dev Med Child Neurol* 2001; **43**: 586–600.

37. Campbell SV, Broderick M, Morton RE. Treating painful dislocated hips in children too vulnerable to undergo surgical procedures. Abstract, British Paediatric Neurology Association Meeting, 2004. *Dev Med Child Neurol* 2004; **Suppl 98**: 21–22.

38. Deshpande S, Gormley ME, Carey JR. Muscle fibre orientation in muscles commonly injected with botulinum toxin: an anatomical study. *Neurotoxic Res* 2006; **9**: 115–120.

Terry Pountney

10

Dislocation of the hip in cerebral palsy

The first report on treatment of hip contractures in cerebral palsy was published in 1880; since that time, hip subluxation and dislocation have been recognised as a common sequelae to cerebral palsy. The process of hip dislocation begins with poor development of the femoral head and acetabulum (dysplasia), subluxation (movement of the femoral head laterally) and finally dislocation of the hip. The most common direction of dislocation is posteriorly with the femoral head moving upwards and posteriorly. Anterior dislocation usually occurs when a child adopts a position where the hips are persistently abducted and externally rotated causing the femoral head to become apparent in the groin.

The reported incidence of hip dislocation varies in the published evidence due to the inclusion of children with different levels of motor ability. Two population studies have found similar incidences of hip dislocation at 35%. However, this figure rises steeply in children with cerebral palsy who are not walking independently at 5 years – reported as 54% in children[1,2] and up to 90%.[3] The study by Soo *et al*.[3] classified their population according to the Gross Motor Function Classification System (GMFCS) and found the overall incidence was 35% rising to 69% and 90%, respectively, in children at levels IV and V on this scale (*i.e.* not walking independently). The mean follow-up in this study was 11.7 years. There is an on-going risk for hip dislocation well into adolescence possibly related to puberty and consequent rapid growth.[4]

The clinical course of hip subluxation and dislocation is well documented and includes pain, impact on function affecting the ability to sit, management of hygiene, and decreasing range of motion.[5] Both or one hip can dislocate; unilateral subluxation is commonly associated with spinal curvature.

Terry Pountney PhD MA MCSP
Research Lead/Physiotherapist, Research Department, Chailey Heritage Clinical Services, North Chailey, East Sussex BN8 4JN, UK
E-mail: terry.pountney@southdowns.nhs.uk

CAUSE

In children with cerebral palsy, the hip appears normal at birth but the effects of delayed motor development lead to hip displacement. Asymmetrical activity of the muscles surrounding the hip and lack of load bearing affect bone development and are the main causes of subluxation and dislocation. Development of hip subluxation begins at a very early stage; typically, developing children achieve symmetry of posture at about 3 months of age. Persisting asymmetry beyond this age can insidiously lead to the long-term gross asymmetry of posture seen in older children with bilateral cerebral palsy. There is a continuing risk of hip subluxation/dislocation into adolescence which is often associated with growth spurts.

ADOPTION OF PERSISTENT ASYMMETRICAL POSTURES

Children with severe cerebral palsy often display stereotypical movements and postures. Initially, these postures may be quite subtle with children exhibiting a very small amount of asymmetry. With growth, however, these minor changes can become marked deformities which impact on a child's function. Typically, children who are at risk of dislocation adopt a wind-swept posture with a rotated, posteriorly tilted and oblique pelvis, legs falling to one side with adduction and internal rotation of one hip and a curved spine (Fig. 1). Persistent postures lead to an imbalance of muscle length across the joints which affects bone shape.

WALKING

Children who do not walk independently have a high risk of subluxation and dislocation. It appears that load bearing through the hip joint is a protective factor for dislocation.[2]

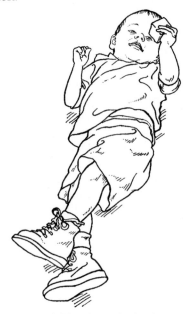

Fig. 1 Wind-swept posture in child with cerebral palsy.

MUSCLE LENGTH CHANGES

Muscle spasticity, particularly of the hip flexors and adductors is often been cited as the first stage of the development of hip dysplasia.[6,8] Spasticity and persistent postures lead to an imbalance of muscle length and strength around the hip joint which disrupts the femoral head contact with the acetabulum causing poor development of the acetabulum and leads to hip subluxation.

As a child grows, spasticity can be confused with muscle and connective tissue shortening. This confusion can lead to a lack of attention to maintaining muscle length and a concentration on managing spasticity.

Many authors suggest that asymmetrical activity of the muscles surrounding the hip is the most influential factor on the direction of growth and shape of the bones and the main cause of dislocation.[6–9]

BONY CHANGES

The effect of asymmetrical muscle activity causes changes in proximal femoral anatomy and altered forces across the growth plate which affect bone growth. Perpendicular forces will cause femoral anteversion, a spiralling deflection of bone growth leading to femoral torsion.[10] Compression causes uneven growth across the growth plates and consequent changes to the direction of growth. Excessive compression on one side of the growth plate can lead to uneven bone growth further hampering the femoral head's ability to achieve congruence with the acetabulum (Figs 2 and 3).[11]

In many children, the femoral neck angle does not decrease to form the femoral neck (coxa valga) which may be due to lengthened and weakened abduct muscles. Coxa valga changes the direction of growth away from the acetabulum (Fig. 3). These changes in the acetabulum and proximal femur have been identified at 18 months of age.[6]

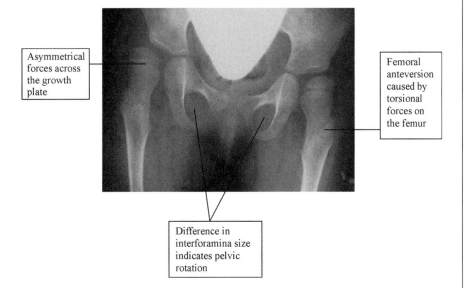

Asymmetrical forces across the growth plate

Femoral anteversion caused by torsional forces on the femur

Difference in interforamina size indicates pelvic rotation

Fig. 2 Changes in bony development as hip subluxation occurs.

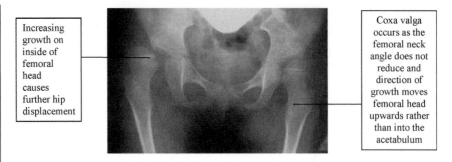

Increasing growth on inside of femoral head causes further hip displacement

Coxa valga occurs as the femoral neck angle does not reduce and direction of growth moves femoral head upwards rather than into the acetabulum

Fig. 3 Coxa valga changes the direction of growth away from the acetabulum.

The imbalance of muscle length and strength between opposing muscle groups and the consequent impact on bony development should be lessened if suitable postural management programmes are implemented at an early stage.

PREVENTION

The population study of Scrutton et al.[2] identified that changes in the hip were apparent at 18 months of age compared to those whose hips do not sublux. This supports the notion that early muscle activity and load bearing may be important for the development of an adequate acetabulum. However, there is debate about how to intervene successfully at an early stage and there is limited evidence to support its success. Suggested options for early intervention include postural management, surgery and botulinum toxin injections.

POSTURAL MANAGEMENT

Postural management programmes primarily aim to promote function and prevent the development of deformity. By providing a range of postures in lying, sitting and standing, muscle length around joints can be maintained and activity promoted. Children who persistently rest in asymmetrical postures, particularly the wind-swept posture, are at greater risk of subluxation. The use of 24-h postural management to control posture is now routinely used including the use of night-time lying supports or sleep systems.

Some limited evidence in the form of cohort studies is available to substantiate this approach.[12,13] A retrospective review of the long-term outcomes of hip migration percentage demonstrated that children who had 24-h postural management intervention prior to hip subluxation were significantly more likely to have neither hip subluxed compared to those receiving it after subluxation or not at all.[13] A pilot study investigating the impact of a sleep system on migration percentage, range of motion and sleep which positioned children in supine with hip abduction of 20° bilaterally found a significant decrease in hip migration percentage over 1 year.[12,13]

A prospective study which introduced positioning equipment to children before the age of 18 months who used the equipment at recommended or moderate levels had a significantly better chance of not having subluxed hips at age 5 years.[14] In light of these findings, a recent consensus statement has recommended that postural management programmes which include positioning equipment for children at GMFCS levels IV and V be instigated as soon as possible after birth to control a child's posture.[15]

BOTULINUM TOXIN

Botulinum toxin injections offer a possible method for controlling hip migration; however, studies to date have demonstrated little impact on displacement although they have been found useful for pain management. Despite the increasing use of botulinum toxin in the management of migration and the reduction of pain in hip subluxation. there are few published studies.

SURGERY

Adductor tenotomies, hamstring releases and obturator neurectomies have been mainstay treatments to prevent further hip displacement and allow remodelling of the femoral head. However, a review by Stott et al.[16] found little evidence of their effectiveness. Of children having this type of surgery, over 60% go on to have a further surgical intervention.[17-19] A prevention programme involving 206 children with cerebral palsy reported that, at 5 years of age, none had developed hip dislocation.[20] However, this was a heterogeneous group many of whom were not at risk of dislocation and achieved by an extensive programme of surgery including 48 soft tissue or bony surgical interventions, 9 selective dorsal rhizotomies and 3 intrathecal Baclofen with 8 awaiting surgery.

Table 1 Gross Motor Function Classification System – motor abilities of children at different levels aged 6–12 years

Level I	Children walk indoors and outdoors and climb stairs without limitation. Children perform gross motor skills including running and jumping, but speed, balance and co-ordination are impaired
Level II	Children walk indoors and outdoors and climb stairs holding onto a railing but experience limitations walking on uneven surfaces and inclines and walking in crowds or confined spaces
Level III	Children walk indoors or outdoors on a level surface with an assistive mobility device. Children may climb stairs holding onto a railing. Children may propel a wheel chair manually or are transported when travelling for long distances or outdoors on uneven terrain
Level IV	Children may continue to walk for short distances on a walker or rely more on wheeled mobility at home and school and in the community
Level V	Physical impairment restricts voluntary control of movement and the ability to maintain antigravity head and trunk postures. All areas of motor function are limited. Children have no means of independent mobility and are transported

Adapted from Palisano et al.[21]

RECOGNITION

There are a range of factors which may indicate that a child is experiencing hip subluxation. A child's physiotherapist and parents are usually the first to notice changes in posture and function, whereas other findings may need to be assessed formally. A pathway to ensure that these are undertaken at the relevant time is useful.

MOTOR ABILITY

The Gross Motor Function Classification System[21] is able to identify a child's motor prognosis from an early age. Severity of motor impairment is a strong indicator of later hip displacement; therefore, classification on this system is ideal for identify children at risk. Children who have a prognosis on the Gross

Table 2 Brief description of Chailey Levels of Ability

SUPINE		
	Level 1	Cannot maintain, rolls into side-lying
	Level 2	Asymmetrical posture
	Level 3	Maintains symmetrical posture
	Level 4	Ability to move in and out of symmetry voluntarily
	Level 5	Able to roll into side-lying
	Level 6	Able to roll into prone
	Level 7	Not applicable
	Level 8	Not applicable
PRONE		
	Level 1	Unable to maintain symmetrical position
	Level 2	Asymmetrical position, beginning to lift head
	Level 3	Moves in and out of symmetry actively
	Level 4	Props on forearms and lifts head
	Level 5	Rolls into supine
	Level 6	Achieves four point kneeling
	Level 7	Not applicable
	Level 8	Not applicable
SITTING		
	Level 1	Cannot be placed in sitting
	Level 2	Can be placed in sitting but cannot maintain position
	Level 3	Maintains sitting position but cannot move
	Level 4	Able to move within sitting base
	Level 5	Able to move outside of sitting base
	Level 6	Able to move out of position
	Level 7	Able to attain sitting
	Level 8	Not applicable
STANDING		
	Level 1	Needs to be fully supported
	Level 2	Fully supported can maintain head upright
	Level 3	Holds on to support if placed
	Level 4	Holds on to support with one hand
	Level 5	Steps within base and able to leave position
	Level 6	Achieve standing position using a support
	Level 7	Stands alone
	Level 8	Assumes standing independently

Motor Function Classification System of not being walking at 5 years (levels IV and V) are at a high risk of hip displacement (Table 1). The use of a postural analysis tool which details the components of posture such as the Chailey Levels of Ability can identify preferred and persistent postures which are predictive of later hip subluxation (Table 2).[22]

CLINICAL PRESENTATION

A child's preferred posture can be indicative of a future hip subluxation. If a child adopts a wind-swept posture as described above or an excessively abducted and external hip position above, there is a risk of changes in muscle length and consequent effect on bones and joints. Apparent shortening of the leg may indicate that the hip is moving upwards and backwards and beginning to sublux (Fig. 1).

A limited range of movement in combined hip extension and abduction (best measured in prone) is cconsidered a risk for subluxation. Limited range may be due to significant spasticity or muscle length changes or both. Correlation between hip abduction only and migration percentage has been found to be weak[17] with migration percentages of 60% showing no evident limitation to range of movement.

PAIN

Pain can be an indication of hip problems and a number of validated tools are available to assess pain. Changing positions and perineal hygiene are key times to note a child's discomfort when hips are moved. For children with complex disability, the Paediatric Pain Profile[23] offers a reliable measure of a child's pain and can be used pre-, during and post-intervention to determine changes in pain levels.

X-RAY MEASUREMENT AND SURVEILLANCE

A programme of hip surveillance was developed from a population-based study and established prognostic factors for hip problems at 5 years.[1] Recommendations include a base-line X-ray for all children with cerebral palsy not walking 10 steps at 30 months and indicated that a migration percentage over 15% was a risk factor for hip problems at 5 years. A recommendation was made for a hip and pelvic X-ray at 18 months but there are concerns that, at this stage, the femoral head may not be fully ossified and X-ray measurement may provide inaccurate data.[2]

Migration percentage

Hip migration percentage is the most reliable and repeatable method of determining the degree of subluxation or dislocation of the hip joint[17] and is measured on an anteroposterior hip and pelvic X-ray (Fig. 4). The percentage of the femoral head lying outside of the acetabulum is measured. A hip is considered to be safe if the migration percentage is less than 33%, subluxed if between 33–80% and dislocated if 80% or greater.[24] Children at 30 months of age with a migration of 15% or greater have a 50% risk of subluxation or

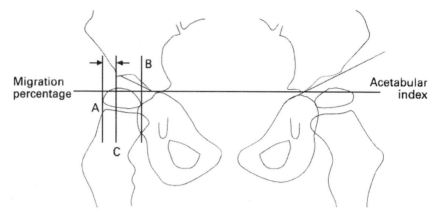

Fig. 4 Measurement of hip migration percentage and acetabular index.

dislocation at 5 years. The rate of, as well as actual, migration are important factors in determining risk and an annual migration of 7% or more was correlated with a later inability to walk.[24,25]

Acetabular index

The acetabular index can also be measured but is not as a reliable as migration percentage as an indicator for later subluxation as it varies with pelvic position.[26,27] This index measures the distance between the femoral head and the acetabulum (Fig. 4). Children with an index of 30° at 30 months all had a subluxation by age 5 years.

Positioning for X-ray

Correct hip and pelvic position at X-ray need to be consistent to ensure sequential X-rays offer reliable data on changes in hip migration (Fig. 5).[17,28,29]

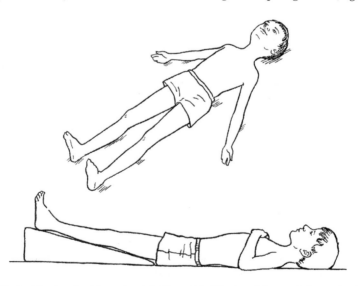

Fig. 5. Positioning for hip and pelvic X-ray. Modified position with legs raised if pelvis is in posterior tilt.

The position of the pelvis (tilt and rotation) can affect measurement as can the position of the hips. Measurements to ensure correct positioning are marked and how migration percentage and acetabular index are measured. The interforamina ratio indicates the level of rotation which needs to lie between 0.5 and 2. The shaft angle should be 10° or less into abduction and 15° or less into adduction for accurate measures to be made.

MANAGEMENT

The range of treatment options for prevention and management of hip dislocation have increased over the past 10 years with the introduction of 24-h postural management programmes and botulinum toxin injections to complement surgical interventions. The following sections will explore each of these options and how a combination of approaches may be appropriate.

ASSESSMENT AND OUTCOMES

A range of outcomes and assessment measures are needed to assess a child's risk of hip dislocation accurately and to identify the most appropriate management for each child. A few examples are described below.

The Gross Motor Function Classification Scale[21,27] offers a clear prognosis for later motor ability and, together with early surveillance programmes, allows clinicians to identify children at risk of dislocation. Together, these can enable postural management interventions to be implemented before subluxation occurs.

Chailey Levels of Ability provides a detailed analysis of a child's postures indicating which components of posture are limiting their ability and need addressing through postural management or surgical intervention.[22]

Pain is a common indicator of hip problems. A range of pain scales are available for children and can be used according to a child's cognitive ability and level of communication. For children who can self-report, scales such as the Brief Pain and Faces scale can be used. Children who are unable to self-report are dependent on their care-givers' observational skills to recognise pain cues and identify a child's level of pain; The Paediatric Pain Profile is a valid and reliable tool for these children.[23]

X-ray surveillance and measurement needs to be continued until a child's hips have stabilised and is recommended until age of 7 years. However, if clinically there is suspicion of further migration, then hips should be X-rayed.

SURGERY

Surgery to the muscles surrounding the hips aims to balance the muscle forces across the hip joint either by unilateral or bilateral surgery and improve location of the femoral head in the acetabulum to prevent further displacement.[5] Surgical release of the muscles surrounding the hips is only likely to be effective when the migration percentage is less than 40%.[30] Several studies have reported the need in over 60% of cases for further surgery following muscle releases.[17,18,31] A review of 27 studies found that evidence for the efficacy of adductor releases was lacking due to the 'small sample sizes,

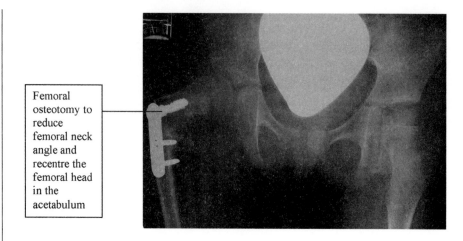

Femoral osteotomy to reduce femoral neck angle and recentre the femoral head in the acetabulum

Fig. 6 Femoral osteotomy to recentre femoral head.

heterogeneous interventions, poorly defined outcome measures and lack of statistical analysis' and identified the need for further research to evaluate this type of surgery.[16]

Bony surgery includes femoral osteotomy, pelvic osteotomy and open reduction which are designed to restructure the proximal femoral and acetabular anatomy to maintain the hip position (Fig. 6). Outcomes from bony surgery are generally good when used to prevent progression of hip subluxation.[5] A long-term review of 63 hips found that femoral osteotomy alone was not sufficient to maintain hip centration and acetabular reconstruction was also advised.[32] Cornell's 1995 review[5] supports this and suggests that the development of the acetabulum is unaffected by femoral osteotomy.

Surgery to only one hip has been reported to cause an alteration in the direction of wind-sweeping and consequent increasing migration of the contralateral hip.[33,34]

Therefore, it is advised that surgery is done unilaterally and that reconstructive surgery involves osteotomies of both the femur and acetabulum.

Many studies on surgery report relatively short follow-up periods and comparison of studies is hampered by the lack of valid functional outcomes, systematically measured pain pre- and post-surgery or the use of a variety and combination of different procedures.[16,30,35–37]

Long-term outcomes of surgery for young adults need to be considered. A cross-sectional study found that 54% of their subjects had a wind-swept deformity despite surgery to the hip.[38] A retrospective study of 60 children and young adults found that the children who had not had hip surgery had a significantly increased chance of having both hips intact than those who did not.[19]

Selective dorsal rhizotomy is a neurosurgical technique to divide the posterior nerve rootlets in the lumbosacral region to reduce the level of spasticity, in particular muscle groups of the lower limb. Its effectiveness on hip migration is inconclusive.[39]

POSTURAL MANAGEMENT PROGRAMMES

The use of positioning equipment in lying, sitting and standing has long been advocated as a method of maintaining muscle length and joint range. Scrutton et al.[2] devised an asymmetric kneeblock to control the hips and pelvis in seating and this has since been developed and is widely used.[22] Orthoses such as hip abduction braces and hip and spinal orthoses are also used, although no studies detailing outcomes have been published.

Twenty-four hour approaches to delivering postural management programmes which combine positioning in lying, sitting and standing to encourage active movement and function and prevent deformity have been developed. The quality of positioning achieved within the equipment is crucial to its success and needs to maintain a neutral pelvic position in terms of tilt, rotation and obliquity and a neutral hip position.[22] Seating systems with a kneeblock and sacral pad combination control hip and pelvic position to maintain pelvic tilt, rotation and obliquity in neutral and the hips in a mid-line position. A consensus statement recommends 24-h postural management from the earliest ages with the use of lying support as soon as possible after birth, seating from 6 months and standing from 12 months.

Figures 7–11 illustrate the effect of postural management equipment including the kneeblock system in a seating to control hip and pelvis position. This aims to reduce wind-swept posture and provide stability for head, upper trunk and limb activity.

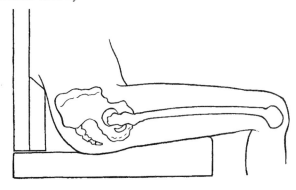

Fig. 7 Child sitting with posteriorly tilted pelvis.

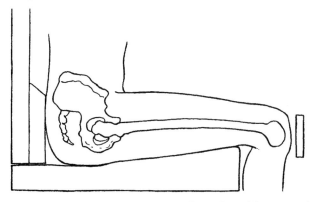

Fig. 8 The effect of the kneeblock and sacral pad to bring the pelvis to an upright position.

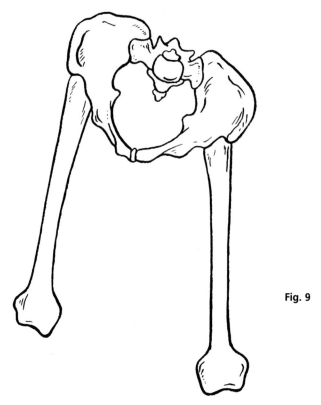

Fig. 9

Figs 9 and 10 The effect of the kneeblock, and sacral pad to control the wind-swept posture.

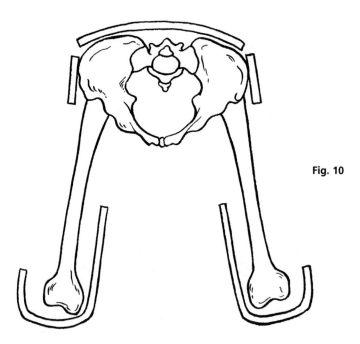

Fig. 10

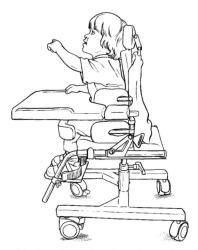

Fig. 11 Child using kneeblock and sacral pad seating system.

PAIN MANAGEMENT

Pain is identified as present during dislocation in a number of studies but with no description of how this is gauged.[18,24] Other studies have identified pain associated with hip dislocation. In the Knapp and Cortess study,[40] 71% of hips were not painful, 11% intermittently painful and only 18% definitely painful whilst others reported hip pain in approximately 40% of interviewees persisting over 20 years and consistent with sites of surgical interventions.[40–42]

Pain needs to recognised and managed in children appropriately. Sites and causes of pain need to be identified and how the pain is relieved. Changes in moving and handling or positioning may be all that is required whilst others will require medication.

Botulinum toxin injections have proved a useful source of pain relief for painful hips. Two studies report dramatic improvements in pain levels following injection and this approach is now used routinely in some centres.[43,44]

Botulinum toxin has also been used to relieve pain in surgical interventions. A randomised, controlled trial on the use of botulinum toxin administered pre-operatively in surgery for hip dislocation was found to reduce pain significantly postoperatively by reducing spasticity.[45]

SELECTING MANAGEMENT APPROACHES

The range of options available for the management of hip dislocation in cerebral palsy should not necessarily be used in isolation and can complement each other. However, decisions regarding which to choose need to be based on clinically reasoned assessment of the best option for each child. Decision making, as to which interventions are most appropriate, needs to consider the whole child and family and the local service provision. Clear criteria for interventions should be defined according to a child's clinical and functional activities, pain levels, hip migration percentage, long-term prognosis and the implications of the interventions in social and emotional terms, financial costs and outcomes. Each option has its own advantages and disadvantages.

Postural management programmes offer conservative options to the management of hip pain and progression to subluxation at the earliest stages of development. They may be used either as a long-term treatment, to delay decision making on surgical options, or postoperatively to maintain improvements gained. However, postural management programmes require sustained input from family and carers. Botulinum toxin injections are quick and simple but unlikely to show ongoing improvements without additional therapy input including postural management equipment and may only be effective for a limited period of time.

Surgery can cause considerable upheaval to the life of a child and the family and requires considerable postoperative rehabilitation.[46] John Fixsen cautions that surgery only 'seeks to adjust at the periphery for the major disturbance of central control' and 'unless it can be clearly shown that there is a reasonable chance that surgery will improve the patient's function, it should not be attempted in the vain hope that it might do some good'.[46]

Less invasive options may offer new approaches to managing hip dislocation but, like surgery, need long-term evaluation using reliable assessment tools. Evaluating the outcomes in this group of children is complicated by their heterogeneity and complex disability. Randomised, controlled trials may not be the most useful way to do this but rather through profiling children to determine most appropriate, possibly multiple, interventions to reduce the levels of hip dislocation.

Key points for clinical practice

- Children who are unable to sit unsupported at any time or walk more than a few paces with the use of aids (Gross Motor Functional Classification System levels IV–V) should start 24-h postural management programmes in lying as soon as appropriate after birth, in sitting from 6 months, and in standing from 12 months.

- All children who cannot walk more than 10 steps by the age of 30 months should have a hip and pelvic radiograph to record the percentage of migration. If hip adduction is pronounced, a radiograph at 18 months may be helpful.

- Repeat radiographs are recommended every 6–12 months until hip migration is stable.

- If migration percentage is greater than 15% at 30 months, positioning equipment to control posture and referral to an orthopaedic surgeon are recommended.

- An integrated approach to prevent hip problems should include postural management, botulinum toxin injections, orthoses and surgery.

- Muscle releases alone should only be used when the migration percentage is under 40% and be bilateral.

- The intervention chosen should have a sound clinical basis taking into account a child's clinical and functional status, pain levels, sleep assessment, percentage of hip migration, and long-term prognosis, together with the implications of these in social and emotional terms.

> ## Key points for clinical practice *(continued)*
>
> - Training in postural care should be given to all people directly involved with the child – health professionals, parents, wheelchair services, education services, and respite carers.
>
> - Outcome measures need to consider the integrity of both hips following interventions as a successful outcome is best represented by both hips being functional and pain-free.
>
> - Multimodal approaches should also be considered such as maintaining improvements of surgical interventions by the use of postural management equipment.

References

1. Scrutton D, Baird G. Surveillance measures of the hips of children with bilateral cerebral palsy. *Arch Dis Child* 1997; **56**: 381–384.
2. Scrutton D, Baird G, Smeeton N. Hip dysplasia in bilateral cerebral palsy: incidence and natural history in children aged 18 months to 5 years. *Dev Med Child Neurol* 2001; **43**: 586–600.
3. Soo B, Howard JJ, Boyd RN *et al.* Hip displacement in cerebral palsy. *J Bone Joint Surg Am* 2006; **88**: 121–129.
4. Miller F, Bagg MR. Age and migration percentage as risk factors for progression in spastic hip disease. *Dev Med Child Neurol* 1992; **37**: 449–455.
5. Cornell MS. The hip in cerebral palsy. *Dev Med Child Neurol* 1995; **37**: 3–18.
6. Baker LD, Dodelin R, Bassett FH. Pathological changes in the hip in cerebral palsy: incidence, pathogenesis and treatment. *J Bone Joint Surg Am* 1962; **44**: 1331–1342.
7. Buckley SL, Sponseller PD, Magid D. The acetabulum in congenital and neuromuscular hip instability. *J Pediatr Orthop* 1991; **11**: 498–501.
8. Fujiwara M, Basmajian JV, Iwamoto M. Hip abnormalities in cerebral palsy: radiological study. *Arch Phys Med Rehabil* 1976; **57**: 278–281.
9. Grenier A. Prevention of early deformations of the hip in brain damaged neonates. *Ann Pediatr* 1988; **35**: 423–427.
10. Arkin AM, Katz JF. The effects of pressure on epiphyseal growth. *J Bone Joint Surg Am* 1956; **38**: 1056–1076.
11. Ralis Z, McKibbin B. Changes in shape of the human hip joint during its development and their relation to its stability. *J Bone Joint Surg Br* 1973; **55**: 780–785.
12. Hankinson J, Morton RE. Use of a lying hip abduction system in children with bilateral cerebral palsy: a pilot study. *Dev Med Child Neurol* 2002; **44**: 177–180.
13. Pountney TE, Mandy A, Green E, Gard P. Management of hip dislocation with postural management. *Childcare Health Dev* 2002; **28**: 179–185.
14. Pountney TE, Green E, Mandy A. To assess the effectiveness of postural management programmes in reducing hip dislocation in children with bilateral cerebral palsy. EACD Abstracts, 2005; 48.
15. Gericke T. Postural management for children with cerebral palsy: consensus statement. *Dev Med Child Neurol* 2006; **48**: 244.
16. Stott NS, Piedrahita L, and AACPDM. Effects of surgical adductor releases for hip subluxation in cerebral palsy : an AACPDM evidence report. *Dev Med Child Neurol* 2004; **46**: 628–645.
17. Reimers J. The stability of the hip in children. *Acta Orthop Scand* 1980; **Suppl 184**: 67.
18. Turker RJ, Lee R. Adductor tenotomies in children with quadriplegic cerebral palsy: longer term follow-up. *J Pediatr Orthop* 2000; **20**: 370–374.
19. Pountney TE. The effect of postural management on hip dislocation and spinal curvature in cerebral palsy. In: *Clinical Research Centre for Health Professions.* PhD Thesis, Eastbourne: University of Brighton, 2002; 244.
20. Hägglund G, Andersson S, Düppe H, Lauge-Pedersen H, Nordmark E, Westbom L. Prevention of dislocation of the hip in children with cerebral palsy. *J Bone Joint Surg Br* 2005; **87**: 95–101.

21. Palisano R, Rosenbaum P, Walter S, Russell D, Wood E, Galuppi B. Development and reliability of a system to classify gross motor function in children with cerebral palsy. *Dev Med Child Neurol* 1997; **39**: 214–223.

22. Pountney TE, *et al*. *Chailey Approach to Postural Management*, 2nd edn. East Sussex: Chailey Heritage Clinical Services, 2004.

23. Hunt A, Goldman A, Seers K *et al*. Clinical validation of the Paediatric Pain Profile. *Dev Med Child Neurol* 2004; **46**: 9–18.

24. Cooperman DR, Bartucci E, Dietrick E, Millar EA. Hip dislocation in spastic cerebral palsy: long term consequences. *J Pediatr Orthop* 1987; **7**: 268–276.

25. Vidal J, Deguillaume P, Vidal M. The antomy of the dysplastic hip in cerebral palsy related to prognosis and treatment. *Int Orthop* 1985; **9**: 105–110.

26. Portinaro NMA, Murray DW, Bhullar TP, Benson MK. Errors in measurement of acetabular index. *J Pediatr Orthop* 1995; **15**: 780–784.

27. Tonnis D. Normal values of the hip joint for the evaluation of X rays. *Clin Orthop* 1976; **119**: 39–46.

28. Parrott J, Boyd RN, Dobson F, Lancaster A, Love S, Oates J. Reliability of radiological measures of hip displacement in children with spastic cerebral palsy. In: *American Academy of Cerebral Palsy and Developmental Medicine*. Toronto: Mac Keith, 2000.

29. Pountney TE, Mandy A, Gard P. Repeatability and limits of agreement in measurement of hip migration percentage in children with bilateral cerebral palsy. *Physiotherapy* 2003; **89**: 276–281.

30. Cottalorda J, Gautheron V, Metton G, Charmet E, Maatougui K, Chavrier Y. Predicting the outcome of adductor tenotomy. *Int Orthop* 1998; **22**: 374–379.

31. Abel MF, Blanco JS, Pavlovich L, Damiano DL. Asymmetric hip deformity and subluxation in cerebral palsy: an analysis of surgical treatment. *J Pediatr Orthop* 1999; **19**: 479–485.

32. Brunner R, Baumannn JU. Long term effects of intertrochanteric varus-derotation osteotomy on femur and acetabulum in spastic cerebral palsy: An 11–18 year follow up study. *J Pediatr Orthop* 1997; **17**: 585–591.

33. Carr C, Gage J. The fate of the non operated hip in cerebral palsy. *J Pediatr Orthop* 1987; **7**: 262–267.

34. Nwaobi OM, Sussman MD. Electromyographic and force patterns of cerebral palsy patients with windblown hip deformity. *J Pediatr Orthop* 1990; **10**: 382–388.

35. Cooke PH, Cole WG, Carey RPL. Dislocation of the hip in cerebral palsy. *J Bone Joint Surg Br* 1989; **71**: 441–446.

36. Houkom JA, Roach JW, Wenger DR, Speck G, Herring JA, Norris EN. Treatment of acquired hip subluxation in cerebral palsy. *J Pediatr Orthop* 1986; **6**: 285–290.

37. Kalen V, Beck EE. Prevention of spastic paralytic hip dislocation. *Dev Med Child Neurol* 1985; **27**: 17–24.

38. Young NL, Wright JG, Lam TP, Rajaratnam K, Stephens D, Wedge JH. Windswept deformity in spastic quadriplegic cerebral palsy. *Pediatr Phys Ther* 1998; **10**: 94–100.

39. Chicoine MR, Park TS, Kaufmnan BA. Selective dorsal rhizotomy and rates of orthopaedic surgery in children with spastic cerebral palsy. *J Neurosurg* 1997; **86**: 43–49.

40. Knapp DRJ, Cortes H. Untreated hip dislocation in cerebral palsy. *J Pediatr Orthop* 2002; **22**: 668–671.

41. Hodgkinson I, Jindrich ML, Duhaut P, Vadot JP, Metton G, Bérard C. Hip pain in 234 non-ambulatory adolescents and young adults with cerebral palsy: a cross-sectional multicentre study. *Dev Med Child Neurol* 2001; **43**: 806–808.

42. Schwartz L, Engel JM, Jensen MP. Pain in persons with cerebral palsy. *Arch Med Rehabil* 1999; **80**: 1243–1246.

43. Deleplanque B, Lagueny A, Flurin V *et al*. Toxine botulinique dans la spasticite des adducteurs de hanche chez les enfants IMC et IMOC non marchants. *Rev Chir Orthop* 2002; **88**: 279–285.

44. Fairhurst CBR. Analgesic effect of botulinum toxin. British Paediatric Neurology Association, London: MacKeith Press, 2004: **46**: 22

45. Barwood S, Baillieu C, Boyd R *et al*. Analgesic effects of botulinum toxin A: a randomized, placebo-controlled clinical trial. *Dev Med Child Neurol* 2000; **42**: 116–121.

46. Fixsen JA. The role of orthopaedic surgery in cerebral palsy. *Semin Orthop* 1989; **4**: 215–219.

Frank Rauch

11

Osteogenesis imperfecta in childhood

Osteogenesis imperfecta (OI), also called 'brittle bone disease', is a heritable disorder of bone formation affecting about 1 in 10,000 people. In most cases, the disease is due to a mutation affecting collagen type I, the most abundant protein in bone.[1] The main characteristic of OI is bone fragility, which is caused by a combination of abnormal bone structure and low bone mass. The severity of the bone fragility is extremely variable, and its consequences range from death *in utero* to almost asymptomatic involvement.

Apart from bone fragility, OI can manifest with a number of extraskeletal features. Clinical examination may reveal blue or grey sclera, dentinogenesis imperfecta (a defect of the tooth enamel that makes the teeth look yellow and crumble easily), hyperlaxity of ligaments and skin, and hearing impairment.[1] However, these findings are quite variable from patient to patient.

On X-rays, long bones of the extremities and ribs often appear thin. In severe cases, there is bowing of the long bones, in particular of the femur and tibia. Spine radiographs can reveal compressed vertebral bodies even in babies (Fig. 1). Skull radiographs may show so-called Wormian bones. These are irregularities in the sutures that produce a mosaic-like pattern, especially in the occipital bone (Fig. 2). Bone mineral density of the lumbar spine is below the age-specific reference range in most OI patients. Blood and urine tests do not show any specific alterations.

The weakness of the bone in OI patients may lead to skull-base abnormalities. These can be diagnosed on lateral skull radiographs, even though magnetic resonance imaging is required for more precise evaluation. Radiographically, detectable skull-base abnormalities may be present in more than a third of adult OI patients suffering from severe bone fragility, but will remain asymptomatic in most of these individuals.[2] Symptoms, if they occur, consist of headaches, lower

Frank Rauch MD
Associate Professor, Department of Paediatrics, McGill University, Canada.
For correspondence: Genetics Unit, Shriners Hospital for Children, 1529 Cedar Avenue, Montréal, Québec H3G 1A6, Canada
E-mail: frauch@shriners.mcgill.ca

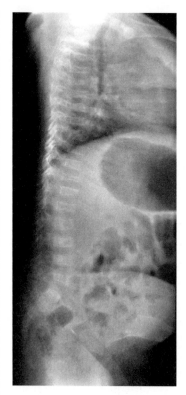

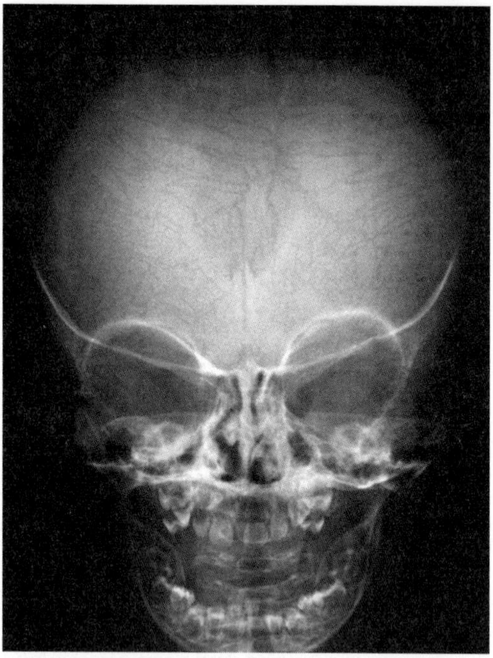

Fig. 2 Anteroposterior skull radiograph of a 3-month-old boy with OI type III. The mosaic-like pattern in the occiput is due to a large number of Wormian bones.

Fig. 1 Lateral spine radiograph of a 2-month-old boy with OI type IV. Most of the vertebral bodies are diminished in height.

cranial nerve dysfunction and hyper-reflexia.[3] In younger children, hydrocephalus may occur.

CLASSIFICATION

OI has been recognised as a disease entity since the 1600s, when it was termed congenital osteomalacia. The term osteogenesis imperfecta was adopted in the late 19th century; by the start of the 20th century, the disorder had been subclassified into congenita (severe) and tarda (mild) forms. As more patients with OI were investigated, a more comprehensive classification distinguishing four types of OI was established, based on clinical findings. However, it is clear that the disorder represents a continuum of severity and that patients do not always fall conveniently into one clinical category.

In the last few years, the application of bone histology to OI has revealed that patients with similar clinical presentation may have quite different changes in their bone architecture.[1] In addition, it was found that collagen type I mutations were absent in some patients who had unusual patterns of bone histology. These new observations have led to further subdivisions of the disorder. Presently, seven subtypes have been defined (Table 1). The severity of bone fragility increases in the order: type I < types IV, V, VI, VII < type III < type II. More than half of all OI patients fall into the type I category. Most of

Table 1 Classification of osteogenesis imperfecta

Type	Clinical severity	Typical features	Typically associated mutations
I	Mild non-deforming OI	Normal height or mild short stature; blue sclera; no DI	Premature stop codon in *COL1A1*
II	Perinatal lethal	Multiple rib and long-bone fractures at birth; marked deformities; broad long bones; low density of skull bones on X-rays; dark sclera	Glycine substitutions in *COL1A1* or *COL1A2*
III	Severely deforming	Very short; triangular face; severe scoliosis; greyish sclera; DI	Glycine substitutions in *COL1A1* or *COL1A2*
IV	Moderately deforming	Moderately short; mild-to-moderate scoliosis; greyish or white sclera; DI	Glycine substitutions in *COL1A1* or *COL1A2*
V	Moderately deforming	Mild-to-moderate short stature; dislocation of radial head; mineralised interosseous membrane; hyperplastic callus; white sclera; no DI	Unknown
VI	Moderately to severely deforming	Moderately short; scoliosis; accumulation of osteoid in bone tissue, fish-scale pattern of bone lamellation; white sclera; no DI	Unknown
VII	Moderately deforming	Mild short stature; short humeri and femora; coxa vara; white sclera; no DI	*CRTAP* splice-site mutation

The 'typically associated mutations' may or may not be detectable in a given patient.
OI, osteogenesis imperfecta; DI, dentinogenesis imperfecta.

the other patients are classified as either OI type III or type IV, as the other types are more rare.

OI TYPE I

OI type I is the mildest and most frequent form of the disease. There are no major bone deformities and most patients have a normal or near-normal height. Patients typically have blue sclera and hyperlaxity of ligaments, but normal-looking teeth. Fractures are not commonly observed at birth, but often begin when the children start to walk and thus have a higher risk of accidents. Vertebral fractures are common and can lead to mild scoliosis, starting in adolescence. The rate of fractures usually decreases after puberty, but may increase again in women after the menopause. Some individuals with OI type I may have few or even no fractures during childhood and adolescence. In such cases, it can occur that the diagnosis of OI is made only later in life, for example during an evaluation for 'postmenopausal osteoporosis'.

OI TYPE II

OI type II is the most severe form of OI. Patients rarely survive for more than a few days after birth. There are multiple intra-uterine rib and long-bone fractures. The cause of death is usually respiratory failure secondary to severe deformation of the thoracic cage. Bone histology reveals a marked decrease in both cortical bone thickness and the amount of trabecular bone.

OI TYPE III

OI type III is the most severe form of OI compatible with survival past the perinatal period. Patients with OI type III often have multiple fractures *in utero* and suffer frequent fractures after birth. The tibia is usually bowed, as it is too weak to resist the pull of the muscles that are located on the posterior aspect of

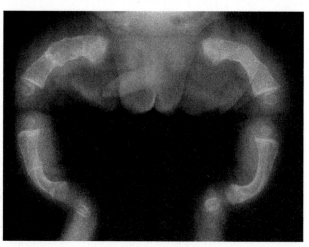

Fig. 3 Lower extremities in a 3-month-old boy with OI type III. The typical posterior bowing of the tibias is evident.

the bone (Fig. 3). Starting in mid-childhood, the chin often appears small whereas the malar bones are wide, resulting in a triangular facial aspect.

Fractures, bone deformities and slow growth result in severe short stature, with adult height typically ranging between 90 cm and 120 cm. Scoliosis affects most patients by the age of 7 years and can lead to respiratory problems, which have been identified as a leading cause of death in this patient group. Dentinogenesis imperfecta is often severe and requires extensive dental work.

OI TYPE IV

OI type IV comprises patients who can not be conveniently classified into either the OI type I or the OI type III groups. As such, their disease severity tends to be intermediate between OI types I and III. Patients are usually short and have dentinogenesis imperfecta. Grey sclera are present in some patients. OI type IV is a very heterogeneous group. The 'newer' OI types V–VII were recognised as distinct entities by careful examination of patients who initially had been diagnosed with OI type IV.

OI TYPE V

OI type V has only recently been described as a separate disorder. Patients suffer from moderate-to-severe bone fragility.[1] Blue sclera and dentinogenesis imperfecta are not present. The patients are characterised by three distinctive features: (i) the presence of hypertrophic callus formation at fracture sites (Fig. 4); (ii) calcification of the interosseous membranes between the bones of the forearm; and (iii) the presence of a radio-opaque metaphyseal band immediately adjacent to the growth plates on X-ray. Upon histological examination, the lamellar organisation of the bone has an irregular mesh-like appearance, which is distinct from the normal lamellar organisation.

The calcified interosseous membrane often severely limits the pronation/supination movement of the hand and may lead to secondary dislocation of the radial head. Importantly, the hyperplastic callus that may develop after fractures or surgical interventions may mimic osteosarcoma. Magnetic resonance imaging and computed tomography can be useful to distinguish hyperplastic callus from osteosarcoma in unclear cases. Patients with OI type V appear to constitute 4–5% of the OI population seen in hospitals.[1]

OI TYPE VI

Type VI OI patients also present with moderate-to-severe skeletal deformity and do not have blue sclera or dentinogenesis imperfecta.[1] The distinctive features of this OI type are the fish scale-like appearance of the bone lamellae and the presence of excessive osteoid upon histological examination. Although the osteoid accumulation suggests a mineralisation defect reminiscent of osteomalacia, there is no abnormality in calcium, phosphate, parathyroid hormone or vitamin D metabolism, and growth plate mineralisation proceeds normally. Inheritance probably is autosomal recessive. OI type VI may be present in about 4% of moderately to severely affected OI patients.[1]

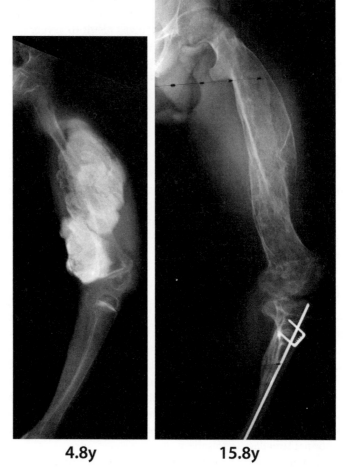

4.8y **15.8y**

Fig. 4 Lateral radiographs of the left femur in a boy with OI type V. At 4.8 years of age, a newly calcified hypertrophic callus lesion is visible. Eleven years later, the lesion has been integrated into the bone structure and the original anatomy has been partly destroyed.

OI TYPE VII

Patients with OI type VII also have moderate-to-severe skeletal deformity and bone fragility, and lack blue sclera and dentinogenesis imperfecta. The distinctive clinical feature of the disease is a rhizomelic shortening of the humerus and femur.[1] Coxa vara may be present even in infancy. So far, this disorder has been observed only in a community of Native Americans in northern Quebec.

GENETIC ASPECTS

Heredity usually follows an autosomal-dominant pattern in OI types I–V. However, spontaneous mutations are frequent. It is, therefore, not uncommon that a child with one of these OI types is born to unaffected parents. OI types VI and VII are transmitted in an autosomal recessive fashion.

In most patients with OI types I–IV, the disease is caused by mutations that directly affect one of the two genes that code for collagen type I α-chains, *COL1A1* and *COL1A2*. A collagen type I molecule comprises three chains (two α-1 and one α-2-chains) which form a triple-helical structure. For the three chains to intertwine correctly, they must have a glycine residue at every third position. The most frequently encountered sequence abnormalities associated with OI are mutations that affect a glycine residue in one of the α-chains. Such mutations typically result in the clinical picture of OI type II, III or IV. In contrast, OI type I is usually caused by mutations that lead to a reduction in α-1-chain synthesis but do not change its amino acid sequence.

Collagen type I mutations are absent in OI types V–VII. The cause of OI type V and VI has not been found yet. Recent research has shown that OI type VII results from a reduction in the expression of the so-called cartilage-associated protein, CRTAP.[4] Subsequently, total absence of CRTAP was found in a few patients who had a clinical diagnosis of OI types II or III.[4,5] CRTAP acts as a co-factor of an enzyme, prolyl-3-hydroxylase, that is involved in the post-translational modification of collagen type I. Mutations in the prolyl-3-hydroxylase enzyme itself can also lead to a clinical picture resembling OI types II or III.[6] Thus, deficiencies in CRTAP and prolyl-3-hydroxylase define new forms of very severe OI with recessive inheritance. In these cases, collagen type I α-chains are not mutated; there is nevertheless a collagen disorder, as the post-translational modification of collagen is disturbed.

DIAGNOSIS

The diagnosis of OI in a child or adult is based primarily on family history, clinical examination and X-ray findings, as described earlier. A few aspects deserve discussion. Dark or bluish sclera are very common in healthy infants; therefore, this finding is not of much diagnostic use in this age group. Dentinogenesis imperfecta is more often clinically evident in primary than in permanent teeth of OI patients. However, even patients whose teeth look normal on inspection frequently have subtle abnormalities in radiological or histological tooth examinations.[7,8]

Noticeable hearing loss is rare in the first two decades of life, even though subtle audiometric abnormalities can be found in a large percentage of children and adolescents with OI.[9,10] About half of patients older than 50 years report hearing loss, and an even higher percentage of adults have clearly pathological audiometric findings.

Diagnosing OI is straight-forward in cases with a positive family history or where several typical features are present, but can be difficult in the absence of affected family members and when bone fragility is not associated with obvious extraskeletal abnormalities. The uncertainty in such cases is compounded by the fact that there are no agreed minimal criteria that establish a clinical diagnosis of OI.

In that situation, genetic testing for collagen type I mutations can be useful. Traditionally, this has been done by protein analysis of type I procollagen molecules that are derived from the patient's cultured skin fibroblasts. This test requires that a skin biopsy is obtained and cells be shipped to the laboratory where the analysis is done. As this is somewhat cumbersome, genetic testing is now more commonly performed by sequence analysis of genomic DNA, which can be extracted from a blood or saliva sample. Both the protein and the DNA approach detect about 90% of all collagen type I mutations. A positive test confirms the diagnosis of OI. However, a negative result does not rule out OI, because it is still possible that a collagen type I mutation is present but was not detected (about 10% of mutations are missed with current techniques) or that the patient has a type of OI that is not associated with collagen type I mutations.

Genetic testing can also be used for prenatal diagnosis. Such testing may be indicated when one of the parents has OI or when the parents are healthy but already have a child with OI. Severe forms of OI often lead to bone deformities *in utero*, which can also be identified on routine ultrasound examination during pregnancy.

DIFFERENTIAL DIAGNOSIS

A number of primary skeletal disorders can be confused with OI. The clinical resemblance of Bruck syndrome and osteoporosis-pseudoglioma syndrome with OI is highlighted by the fact that these disorders have previously been called 'OI with congenital joint contractures' and 'ocular form of OI', respectively.[11,12] Panostotic fibrous dysplasia is an extreme form of polyostotic fibrous dysplasia where all bones are affected, which can mimic severe OI.[13] However, alkaline phosphatase levels are elevated in panostotic fibrous dysplasia but not in OI. Similarly, the severe bone deformities occurring in idiopathic autosomal recessive hyperphosphatasia (previously also called juvenile Paget's disease) can resemble severe OI, but is usually easily distinguishable on the basis of extremely high serum alkaline phosphatase activity.[14] Hypophosphatasia is very variable in clinical expression, ranging from still-birth without mineralised bone to pathological fractures which develop only late in adulthood.[15] Low serum activity of alkaline phosphatase separates hypophosphataemia from OI. Cole–Carpenter syndrome is a very rare disorder with severe bone fragility and a characteristic facial aspect.

Idiopathic juvenile osteoporosis, a transient, non-hereditary form of bone fragility in childhood, may be difficult to distinguish from OI type I. However, in idiopathic juvenile osteoporosis there is no extraskeletal involvement and collagen type I studies do not reveal any abnormalities.[16] In unclear cases, an iliac bone biopsy may provide the diagnostic clue, as bone turnover is low in idiopathic juvenile osteoporosis but not in OI.

The diagnostic dilemma most frequently encountered in clinical practice is the distinction between OI type I and child abuse. Child abuse is a frequent cause of fractures, with the highest incidence in the first year of life.[17] The clinical differentiation of OI type I from child abuse can be difficult at times, especially if the family history is negative for OI and the sclera have a normal appearance. The finding of thin bones on X-rays and a low bone mineral density result strengthen the case for a diagnosis of OI. Collagen type I analysis can be very useful when the test is unequivocally positive, thus proving OI.[18] However, a negative collagen type I analysis evidently does not prove child abuse. Thus, in some cases, the distinction between mild OI and child abuse still relies entirely on careful evaluation by an experienced clinician.

FOLLOW-UP

There are no established guidelines for follow-up of OI patients. However, most patients with one of the more severe forms of OI frequently require orthopaedic interventions and rehabilitative measures and, therefore, should be followed in specialised centres. Patients with mild forms of OI may not seek medical attention for their condition. Nevertheless, children and adolescents with mild OI can have vertebral compression fractures even without a clear history of prolonged back pain, and may develop scoliosis. Therefore, it is useful to have such paediatric OI patients examined in a specialised institution once per year. Adults with OI should have a bone density test at least once. It is also recommended that OI patients above the age of 10 years undergo audiometry every 2–3 years.

TREATMENT

Some patients with mild forms of OI may not need treatment for their condition other than occasional fracture management. More severely affected patients require a multidisciplinary approach including specialists in physiotherapy, rehabilitation, orthopaedic surgery and metabolic bone disorders.[19] Therapeutic efforts aim at maximising mobility and other functional capabilities. Physical activity programmes are encouraged (as far as is compatible with the increased risk of fracture) to prevent contractures and immobility-induced bone loss. In children, orthoses are used to protect the lower limbs during the earlier phases of mobilisation. Standing and walking can often only be achieved after femora and tibiae have been straightened using intramedullary rods.

BISPHOSPHONATE TREATMENT

The more severe forms of OI have long been a source of frustration to care-givers, because the weakness of the bones made surgical interventions and rehabilitation difficult. This situation has improved in the past few years thanks to the introduction of bisphosphonate therapy. Bisphosphonates are potent anti-resorptive agents that inhibit osteoclast function. The hypothesis initially underlying the use of an anti-osteoclast medication in an osteoblast disorder such as OI was that a decrease in the activity of the bone resorbing system might compensate for the weakness of the bone forming cells. The use of these drugs in OI became wide-spread after the 1998 publication of a series of children and adolescents with OI who had been treated with cyclical intravenous pamidronate.[20]

The majority of OI patients who were described in published reports received cyclical intravenous pamidronate. None of these studies compared various dosing regimens against each other; therefore, the optimal dose of pamidronate and the best treatment interval are unknown. Nevertheless, investigators agreed that intravenous pamidronate infusions, given every 1–4 months, led to a marked and rapid decrease of chronic bone pain, an increased sense of well-being and a rapid rise in vertebral bone mineral mass. Collapsed vertebral bodies were also noted to regain a more normal size and shape.[21] The two largest studies reported improved mobility in more than half of the patients.[22,23] It is unknown, at present, whether pamidronate treatment prevents long-bone deformities or delays the progression of scoliosis.

It is unclear whether oral bisphosphonates are as effective as intravenous pamidronate. A double-blind, placebo-controlled trial in 139 children and adolescents found that 2 years of oral alendronate significantly decreased bone turnover, increased spine bone mineral density, and was generally well tolerated.[24] However, no significant effect on the incidence of fractures, bone pain or functional status was evident. Sakkers et al.[25] tested oral olpadronate at a daily dose of 10 mg/m^2 body surface area in a randomised, placebo-controlled study that comprised 34 children and adolescents with OI. After a treatment period of 2 years, the group receiving active therapy had a higher lumbar spine areal bone mineral density and a lower incidence of long-bone fractures. No difference in functional outcome such as mobility and muscle force was detected.

The effect of bisphosphonates on the skeleton is largest during growth. Adult OI patients, therefore, derive much less, if any, benefit from the treatment than children and adolescents. There are also caveats for the use of bisphosphonates in children, as the optimal treatment regimen and the long-term consequences of this treatment are unknown. Given these uncertainties, treatment with bisphosphonates should only be given in collaboration with a specialised centre. Also, there is no consensus verdict on whether such drugs are of benefit in children and adolescents suffering from milder forms of OI. Patients with mild OI have less to gain from the treatment but have more to lose from potential side-effects than more severely affected patients. In particular, it is unclear whether there is any benefit in treating young and asymptomatic OI patients whose only 'problem' is low bone density.

It is an inevitable drawback of antiresorptive drugs such as bisphosphonates to decrease the activity of bone remodelling and modelling (shaping). A sustained suppression in remodelling activity during growth may be harmful, as it can lead to the accumulation of growth plate residues within trabecular bone tissue. Low remodelling activity might also delay bone healing after injury. In fact, pamidronate treatment delayed the healing of osteotomy sites after intramedullary rodding procedures.[26] This can lead to pain and fracture at the affected site and may necessitate further surgical procedures. Bisphosphonates are known to persist in bone tissue for many years.[27] Therefore, bisphosphonate treatment of girls and premenopausal women might have an effect on future pregnancies.

When bisphosphonate therapy is discontinued in growing children and adolescents, lumbar spine areal bone mineral density tends to decrease.[28] In addition, the new bone that is added by longitudinal growth after treatment is stopped has never been exposed to the drug, which may create zones of localised bone weakness.[29] Some patients also complain about a lack of stamina and recurrence of bone pain after they had been off pamidronate for several months. These observations provide arguments for continuing some form of bisphosphonate therapy during the growing years.

MEDICAL THERAPIES OTHER THAN BISPHOSPHONATES

Growth hormone has long been proposed as a possible treatment for OI. Small studies suggest that growth hormone treatment may accelerate short-term height velocity in some patients.[30] Increased bone turnover during growth hormone therapy was also found in histomorphometric studies of iliac bone samples.[30] As bone turnover is already abnormally high in untreated children with OI, further stimulation does not appear to be a desirable goal. Possibly, growth hormone would be more useful in combination with bisphosphonate therapy, but this remains to be tested.

Parathyroid hormone is a potent bone anabolic agent and has been shown to reduce the fracture incidence in postmenopausal osteoporosis. These results made parathyroid hormone look like an attractive candidate for treating children with OI. However, a substantial proportion of young rats receiving parathyroid hormone subsequently developed osteosarcoma.[31] It cannot be excluded that a similar effect could happen in humans. Thus, parathyroid hormone should probably not be used in children until these issues have been resolved.

POTENTIAL FUTURE THERAPIES

Bone marrow stromal cells can differentiate into a variety of cell lineages, including osteoblasts.[32] This observation led to the straight-forward hypothesis that transplanting bone marrow stromal cells from healthy subjects might improve the clinical course of OI. Bone marrow transplantation has indeed been attempted in a few children with severe OI,[33,34] but the benefit to the patient was not clear. Gene-based therapy offers the hope for a curative treatment of OI, but remains at present in the early stages of preclinical research.

Key points for clinical practice

- Osteogenesis imperfecta is a hereditary bone fragility disorder with low bone mass, disorganised bone structure and variable extraskeletal findings. These include dentinogenesis imperfecta, blue or greyish sclera and joint hyperlaxity.

- Typical radiological findings are Wormian bones (suture irregularities in the skull), reduced bone diameter, compression fractures of vertebral bodies and lower-limb deformities.

- Blood and urine tests do not show any specific alterations.

- Complications of osteogenesis imperfecta include hearing impairment (especially after the third decade of life) and skull-base abnormalities (predominantly in patients with severely fragile bones).

- At present, seven types of osteogenesis imperfecta are distinguished, mostly based on clinical, radiological and bone histological findings. Among these, osteogenesis imperfecta type I is the mildest and most frequent form.

- In the large majority of osteogenesis imperfecta types I to IV, the disease is caused by mutations affecting one of the two genes that code for collagen type I α- chains. The genetic defects causing osteogenesis imperfecta types V and VI have not been elucidated, but osteogenesis imperfecta type VII is due to a defect in the post-translational modification of collagen type I.

Key points for clinical practice *(continued)*

- Osteogenesis imperfecta types I to V are usually transmitted in an autosomal-dominant fashion, even though recessive inheritance is present in rare cases. Osteogenesis imperfecta types VI and VII are recessive disorders.

- The diagnosis of osteogenesis imperfecta types I to IV can be confirmed by sequencing the collagen type I encoding genes in genomic DNA or by biochemical analysis of skin fibroblasts. However, a negative test result does not exclude osteogenesis imperfecta.

- A number of rare bone disorders can resemble osteogenesis imperfecta. Most disorders can be distinguished from osteogenesis imperfecta on the basis of clinical findings, standard serum biochemistry, or molecular testing, but sometimes a bone biopsy is necessary to establish the diagnosis.

- Treatment of osteogenesis imperfecta aims at maximising mobility and at reducing the number of fractures. Physical activity programmes are encouraged to prevent immobility-induced bone loss.

- Bisphosphonates can improve the clinical status of patients suffering from moderate to severe osteogenesis imperfecta. In contrast, children and adolescents with osteogenesis imperfecta who have few fractures and no functional limitations have less to gain from treatment.

- Bisphosphonate therapy does not constitute a cure of osteogenesis imperfecta, but rather is an adjunct to physiotherapy, rehabilitation and orthopaedic care.

- The optimal medical treatment strategy and duration of bisphosphonate treatment have not been established. Medical treatment of osteogenesis imperfecta patients should, therefore, be supervised by a specialised centre.

ACKNOWLEDGEMENTS

The author's research is supported by the Fonds the la Recherche en Santé du Québec and the Shriners of North America.

References

1. Rauch F, Glorieux FH. Osteogenesis imperfecta. *Lancet* 2004; **363**: 1377–1385.
2. Kovero O, Pynnonen S, Kuurila-Svahn K, Kaitila I, Waltimo-Siren J. Skull base abnormalities in osteogenesis imperfecta: a cephalometric evaluation of 54 patients and 108 control volunteers. *J Neurosurg* 2006; **105**: 361–370.
3. Sawin PD, Menezes AH. Basilar invagination in osteogenesis imperfecta and related osteochondrodysplasias: medical and surgical management. *J Neurosurg* 1997; **86**: 950–960.

4. Morello R, Bertin TK, Chen Y *et al.* CRTAP is required for prolyl 3-hydroxylation and mutations cause recessive osteogenesis imperfecta. *Cell* 2006; **127**: 291–304.

5. Barnes AM, Chang W, Morello R *et al.* Deficiency of cartilage-associated protein in recessive lethal osteogenesis imperfecta. *N Engl J Med* 2006; **355**: 2757–2764.

6. Marini JC, Forlino A, Cabral WA *et al.* Consortium for osteogenesis imperfecta mutations in the helical domain of type I collagen: regions rich in lethal mutations align with collagen binding sites for integrins and proteoglycans. *Hum Mutat* 2007; **28**: 209–221.

7. Lund AM, Jensen BL, Nielsen LA, Skovby F. Dental manifestations of osteogenesis imperfecta and abnormalities of collagen I metabolism. *J Craniofac Genet Dev Biol* 1998; **18**: 30–37.

8. Malmgren B, Norgren S. Dental aberrations in children and adolescents with osteogenesis imperfecta. *Acta Odontol Scand* 2002; **60**: 65–71.

9. Kuurila K, Grenman R, Johansson R, Kaitila I. Hearing loss in children with osteogenesis imperfecta. *Eur J Pediatr* 2000; **159**: 515–519.

10. Kuurila K, Kaitila I, Johansson R, Grenman R. Hearing loss in Finnish adults with osteogenesis imperfecta: a nationwide survey. *Ann Otol Rhinol Laryngol* 2002; **111**: 939–946.

11. McPherson E, Clemens M. Bruck syndrome (osteogenesis imperfecta with congenital joint contractures): review and report on the first North American case. *Am J Med Genet* 1997; **70**: 28–31.

12. Beighton P, Winship I, Behari D. The ocular form of osteogenesis imperfecta: a new autosomal recessive syndrome. *Clin Genet* 1985; **28**: 69–75.

13. Cole DE, Fraser FC, Glorieux FH *et al.* Panostotic fibrous dysplasia: a congenital disorder of bone with unusual facial appearance, bone fragility, hyperphosphatasemia, and hypophosphatemia. *Am J Med Genet* 1983; **14**: 725–735.

14. Cundy T, Hegde M, Naot D *et al.* A mutation in the gene *TNFRSF11B* encoding osteoprotegerin causes an idiopathic hyperphosphatasia phenotype. *Hum Mol Genet* 2002; **11**: 2119–2127.

15. Whyte MP, Obrecht SE, Finnegan PM *et al.* Osteoprotegerin deficiency and juvenile Paget's disease. *N Engl J Med* 2002; **347**: 175–184.

16. Rauch F, Bishop N. Juvenile osteoporosis. In: Favus MJ. (ed) *Primer on the metabolic bone diseases and disorders of mineral metabolism*, 6th edn. Washington, DC: American Society for Bone and Mineral Research, 2006; 293–296.

17. Nimkin K, Kleinman PK. Imaging of child abuse. *Radiol Clin North Am* 2001; **39**: 843–864.

18. Marlowe A, Pepin MG, Byers PH. Testing for osteogenesis imperfecta in cases of suspected non-accidental injury. *J Med Genet* 2002; **39**: 382–386.

19. Zeitlin L, Fassier F, Glorieux FH. Modern approach to children with osteogenesis imperfecta. *J Pediatr Orthop B* 2003; **12**: 77–87.

20. Glorieux FH, Bishop NJ, Plotkin H, Chabot G, Lanoue G, Travers R. Cyclic administration of pamidronate in children with severe osteogenesis imperfecta. *N Engl J Med* 1998; **339**: 947–952.

21. Rauch F, Glorieux FH. Bisphosphonate treatment in osteogenesis imperfecta: which drug, for whom, for how long? *Ann Med* 2005; **37**: 295–302.

22. Astrom E, Soderhall S. Beneficial effect of long term intravenous bisphosphonate treatment of osteogenesis imperfecta. *Arch Dis Child* 2002; **86**: 356–364.

23. Land C, Rauch F, Montpetit K, Ruck-Gibis J, Glorieux FH. Effect of intravenous pamidronate therapy on functional abilities and level of ambulation in children with osteogenesis imperfecta. *J Pediatr* 2006; **148**: 456–460.

24. Glorieux FH, Rauch F, Ward LM *et al.* Alendronate in the treatment of pediatric osteogenesis imperfecta. *J Bone Miner Res* 2004; **19**: S12.

25. Sakkers R, Kok D, Engelbert R *et al.* Skeletal effects and functional outcome with olpadronate in children with osteogenesis imperfecta: a 2-year randomised placebo-controlled study. *Lancet* 2004; **363**: 1427–1431.

26. Munns CF, Rauch F, Zeitlin L, Fassier F, Glorieux FH. Delayed osteotomy but not fracture healing in pediatric osteogenesis imperfecta patients receiving pamidronate. *J Bone Miner Res* 2004; **19**: 1779–1786.

27. Papapoulos SE, Cremers SC. Prolonged bisphosphonate release after treatment in children. *N Engl J Med* 2007; **356**: 1075–1076.

28. Rauch F, Munns C, Land C, Glorieux FH. Pamidronate in children and adolescents with osteogenesis imperfecta: effect of treatment discontinuation. *J Clin Endocrinol Metab* 2006; **91**: 1268–1274.

29. Rauch F, Cornibert S, Cheung M, Glorieux FH. Long-bone changes after pamidronate discontinuation in children and adolescents with osteogenesis imperfecta. *Bone* 2007; **40**: 821–827.

30. Marini JC, Hopkins E, Glorieux FH *et al.* Positive linear growth and bone responses to growth hormone treatment in children with types III and IV osteogenesis imperfecta: high predictive value of the carboxy-terminal propeptide of type I procollagen. *J Bone Miner Res* 2003; **18**: 237–243.

31. Vahle JL, Sato M, Long GG *et al.* Skeletal changes in rats given daily subcutaneous injections of recombinant human parathyroid hormone (1–34) for 2 years and relevance to human safety. *Toxicol Pathol* 2002; **30**: 312–321.

32. Bianco P, Gehron Robey P. Marrow stromal stem cells. *J Clin Invest* 2000; **105**: 1663–1668.

33. Horwitz EM, Prockop DJ, Fitzpatrick LA *et al.* Transplantability and therapeutic effects of bone marrow-derived mesenchymal cells in children with osteogenesis imperfecta. *Nat Med* 1999; **5**: 309–313.

34. Horwitz EM, Prockop DJ, Gordon PL *et al.* Clinical responses to bone marrow transplantation in children with severe osteogenesis imperfecta. *Blood* 2001; **97**: 1227–1231.

Suresh Kotagal

12

Obstructive sleep apnoea

About 25% of children experience some type of sleep problem during childhood.[1] This may vary from a transient, self-limiting disturbance to a significant and chronic problem such as sleep disordered breathing. The spectrum of sleep disordered breathing in childhood ranges from primary snoring (supposedly with little or no impact on day-time or night-time function) to classic obstructive sleep apnoea, which significantly impairs the quality of life. Based upon the current International Classification of Sleep Disorders nomenclature (ICSD-2),[2] the upper airway resistance syndrome is considered under the obstructive sleep apnoea syndrome (OSAS). The American Thoracic Society[3] has defined OSAS as a 'disorder of breathing during sleep characterized by prolonged partial upper airway obstruction and/or intermittent complete obstruction (obstructive apnea) that disrupts normal ventilation during sleep and normal sleep patterns'. This chapter provides a synopsis of the childhood obstructive sleep apnoea syndrome.

EPIDEMIOLOGY AND RISK FACTORS

Habitual snoring represents the mildest form of sleep disordered breathing. Questionnaires that can reliably screen for snoring and sleep apnoea have now been developed.[4–6] In a survey of 895 children of 3–11 years of age, Brunetti *et al.*[6] found that habitual snoring was present in 4.9% of the subjects. A meta-analysis of six surveys of children which had employed questionnaires found the prevalence of habitual snoring to range from 3.2% to 14.3%.[7] The subjects were 0.5–13 years of age. Most studies show a slight male predominance for habitual snoring.

Suresh Kotagal MD
Consultant, Departments of Neurology and Pediatrics, Division of Child Neurology, Mayo Clinic, 200
First Street SW, Rochester, MN 55905, USA
E-mail: kotagal.suresh@mayo.edu

Brunetti et al.[6] also evaluated habitual snorers using ambulatory sleep studies. When they applied an apnoea–hypopnoea index (respiratory events/hours of sleep) of three or more as the diagnostic criterion for OSAS, they found a prevalence rate of 1%. Rosen et al.[8] studied 907 children of 8–11 years age in the Cleveland Children's Sleep and Health Study. They employed a design similar to that of Brunetti et al.[6] and found a childhood obstructive sleep apnoea prevalence rate of 2.2%. Sleep disordered breathing was 4–6 times more common in black children than in white children, and 3–5 times more likely to occur in children born prior to term than those born at term. In a subsequent study, Rosen et al.[9] also established that living in a socio-economically disadvantaged area further increased the likelihood of OSAS, perhaps due to increased exposure to inhaled irritants and allergens. Children with adenotonsillar hypertrophy, craniofacial anomalies, neuromuscular disorders, obesity, subglottic stenosis, gastro-oesophageal reflux, cerebral palsy and those with congenital craniofacial anomalies are at most risk for developing OSAS. The incidence of OSAS peaks at 2–6 years of age, co-inciding with the period of most prominent lymphoid hyperplasia in the upper airway. There might also be a genetic predisposition.[10]

Some special groups of children exhibit an increased risk for OSAS; Down syndrome is one such example.[11,12] de Miguel-Diez et al.[12] have prospectively evaluated the prevalence of sleep disordered breathing in 108 children with Down syndrome. Their study used history, clinical examination, lateral radiographs of the nasopharynx and overnight cardiorespiratory polysomno-graphy. While using three or more apnoea–hypopnoea events per hour of sleep as cut-off, they found a 54% prevalence of sleep disordered breathing – in boys it was significantly higher (64.7%) as compared to girls (38.5%; $P < 0.05$). The group with sleep disordered breathing was significantly younger (mean age, 6.4 years) than those with normal polysomnograms (mean age, 9.6 years). The exact prevalence in children with neuromuscular disorders has not been established, though close to 75% of subjects are suspected to have sleep disordered breathing.[13–15] Children with sickle cell anaemia are also at increased risk for OSAS which, in turn, might exacerbate their tendency for vaso-occlusive episodes. In a study based upon clinical assessment and blinded review of overnight multichannel respiratory monitoring, Samuels et al.[16] found sleep-related upper airway obstruction in 18 of 53 (36%) sickle cell anaemia patients, whose age ranged from 1.9–16.5 years. Obesity, with its steadily rising incidence in adolescents (currently estimated at around 30%), also shows a moderate association with OSAS.[17] Also of concern is the relationship between passive exposure to cigarette smoke and sleep disordered breathing – a dose–response effect between smoking and habitual snoring was found by Ali and Stradling.[7] After controlling for social class as a confounding factor, they observed that children whose mothers smoked were 4.4 times more likely to exhibit habitual snoring as compared to children whose mothers did not smoke (95% confidence interval, 1.5–13.1). Paternal smoking habits had a weaker relationship, presumably because of less time spent by smoking fathers with their children as compared to the mothers. The inflammation associated with allergic rhinitis also promotes upper airway occlusion. Following a review of the literature on allergic rhinitis, Ng et al.[18] concluded that allergies affect close to 40% of children with OSAS, and thus constitute a significant risk factor.

PATHOPHYSIOLOGY

There is an intricate relationship between the upper airway skeleton and its soft tissue components such as muscles, ligaments, mucous membranes, and adipose tissue which determines the ultimate shape, patency and function of the upper airway. Neural control of the upper airway musculature also modulates upper airway patency.[19] Abnormal development of the upper airway is also influenced partially by genetic factors; the small jaw of the child with Pierre Robin syndrome exemplifies this. Acquired intra-uterine conditions (e.g. deformation of the mandible as a result of a malpresentation with resultant mandibular hypoplasia) may play a role as well.[20] Cleft palate is frequently accompanied by maxillary hypoplasia. Acquired post-natal factors that can narrow the airway include trauma, nasal allergies, post-inflammatory pharyngeal oedema consequent to gastro-oesophageal reflux; also deviated nasal septum, pharyngeal flap surgery for cleft palate repair and the macroglossia of storage disorders such as the mucopolysaccharidoses, of which the Hurler syndrome is prototypic. The local release of cytokines such as tumour necrosis factor-α and interleukin-6 can play a role in exacerbating mucosal inflammation, oedema, and narrowing of the airway lumen.[21,22] In children with Prader-Willi syndrome who are being treated with growth hormone, the issue of whether growth hormone itself contributes to obstructive sleep apnoea by enhancing oropharyngeal soft tissue proliferation needs consideration.[23,24]

Is the airway of children with OSAS unusually prone to collapse during sleep? Marcus et al.[25] had evaluated the mean critical pressure (pCrit) at which the airway lumen collapses in children with severe OSAS, and compared it to that of primary snorers; they found that the pCrit was indeed higher in the former group. Some critiques of their study have been that their OSAS group had severe symptoms and was drawn from the specialised population of a sleep centre, thus likely not representative of the broader range of childhood sleep disordered breathing.[26] To address this concern, Fregosi et al.[26] evaluated the pCrit in a population of children with mild sleep disordered breathing (mean age, 10.6 ± 0.5 years) and compared it to that of 10 control subjects (mean age, 9.4 ± 0.5 years). Airway collapsibility was measured by brief (lasting two breaths) and sudden reductions in pharyngeal pressure while the breathing mask was connected to a negative-pressure source. Once again, the pCrit was significantly higher in OSAS than controls even though the former had only mild sleep disordered breathing (pCrit, −10.8 ± 2.8 cmH$_2$O versus −15.7 ± 1.2 cmH$_2$O in the controls). The upper airway of children with Down syndrome tends to collapse at multiple levels during sleep. Neuromuscular disorders like myotonic dystrophy and cerebral palsy can be associated with insufficient or incordinated activity of the upper airway dilator muscles like the genioglossus, and predispose to airway collapse, especially during the hypotonia that normally accompanies rapid eye movement (REM) sleep.

In general, children with OSAS exhibit partial upper airway occlusion more often and have less of the frank obstructive apnoea episodes that are characteristically seen in adults. The duration of obstructive events in children is brief, generally lasting 5–10 s, whereas adults show obstructive events of 10 s or more duration. Blunting of the central ventilatory drive and genetic predisposition to OSAS also play a role in some patients.

The autonomic consequences of the airway occlusion and/or recurrent hypoxemia include sympathetic activation, tachycardia and transient arousals at the cerebral cortical or subcortical levels. Repeated arousals from sleep tend to disrupt the function of the prefrontal cortex, with consequent day-time behavioural disinhibition in the form of inattentiveness, impulsivity and hyperactivity.[27] O'Brien et al.[28] have recently described the neurobehavioural sequelae of childhood OSAS in 35 children (mean age, 6.7 years). They compared the results with that of 35 age-, gender-, and ethnically-matched controls, and found that the OSAS group had significant deficits in attention span, executive functioning, phonological processing, visual attention and general conceptual ability. Phonological processing is, of course, the basic building block for the development of reading skills. Therefore, one wonders about the potential negative impact of untreated, long-standing OSAS on childhood learning and academic performance. It is now felt that even primary snoring (characterised by concurrent apnoea, hypopnoea, or oxygen desaturation) is not harmless, and likely associated with neurobehavioural disturbances,[29] that result from the increased tendency to sleep fragmentation.

OSAS can be associated with increased likelihood of systemic and pulmonary hypertension. Amin et al.[30] have reported that about 15% of children with primary snoring and 39% of children with OSAS may show abnormal left ventricular geometry. This is probably partly related to recurrent hypoxemia, sympathetic over-activity and systemic and pulmonary vasospasm.[30] The percentage of Stage III/IV NREM sleep (also termed slow-wave sleep) and the slow-wave sleep-linked release of nocturnal growth

Table 1 A comparison of adult and paediatric obstructive sleep apnoea

	Child	Adult
Peak age of onset	2–6 years	3rd to 6th decade
Aetiology	Adenotonsillar hypertrophy Craniofacial anomalies Neuromuscular disorders Obesity	Obesity Craniofacial anomalies Hypothyroidism Acromegaly
Day-time features	Irritability, inattentiveness, hyperactivity	Daytime sleepiness, fatigue, hypertension, insomnia, feeling of choking, headaches
Nocturnal polysomnography	Hypopnoeas predominate, obstructive apnoeas are of 5–10 s duration, frequent arousals triggered by snoring, apnoea–hypopnoea index > 1 when accompanied by symptoms	Obstructive apnoeas predominate, are usually of 10 s or more duration, apnoea– hypopnoea index > 5 when accompanied by symptoms
Treatment strategies	Adenotonsillectomy Orthodontic appliances Positive pressure breathing Weight reduction	Positive pressure breathing Weight reduction Uvulopalatopharyngo plasty in mild cases

hormone might also be impaired in severe childhood OSAS as there is a rebound surge in nocturnal growth hormone levels following treatment of OSAS with adenotonsillectomy.[31] Distinctions between adult and paediatric OSAS are listed in Table 1.

CLINICAL FEATURES

SNORING

Snoring is the vibratory sound generated by the upper airway muscles when air moves across a narrow passage. In mild OSAS, snoring may be present only in the supine position; with progression in severity, the snoring is present in both the supine and the lateral decubitus. In spite of having significant narrowing of the upper airway, infants may not be able to generate sufficient forceful negative pressure during inspiration to generate audible snoring. In older children, though, habitual snoring is commonly observed with OSAS.[32] Characteristic of OSAS are periods of snoring that are punctuated by silent pauses that represent apnoea, which then terminate with snorting sounds. There is, however, no correlation between how loudly a child snores and the severity of OSAS. Children with nasal obstruction may show a tendency for mouth breathing as well and complain of a dry mouth. The 'adenoid facies' is a useful marker for habitual snoring, and possible OSAS.[32]

SLEEP FRAGMENTATION

Recurrent episodes of oxygen desaturation may lead to autonomic dysfunction that is manifested in the form of frequent arousals, restless sleep, bed wetting, and excessive sweating. The frequent partial arousals may also trigger parasomnias like sleep walking and confusional arousals, in which there is activation of the motor and autonomic systems while the patient is still stuck in the deeper stages of non-rapid eye movement sleep. Children with OSAS wake up in the morning feeling tired and unrefreshed as a consequence of nocturnal sleep fragmentation.

ABNORMAL POSTURES

In a subconscious effort to increase the anteroposterior diameter of the upper airway, children may keep the neck hyperextended. Patients with associated gastro-oesophageal reflux may show episodes of tonic extension of the trunk (Sandifer syndrome). One peculiar, but characteristic, position is sleeping in the prone position, with the knees and elbows tucked under the trunk and the bottom raised up.

ALTERED DAYTIME BEHAVIOUR

Parents may notice fatigue and moodiness upon awakening in the morning. Daytime inattentiveness, hyperactivity, impulsivity, aggressive behaviour and academic under-achievement seem to show a 3-fold increase. The clinical profile often fits that of the attention deficit hyperactivity disorder. School-age children and adolescents with OSAS may exhibit frank daytime sleepiness that can be documented objectively on the Multiple Sleep Latency test, which measures the speed with which one falls asleep at multiple times of the day in a darkened, quiet room.[33] Some children may admit to fighting hard to stay awake in the classroom, taking habitual involuntary naps and increased use of stimulants like caffeine and nicotine. The sleepy appearance may be apparent on facial inspection even during the course of the office visit. The sleepiness tends to resolve after successful treatment of OSAS with adenotonsillectomy.

SYSTEMIC MANIFESTATIONS

Older children and adolescents with sleep disordered breathing may be obese. Failure to thrive, perhaps as a consequence of impaired growth hormone release or increased energy expenditure during sleep, was a common manifestation in infants and young children two decades ago. It is now encountered less often, perhaps due to the increasing early recognition and treatment of OSAS. Adenotonsillectomy for OSAS has been reported to be followed by a significant increase in slow-wave sleep, weight and circulating levels of insulin-like growth factor-1,[31] which, once again, attests to its adverse effect on growth. Children with OSAS are also heavy consumers of healthcare resources. In a study of 287 consecutive children from Southern Israel with OSAS (who were compared with a control group of 1149 age, gender and geographically matched children), Reuveni et al.[34] noted a 226% increase in healthcare resource utilisation in the former group. OSAS children under 5 years of age consumed more resources than older children. Overall, the OSAS children used more hospital days, drugs and emergency room visits.

NOSE AND THROAT FINDINGS

Tonsils and adenoids may be enlarged, but a consistent relationship between the size of tonsils or adenoids and the severity of sleep apnoea is not seen.[32] The examiner should look for craniofacial anomalies that predispose to OSAS such as retrognathia, macroglossia, maxillary hypoplasia, high arched palate, deviated nasal septum, elongated and inflamed uvula or soft palate. Tonsil size should be graded on a I–IV scale, with grade I being minimal enlargement, grade IV representing tonsils that are almost kissing in the midline. Thyromegaly may be a clue to underlying hypothyroidism.

WHAT IS THE UTILITY OF THE CLINICAL ASSESSMENT?

There has been some debate about the lack of correlation between sleep history and clinical examination findings of OSAS with objective, polysomnographic findings. Specifically, it has been felt that, though clinical features may suggest OSAS, there may or may not be evidence of sleep disordered breathing on nocturnal polysomnography. The weakness of this argument is that at least two of the studies on which it is based had used polysomnogram methodology that would today be considered relatively insensitive from the standpoint of detection of sleep disordered breathing. For example, Brooks et al.,[35] in 1998, used thermocouples for measuring nasal respiration whereas today the gold standard is the nasal pressure transducer. Similarly, Carroll et al.,[36] in 1995, used strain gauges for measuring chest and abdominal respiratory effort plus thermistors for recording nasal respiration, whereas today the gold standard is respiratory inductance plethysmography for breathing effort and pressure transducers for nasal respiration.[37,38] It is the author's opinion that a careful history and physical examination can indeed provide valuable information about the likelihood of OSAS, and may indeed correlate with polysomnographic findings, especially in cases of moderate-to-severe OSAS. Attention should be paid to the height and weight, body mass index, adenoid facies, tonsil size, oropharyngeal diameter, enlargement of the tongue base, deviated nasal septum, nasal inflammation, maxillary and mandibular hypoplasia. The child's attention span and behaviour may also provide vital clues.

Further validation of the role of history and clinical assessment in childhood OSAS is provided by a recent study of Chervin et al.[5] They reported on the usefulness of a 22-item, sleep-related breathing disturbance subscale of their Paediatric Sleep Questionnaire.[5] The patients also underwent polysomnography, adenotonsillectomy and follow-up 1 year later. Subjects were 5–12.9 years old. When the baseline questionnaire showed a sleep-related breathing disturbance score that was greater than one standard deviation above the mean, there was an almost 3-fold risk of OSAS that was confirmed on polysomnography (odds ratio, 2.80; 95% confidence interval, 1.68–4.68). The subscale showed a diagnostic sensitivity of 78% and specificity of 72% for OSAS, and can thus play a role in screening for childhood sleep apnoea. Many of the questions pertain to items that have been discussed above.

INVESTIGATIONS

PORTABLE OXIMETRY

When tonsillar hypertrophy is significant and the history characteristic of OSAS, the documentation of recurrent episodes of oxygen desaturation on overnight oximetry is sufficient to establish the diagnosis.[39] Between 12–15 episodes of oxygen desaturation of 4% or more is considered normal. In a study of 349 children of 2.9–7 years with sleep disordered breathing, Brouilette et al.[39] found abnormal oximetry trend analysis studies in 93, negative studies in 95 subjects, and inconclusive studies in 161 subjects. The positive predictive value of oximetry for OSAS was 97%; the median obstructive apnoea–hypopnoea index in this subgroup was 16.4. Advantages of oximetry are that it is inexpensive, readily available, and the data can be obtained even in the home environment. A 'normal' overnight oximetry study does not rule out the possibility of mild or moderate OSAS, in which case polysomnography would still be indicated.

NOCTURNAL POLYSOMNOGRAPHY

Multiple physiological parameters are monitored in sleep during this procedure, which is considered the gold standard for OSAS diagnosis. Technical guidelines for polysomnography have been published by the American Thoracic Society.[3] Nasal airflow/pressure, thoracic and abdominal respiratory effort, oxygen saturation, end-tidal CO_2, electrocardiogram, eye movements, chin and leg electromyogram, and electroencephalogram are recorded simultaneously in a sleep laboratory under the supervision of a sleep technologist. Owing to their tendency to exhibit shallow breathing, it is especially important to include end-tidal CO_2 monitoring when evaluating children with Down syndrome, neuromuscular disease or obesity. The data are stored on computerised polygraph, analysed manually and reported by a sleep specialist. Childhood obstructive apnoea events are characterised by loss of

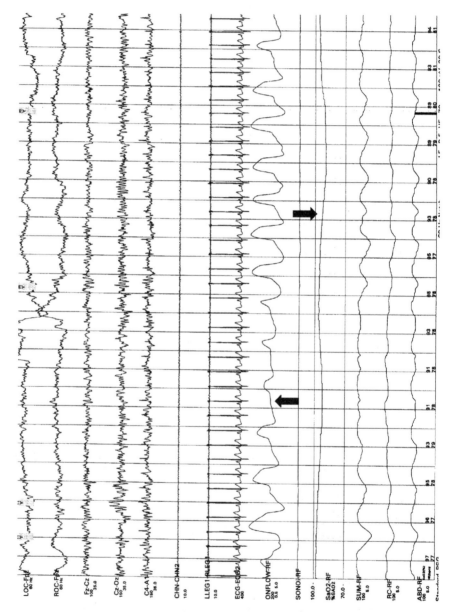

Fig. 1 A 30-s segment of a polysomnogram, showing a hypopnoea, characterised by reduction in amplitude of the nasal respiration (up arrow), together with oxygen desaturation (down arrow).

nasal airflow/pressure signal despite the persistence of thoracic and abdominal respiratory effort that is combined with a 3–4% drop in oxygen saturation. Obstructive apnoea events in children need only to be longer than

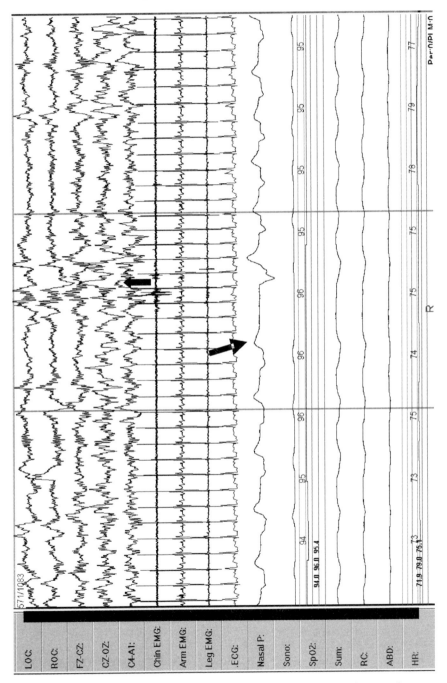

Fig. 2 A 30-s segment of a polysomnogram, showing a subtle upper airway resistance event, characterised by blunting of the signal of the nasal pressure tracing (down arrow) that is followed by disruption of the electroencephalogram in the form of a cortical arousal (up arrow).

5 s in duration, rather than the 10 s rule established for adults. Periods of crescendo snoring or apnoea may trigger transient shifts in the EEG pattern from sleep to wakefulness, along with body movement, eye movements and acceleration of heart rate (respiratory event related arousals). Children frequently fail to show classic obstructive sleep apnoea, but may manifest only partial airway obstructions or hypopnoeas (Fig. 1). Nasal pressure transducers can detect episodes of upper airway resistance, which appear as periods of flow limitation leading to electro-encephalographic arousal without simultaneous drop in oxygen saturation (Fig. 2). Whenever therapy of OSAS with positive pressure is being contemplated, it is appropriate to repeat a second night of polysomnography during which the mask size and fit and appropriate pressure settings are determined for application ultimately in the home environment.

CLINICAL DECISION MAKING

Though nocturnal polysomnography is considered the gold standard for evaluation of sleep apnoea, it is a labour-intensive and expensive procedure that is best conducted by paediatric sleep technologists and sleep specialists. Access to such a service may be limited; thus, overnight oximetry serves as a useful initial screen for childhood OSAS. Polysomnography can be resorted to if oximetry is non-diagnostic and when one needs to determine if therapeutic measures (e.g. positive-pressure breathing) will be helpful.

MISCELLANEOUS DIAGNOSTIC PROCEDURES

Electrocardiography is not recommended routinely for patients with OSAS, but warranted for those with long-standing and severe OSAS. Audiotaping of snoring in the home environment may, at times, provide useful information. Sounds of struggle have been felt to be more predictive of OSAS than periods of silent pauses.[32] The positive predictive value for audiotaping has ranged from 50%[40] to 75%,[41] while the negative predictive value is 73–88%. Small children or those with weak chest walls do not always snore, and this limits the utility of audiotapes.

MANAGEMENT

ADENOTONSILLECTOMY

Patients with enlarged adenoids and/or tonsils show significant resolution of their sleep disordered breathing following this procedure.[32] Children under the age of 3 years and those with severe OSAS or craniofacial anomalies are at greater risk for postoperative complications like upper airway oedema and its occlusion, and should, therefore, be monitored closely in the hospital setting prior to discharge.[27] In a prospective study of 23 children that had evaluated behaviour at baseline and 6, 9 and 18 months after adenotonsillectomy, there was an improvement in aggression, depression and hyperactivity that remained sustained till 18 months after surgery.[42] Not all subjects with childhood OSAS are likely to show such improvements, and those with underlying craniofacial syndromes, Down syndrome, obesity, and very high baseline apnoea–hypopnoea indices need postoperative follow-up in order to exclude the persistence of residual sleep disordered breathing. Serial follow-up of children with complicated OSAS in a multidisciplinary setting that involves the sleep specialist, otorhinolaryngologist, pulmonologist, paediatrician, nursing, nutritional expert and social services is key to ensuring that children with a treatable disorder such as OSAS do not 'fall through the cracks'.

MEDICAL THERAPY

The administration of intranasal corticosteroids helps reduce mucosal inflammation and swelling and enhances airway patency. In a prospective, open-label study of 22 children with residual OSAS following adenotonsillectomy, Kheirandish and Gozal[43] found that the leukotriene antagonist monteleukast, when combined with intranasal budesonide, led to a significant improvement in the apnoea–hypopnoea index and oxygen saturation nadir as compared to controls who did not receive this drug combination. Similarly, treatment of associated asthma may be helpful.

POSITIVE PRESSURE BREATHING

Patients who continue to demonstrate clinical and polysomnographic evidence of OSAS despite adenotonsillectomy and the above medical measures should be treated with a continuous positive airway pressure (CPAP) device[44] or a bi-level airway pressure breathing device (BiPAP).[45] The humidified air under pressure for CPAP/BiPAP is provided through an electronic blower device using a customised mask that fits over the face. The air pressure 'splints' the upper airway and prevents its collapse during sleep. In contrast to the fixed pressure of CPAP, in BiPAP the inspiratory pressure setting can be set at a higher level in inspiration (usually 4–10 cmH$_2$O) than in expiration (generally 4–8 cmH$_2$O). BiPAP may be more effective than CPAP in those with Down syndrome and neuromuscular disorders. Children are often anxious about having the mask placed over their face during sleep, and acceptance of positive pressure breathing by the child and the family may take weeks, during which time encouragement and positive reinforcement of the child and family members by the sleep centre nursing staff is crucial. Approximately one-third of children drop out of positive airway pressure therapy.[46]

GENERAL MEASURES

Weight reduction is a critical step in the management of obesity-related childhood OSAS and may necessitate consultation with a nutritional expert and social services. An emotional buy-in on the part of the child and the entire family is critical for this measure to succeed. Parental education is needed for avoidance of exposure to passive smoke and indoor allergens. Regular exercise helps keep the child more alert and counters the tendency for weight gain. In infants and in those with severe OSAS that is unresponsive to positive pressure breathing, nocturnal oxygen therapy may alleviate the hypoxemia, but should be used with care for fear of worsening the tendency towards hypoventilation.

WHAT DOES THE FUTURE HOLD?

Sleep medicine is now being included in the curriculum of an increasing number of medical schools world-wide. The awareness of childhood OSAS as an important treatable disorder of childhood with multisystem ramifications will thus continue to increase. Emphasis on prevention of exposure to risk factors like cigarette smoke and inhaled allergens may lessen the incidence to a slight extent. Paediatricians will have an increasing role in the diagnosis and treatment. Some technology has been developed for unattended, in-home polysomnography. Whilst it may play a role in the ambulatory, in-home assessment of some children with suspected OSAS, the field will continue to struggle in coming up with a low-cost alternative to polysomnography that will also be sensitive and specific towards its diagnosis. Technology and techniques to administer positive pressure breathing successfully are likely to improve. As developing nations become more industrially oriented and prosperous, children in these countries will also likely encounter risk factors for OSAS, such as environmental pollution and obesity.

Key points for clinical practice

- The prevalence rate for habitual snoring is between 3–14%. About 1–2% of children have obstructive sleep apnoea.

- The most common aetiologies for obstructive sleep apnoea are adenotonsillar hypertrophy, craniofacial anomalies, neuromuscular disorders and obesity.

- Prematurity, gastro-oesophageal reflux, allergic rhinitis and exposure to second-hand smoke may also predispose to sleep-disordered breathing.

- Habitual snoring, mouth breathing, periods of observed apnoea, restless sleep, enuresis, day-time fatigue, hypersomnolence, inattentiveness, and hyperactivity are common clinical manifestations.

- Long-standing, untreated obstructive sleep apnoea may lead to somatic growth impairment, pulmonary hypertension and right heart failure.

- Obesity and neuromuscular disorders may predispose to sleep-related hypoventilation, which elevates levels of end-tidal carbon dioxide levels and the tendency to early morning headaches.

- When the history and clinical features are characteristic, overnight oximetry can serve as an inexpensive, diagnostic screen by capturing recurrent episodes of oxygen desaturation.

- Normal oximetry, however, does not exclude the possibility of mild-to-moderate obstructive sleep apnoea. In these cases, one may need to resort to nocturnal polysomnography – the definitive diagnostic procedure.

Key points for clinical practice *(continued)*

- Adenotonsillectomy is the most common treatment. Children younger than age 3 years or those with craniofacial anomalies and severe obstructive apnoea are at increased risk for postoperative airway occlusion and need close monitoring for a transient increase in breathing difficulty.

- Positive pressure breathing, orthodontic appliances, treatment of gastro-oesophageal reflux and nasal allergies are some additional therapeutic measures.

- Primary care health providers should keep a high index of suspicion for this treatable, multisystem disorder.

References

1. Owens J. Epidemiology of sleep disorders during childhood. In: Sheldon SH, Ferber R, Kryger MH. (eds) *Principles and Practice of Pediatric Sleep Medicine*. Philadelphia, PA: Elsevier Saunders, 2005; 27–33.
2. American Academy of Sleep Medicine. *International classification of sleep disorders, 2nd edn, pocket version: Diagnostic and coding manual*. Westchester, IL: American Academy of Sleep Medicine, 2006; 127–135.
3. American Thoracic Society. Standards and indications for cardiopulmonary sleep studies in children. *Am J Respir Crit Care Med* 1996; **153**: 866–878.
4. Li AM, Cheung A, Chan D *et al*. Validation of a questionnaire instrument for prediction of obstructive sleep apnea in Hong Kong Chinese children. *Pulmonology* 2006; **41**: 1153–1160.
5. Chervin RD, Weatherly RA, Garetz SL *et al*. Pediatric sleep questionnaire: prediction of sleep apnea and outcomes. *Arch Otolaryngol Head Neck Surg* 2007; **133**: 216–222.
6. Brunetti L, Rana S, Lospalluti ML *et al*. Prevalence of obstructive sleep apnea syndrome in a cohort of 1,207 children of southern Italy. *Chest* 2001; **120**: 1930–1935.
7. Ali NJ, Stradling JR. Epidemiology and natural history of snoring and sleep disordered breathing in children. In: Loughlin GM, Carroll JL, Marcus CL. (eds) *Sleep and Breathing. A Developmental Approach*. New York: Marcel Dekker, 2000; 555–574.
8. Rosen CL, Larkin EK, Kirchner HL *et al*. Prevalence and risk factors for sleep-disordered breathing in 8- to 11-year-old children association with race and prematurity, *J Pediatr* 2003; **142**: 383–389.
9. Spilsbury JC, Storfer-Isser A, Kirchner HL *et al*. Neighborhood disadvantage as a risk factor for pediatric obstructive sleep apnea. *J Pediatr* 2006; **149**: 342–347.
10. Brooks LJ. Genetic syndromes affecting breathing during sleep. In: Loughlin GM, Carrol JL, Marcus CL. (eds). *Sleep and Breathing in Children. A Developmental Approach*. New York: Marcel Dekker, 2000; 737–754.
11. Shott SR, Amin R, Chini B *et al*. Obstructive sleep apnea. Should all children with Down syndrome be tested? *Arch Otolaryngol Head Neck Surg* 2006; **132**: 432–436.
12. De Miguel-Diez J, Villa-Assensi J, Alvarez-Sala JL. Prevalence of sleep-disordered breathing in children with Down syndrome: polygraphic findings in 108 children. *Sleep* 2003; **26**: 1006–1009.
13. Giannini A, Pinto AM, Rossetti G *et al*. Respiratory failure in infants due to spinal muscular atrophy with respiratory distress type 1. *Intensive Care Med* 2006; **32**: 1851–1855.
14. Hess DR. Noninvasive ventilation in neuromuscular disease: equipment and application. *Respir Care* 2006; **51**: 896–911.
15. Quera Salva MA, Blumen M, Jacquette A *et al*. Sleep disorders in childhood myotonic

dystrophy type 1. *Neuromuscul Disord* 2006; **16**: 564–570.

16. Samuels MP, Stebbens VA, Davies SC *et al.* Sleep related upper airway obstruction and hypoxemia in sickle cell disease. *Arch Dis Child* 1992; **67**: 925–929.

17. Ievers-Landis CE, Redline S. Pediatric sleep apnea: implications of the epidemic of childhood overweight. *Am J Respir Crit Care Med* 2007; **175**: 436–441.

18. Ng DK, Chan CH, Hwang GY, Chow PY, Kwok KL. A review of the roles of allergic rhinitis in childhood obstructive sleep apnea syndrome. *Allergy Asthma* 2006; **27**: 240–242.

19. Ferraro NF. Craniofacial development and the upper airway during sleep. In: Loughlin GM, Carrol JL, Marcus CL. (eds) *Sleep and Breathing in Children. A Developmental Approach.* New York: Marcel Dekker, 2000; 293–309.

20. Wills LM, Swift JQ, Moller KT. Craniofacial syndromes and sleep disorders. In: *Sleep: A Comprehensive Handbook.* Hoboken, NJ: Wiley, 2006; 551–560.

21. Mills PJ, Dimsdale JE. Sleep apnea: a model for studying cytokines, sleep and sleep disruption. *Brain Behav Immunity* 2004; **8**: 298–303.

22. Gozal D, Kheirandish L. Oxidant stress and inflammation in the snoring child: confluent pathways to upper airway pathogenesis and end-organ morbidity. *Sleep Med Rev* 2006; **10**: 83–96.

23. Festen DAM, de Weerd W, van den Bossche RAS *et al.* Sleep-related breathing disorders in prepubertal children with Prader-Willi syndrome and effects of growth hormone treatment. *J Clin Endocrinol Metab* 2006; **91**: 4911–4995.

24. Einfeld SL, Kavanagh SJ, Smith A *et al.* Mortality in Prader-Willi syndrome. *Am J Ment Retard* 2006; **111**: 193–198.

25. Marcus CL, Gozal D, Arens R *et al.* Ventilatory responses during wakefulness in children with obstructive sleep apnea. *Am J Respir Crit Care Med* 1994; **149**: 715–721.

26. Fregosi RF, Quan SF, Morgan WL *et al.* Pharyngeal critical pressure in children with mild sleep-disordered breathing. *J Appl Physiol* 2006; **101**: 734–739.

27. Kotagal S. Childhood obstructive sleep apnoea. *BMJ* 2005; **330**: 978–979.

28. O'Brien LM, Mervis CB, Holbrook CR *et al.* Neurobehavioral correlates of sleep-disordered breathing in children. *J Sleep Res* 2004; **2**: 165–172.

29. O'Brien LM, Mervis CB, Holbrook CR *et al.* Neurobehavioral implications of habitual snoring in children. *Pediatrics* 2004; **114**: 44–49.

30. Amin RS, Kimball TR, Bean JA *et al.* Left ventricular hypertrophy and abnormal ventricular geometry in children and adolescents with obstructive sleep apnea. *Am J Respir Crit Care Med* 2002; **165**: 1395–1399.

31. Bar A, Tarasiuk A, Segev Y, Phillip M, Tal A. The effect of adenotonsillectomy on serum insulin-like growth factor-I and growth in children with obstructive sleep apnea syndrome. *J Pediatr* 1999; **135**: 76–80.

32. Section on Pediatric Pulmonology, Subcommittee on Obstructive Sleep Apnea Syndrome. Clinical practice guideline: diagnosis and management of childhood obstructive sleep apnea syndrome. *Pediatrics* 2002; **109**: 704–712.

33. Chervin RD, Ruzika DL, Giordani BJ *et al.* Sleep-disordered breathing, behavior, and cognition in children before and after adenotonsillectomy. *Pediatrics* 2006; **117**: e769–e778.

34. Reuveni H, Simon T, Tal A, Elhayany A, Tarasiuk A. Health care services utilization in children with obstructive sleep apnea syndrome. *Pediatrics* 2002; **110**: 68–72.

35. Brooks LJ, Stephens BM, Bacevice AM. Adenoid size is related to severity but not the number of episodes of obstructive apnea in children. *J Pediatr* 1998; **132**: 682–686.

36. Carroll J, McColley SA, Marcus CL, Curtis S, Loughlin GM. Inability of clinical history to distinguish primary snoring from obstructive sleep apnea syndrome in children. *Chest* 1995; **108**: 610–618.

37. Trang H, Leske V, Gaultier C. Use of nasal cannula for detecting sleep apneas and hypopneas in infants and children. *Am J Respir Crit Care Med* 2002; **166**: 464–468.

38. Griffiths A, Maul J, Wilson A, Stick S. Improved detection of obstructive events in childhood sleep apnea with the use of the nasal cannula and the differentiated sum signal. *J Sleep Res* 2005; **14**: 431–436.

39. Nixon GM, Brouilette RT. Diagnostic techniques for obstructive sleep apnea: is polysomnography necessary? *Paediatr Respir Rev* 2002; **3**: 18–24.

40. Goldstein NA, Sculerati N, Walsleben JA, Bhatia N, Friedman DM, Rappoport DM.

Clinical diagnosis of pediatric obstructive sleep apnea validated by polysomnography. *Otolaryngol Head Neck Surg* 1994; **111**: 611–617.

41. Lamm C, Mandeli J, Kattan M. Evaluation of home audiotapes as an abbreviated test for obstructive sleep apnea (OSAS) in children. *Pediatr Pulmonol* 1999; **27**: 267–272.

42. Mitchell RB, Kelly J. Long-term changes in behavior after adenotonsillectomy for obstructive sleep apnea syndrome in children. *Otolaryngol Head Neck Surg* 2006; **134**: 374–378.

43. Kheirandish L, Gozal D. Intranasal steroids and oral leukotriene modifier therapy in residual sleep-disordered breathing after tonsillectomy and adenoidectomy in children. *Pediatrics* 2006; **117**: e61–e66.

44. Marcus CL, Ward SL, Mallory GB *et al*. Use of nasal continuous positive airway pressure as treatment of childhood obstructive sleep apnea. *J Pediatr* 1995; **127**: 88–94.

45. Johnstone SJ, Tardif HP, Barry RJ, Sands T. Nasal bilevel positive airway pressure therapy in children with a sleep-related breathing disorder and attention-deficit hyperactivity disorder: effects on electrophysiological measures of brain function. *Sleep Med* 2001; **2**: 407–416.

46. Marcus CL, Rosen G, Ward SL *et al*. Adherence to and effectiveness of positive airway pressure therapy in children with obstructive sleep apnea. *J Pediatr* 2006; **117**: e442–e451.

Steven M. Donn Sunil K. Sinha

13

Ventilator-induced lung injury in preterm newborns

The advent of modern-day neonatal intensive care has extended survival to infants as premature as 23–24 weeks of gestation. These infants, deprived of the final months of intra-uterine development, are at extremely high risk for sustaining complications from the very therapy that is necessary to save their lives. It is, indeed, a delicate balance.

Box 1 Abbreviations used	
VILI	ventilator-induced lung injury
CLD	chronic lung disease
BPD	bronchopulmonary dysplasia
RDS	respiratory distress syndrome
VLBW	very low birth-weight
PEEP	positive-end-expiratory pressure
ECMO	extracorporeal membrane oxygenation
CPAP	continuous positive airway pressure
PTV	patient-triggered ventilation
IMV	intermittent mandatory ventilation
SIMV	synchronised intermittent mandatory ventilation
A/C	assist/control
PSV	pressure support ventilation
HFV	high-frequency ventilation
HFJV	high-frequency jet ventilation
HFOV	high-frequency oscillatory ventilation

Steven M. Donn MD (for correspondence)
Professor of Pediatrics, Director, Division of Neonatal-Perinatal Medicine (F5790), C.S. Mott Children's Hospital, University of Michigan Health System, 1500 E. Medical Center Drive, Ann Arbor, MI 48109-0254, USA
E-mail: smdonnmd@med.umich.edu

Sunil K. Sinha MD PhD
Professor of Paediatrics and Neonatology, The James Cook University Hospital, University of Durham, Middlesbrough, UK

The lungs are among the last organs to develop and also represent the initial threat to survival. Dramatic advances in the past quarter century, including antenatal corticosteroid therapy, exogenous surfactant replacement, and microprocessor-based mechanical ventilation, have dramatically altered the demographics of the surviving population. Yet, it underscores the need to understand and to prevent ventilator-induced lung injury (VILI), which affects 30–40% of infants weighing < 1500 g, inflicts significant medical and developmental hardships, and consumes countless healthcare resources.

BRONCHOPULMONARY DYSPLASIA – THE OLD BPD

The term chronic lung disease (CLD), initially referred to as broncho-pulmonary dysplasia (BPD), and was first coined by Northway et al.[1] in 1967. They described the radiographic and clinical features of the disorder in a group of 13 infants who survived mechanical ventilation for respiratory distress syndrome (RDS). These infants ranged from 30–39 weeks' gestation and 1474–3204 g birth weight. Most had required high airway pressures and significant concentrations of supplemental oxygen. Their chest radiographs demonstrated overinflation and cystic emphysema, and pulmonary histopathology revealed small airway disease, extensive inflammation, interstitial and alveolar oedema, and fibrosis.[1] Over the ensuing decade, the mechanisms of BPD became better understood. Philip[2] described the aetiology of BPD as 'oxygen plus pressure plus time'.

CHRONIC LUNG DISEASE – THE NEW BPD

A quarter of a century later, surviving infants are considerably more immature than those described by Northway et al.[1] The 'old BPD' described by Northway and Philip has been replaced by the 'new BPD' described by Jobe.[3] The disorder is now seen primarily in very low birth-weight (VLBW, < 1500 g) infants requiring only modest supplemental oxygen and ventilatory support. The new BPD is also very different. It is characterised by diffuse haziness and a fine, lacy pattern on radiography, and by minimal small airway disease, less inflammation and fibrosis, and, importantly, by decreased alveolarisation on histopathology. Unfortunately, there is, as yet, no universally accepted definition of CLD; therefore, its incidence has varied according to definition. Recent work has suggested that a physiological definition be adopted, where oxygen dependency is proven by attempts to wean to room air.[4]

Although the past three decades have brought dramatic advances in the treatment of RDS, the prevalence of CLD in survivors remains unacceptably high. While recognising that the demographics of CLD have changed, and that CLD may not be entirely avoidable, VILI remains a significant component of its pathophysiology, and its incidence appears to be inversely proportional to gestational age.

THE PULMONARY INJURY SEQUENCE

VILI is multifactorial.[5,6] Comprehension of the pulmonary injury sequence (Fig. 1) leads one to the realisation that some lung damage might be

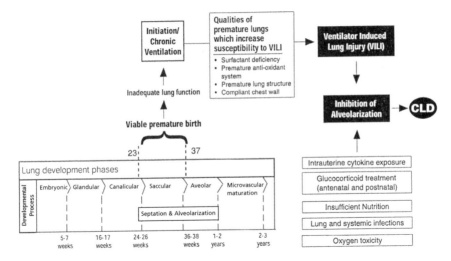

Fig. 1 The pulmonary injury sequence. (Reprinted from Attar MA, Donn SM. Mechanism of ventilator-induced lung injury in premature infants. *Semin Neonatol* 2002; **7**: 353–360, with permission from Elsevier.)

ameliorated by using ventilator (and adjunctive) strategies to circumvent the cascade.

As shown in Figure 1, there are two prominent pathways leading to CLD. The first is intrinsic. Preterm infants delivered at 23–37 weeks' gestation are in either the canalicular or saccular phases of lung development, and there is little alveolarisation occurring. This results in inadequate lung function, often requiring the initiation of chronic ventilation. Qualities of the preterm lung increase the susceptibility to VILI, and include surfactant deficiency, premature anti-oxidant defences, the premature structure of the lung at this gestational age, and a very compliant chest wall. Extrinsic factors, which also inhibit alveolarisation, include intra-uterine cytokine exposure, antenatal and postnatal glucocorticoid treatment (which inhibit lung growth), insufficient nutrition, lung and systemic infections, and exposure to high concentrations of oxygen.

Various terms have been used to describe the individual components of ventilator trauma, but these are probably inter-related and likely act synergistically. Barotrauma, or excessive pressure, may disrupt airway epithelium and alveoli. Volutrauma refers to injury related to overdistension or stretching of the lung units by delivering too much gas. Atelectotrauma refers to the damage caused by the repetitive opening and closing of lung units (also referred to as the cycle of recruitment and subsequent derecruitment). Biotrauma is a collective term to describe infection and inflammation and their relationship to lung injury and the role of oxidative stress on the delicate tissue of the developing lung. Rheotrauma refers to damage evoked by inappropriate airway flow (Fig. 2). If flow is excessive, inefficient gas exchange, inadvertent positive-end-expiratory pressure (PEEP), turbulence, and lung overinflation may occur; if flow is inadequate, it may lead to air hunger (flow starvation) and increased work of breathing. Avoidance of these components might mitigate VILI and clinicians are continuously seeking lung protective strategies.

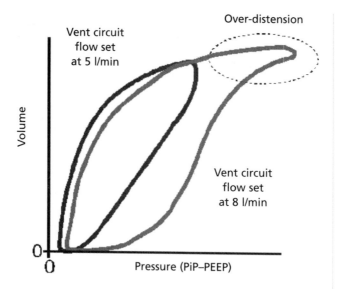

Fig. 2 Pressure–volume loops showing the effects of ventilator circuit flow on the elastic load. Note the overdistension occurring at the higher flow rate, which can be normalised when flow is decreased. (Courtesy of V.K. Bhutani, with permission from *Archives of Diseases in Childhood*.)

LUNG PROTECTIVE STRATEGIES

Lung protective strategies can actually commence before the birth of the infant. It is now a nearly universal practice to administer corticosteroids to pregnant women at risk for delivering preterm infants at, or before, 32 weeks' completed gestation. Antenatal corticosteroid therapy has clearly decreased the incidence and severity of RDS and thus CLD,[7] although it may be argued that improved survival of extremely preterm infants resulting from this has caused a demographic shift, and the overall incidence of CLD has actually increased among the smallest survivors. Similarly, there is little doubt about the role of exogenous surfactant therapy on the outcome RDS resulting in increased survival,[8] but without a concomitant decrease in CLD. It seems, therefore, that the task of improving the incidence and severity of CLD must be approached by the use of appropriate ventilatory strategies aimed at reducing or avoiding VILI, augmented by nutritional and pharmacological adjuncts.

RESPIRATORY DISTRESS SYNDROME

RDS is a disorder of the lung of the preterm infant. Although exogenous surfactant treatment can compensate for the biochemical deficits to a significant extent, the anatomical and morphological features must be addressed, for they are important contributory factors in the pathogenesis of VILI. Historically, RDS has been considered the forerunner of BPD/CLD. The lung has insufficient alveolarisation and, therefore, inadequate functional surface area for gas exchange. The distance from the alveolus to its adjacent capillary is increased, and there is deposition of fibrin in the air spaces; both impair gas diffusion. The fibrin may also inactivate surfactant. Pulmonary

Table 1 Goals of mechanical ventilation

- Maximise patient comfort
- Achieve adequate pulmonary gas exchange
- Decrease the patient work of breathing
- Overcome alveolar atelectasis
- Avoid ventilator-induced lung injury

vascular resistance may be elevated as a result of arteriolar muscularisation and it may lead to diminished pulmonary blood flow, often accompanied by right-to-left shunting (also referred to as pulmonary hypertension).

STRATEGIES TO REDUCE VENTILATOR-INDUCED LUNG INJURY

OXYGEN + PRESSURE + TIME

Table 1 lists the general goals of mechanical ventilation. These should be considered no matter what ventilatory device, mode, or modality is chosen. Other means of providing artificial respiratory support range from the least invasive (supplemental oxygen, CPAP) to the most invasive (extracorporeal membrane oxygenation, ECMO), occasionally used in premature infants > 34 weeks' gestation who have intractable but potentially reversible respiratory failure.[9]

CONTINUOUS POSITIVE AIRWAY PRESSURE

Continuous positive airway pressure (CPAP) was first introduced into neonatal practice by Gregory and colleagues in 1971. It is a type of continuous distending pressure applied to the upper airway to maintain some degree of alveolar inflation during expiration. CPAP takes advantage of LaPlace's law. The partially distended alveolus has a larger radius of curvature than a deflated alveolus, and thus requires less pressure to overcome the surface tension hindering its further inflation. In this way, CPAP decreases the work of breathing.

CPAP as a primary strategy for respiratory distress syndrome

CPAP as a primary strategy for the treatment of RDS has been advocated by Wung and colleagues,[10] who demonstrated an impressive decrease in CLD compared to neonatal centres where mechanical ventilation is used instead. Wung and co-workers emphasised that this approach depends upon the maintenance of spontaneous breathing, the avoidance of sedatives and paralytics, and the acceptance of blood gas and pH values that many consider non-physiological. The results of a recently completed randomised controlled trial (The COIN trial), only available in abstract form, suggest that babies born at 25–28 weeks' gestation, who breathe after birth, can be treated with CPAP from birth with similar outcomes to those treated with mechanical ventilation.[11] While this remains an attractive proposal, there is still a debate over the usefulness and safety of CPAP as a primary modality of treatment, as there were more babies with pneumothoraces in the CPAP group, and long-term results are not yet available. This approach of early CPAP treatment as an alternative to mechanical ventilation is conceptually different from use of CPAP after extubation, where it is helpful by reducing the need for re-intubation and resumption of invasive ventilation.[12] The relationship of CPAP and exogenous surfactant treatment also needs to be evaluated. It is plausible that the use of CPAP and the avoidance of intubation might diminish the effectiveness of surfactant in those infants who subsequently require it. There are other considerations, too. The work of breathing and caloric expenditure during CPAP might be higher than during a brief course of mechanical ventilation following surfactant administration. The long-term neurological outcomes for infants treated by primary CPAP as suggested by Wung *et al.* have never been reported. Data are also not available with respect to comparison of different devices, such as bubble CPAP, fluidic CPAP, short prongs, long prongs, and CPAP produced by high-flow nasal cannulas.

PERMISSIVE HYPERCAPNIA

The idea of permissive hypercapnia, allowing an elevated arterial carbon dioxide tension, was based on the retrospective observation of Kraybill *et al.*[13] in 1989. Infants with the highest levels of carbon dioxide had the lowest incidence of CLD.

The rationale for permissive hypercapnia as a protective lung strategy is that it may diminish volutrauma, reduce the duration of positive-pressure ventilation, decrease alveolar ventilation, lessen complications associated with hypocapnia (such as periventricular leukomalacia), and enhance oxygen unloading from haemoglobin at the tissue level.

There have been two prospective, controlled trials, both published in 1999.[14,15] Although there was a reduction in the duration of positive pressure ventilation, it failed to decrease in the incidence of CLD. Although this is another attractive hypothesis, further study is necessary. In addition, permissive hypercapnia is difficult to achieve with patient-triggered ventilation (PTV) when chemo-receptors are intact.

CONVENTIONAL VENTILATION

The initial experience with intermittent mandatory ventilation (IMV), not surprisingly, resulted in many infants with BPD. Patient–ventilator asynchrony was associated with several complications, including inefficient gas exchange, gas trapping and thoracic air leaks, and irregular cerebral blood flow velocity patterns.[16] Much effort has gone into enhancing the interaction between the ventilator and the baby by improving patient–ventilator synchrony during initiation of breathing through flow triggering, limiting inspiratory gas flow by volume-controlled (volume-targeted) ventilation, providing variable inspiratory flow to match patient demand, and enabling the baby to control inspiratory time by the use of flow cycling.

PATIENT-TRIGGERED VENTILATION

The advent of tiny transducers and sophisticated microprocessor-based ventilators introduced the era of PTV and the development of newer modes of ventilation, including synchronised intermittent mandatory ventilation (SIMV), assist/control

(A/C), pressure support ventilation (PSV) and even hybrid modes, such as volume assured pressure support.[17] It was hoped that, by establishing synchronous breathing between the baby and the ventilator, many of these complications could be eliminated and the incidence of CLD could be reduced. PTV takes advantage of a signal derived from the patient, which represents spontaneous respiratory effort and allows synchronisation of the mechanical to the spontaneous breath. A breath may also be terminated by taking advantage of the decelerating inspiratory airway flow signal. Establishing synchronous breathing might result in lower pressures, augment weaning by making pressure the primary weaning variable, and significantly reduce gas trapping and air leaks. In addition, the recent availability of PSV enables variable levels of synchronised support of spontaneous breathing during mechanical ventilation.

Unfortunately, clinical trials of PTV have thus far been disappointing. Most of the trials have been underpowered to measure the impact on CLD, although short-term benefits, such as fewer air leaks and reduced ventilator days, have been demonstrated.[18] The concept of PTV makes good physiological sense, but additional investigation is warranted.

VOLUME-TARGETED VENTILATION

Volume-targeted ventilation, in which the clinician selects a volume of gas to be delivered to the patient and the ventilator pressure is varied to deliver this volume, has received recent attention. Theoretically, this modality should result in a more consistent delivery of tidal volume because, regardless of the patient's lung compliance, volume delivery will be controlled, or limited, reducing volutrauma. A meta-analysis of randomised controlled trials showed potential advantages of volume-controlled ventilation in terms of reducing the duration of assisted ventilation and complications.[19] In addition, a recently published randomised clinical trial also demonstrated a significant reduction in time for weaning and duration of ventilation in infants weighing 600–1000 g treated with volume-controlled ventilation. The smaller infants enrolled in this trial also had a significant reduction in CLD compared to those managed with pressure-limited ventilation.[20] The concept of targeting tidal volume is gaining support within the neonatal community and further studies are in progress.

PROPORTIONAL ASSIST VENTILATION

Another novel idea is proportional assist ventilation, a form of ventilation based on the individual pulmonary mechanics and the resistive and elastic loading and unloading of respiratory musculature to servo-regulate the ventilator (adaptive ventilation). In 2001, Schulze and colleagues[21] reported a small clinical trial showing lower mean and peak transpulmonary pressures compared to those generated by conventional ventilation. This may help ameliorate barotrauma, and further study seems worthwhile.

HIGH-FREQUENCY VENTILATION

High-frequency ventilation (HFV) emerged in the 1980s as an alternative method to provide non-tidal ventilation. Two forms of HFV have been in clinical use – high-frequency jet ventilation (HFJV), and high-frequency oscillatory ventilation (HFOV). The basic concept of all HFV is the use of tiny gas volumes, less than the anatomical dead-space, moved in and out of the lung at very rapid rates. Ventilation can be accomplished at lower pressures, as minute ventilation becomes a function of the square of tidal volume. HFOV differs from HFJV in that it also creates active exhalation, where gas is actively withdrawn from the lung during expiration. Usual frequencies used during HFJV range from 150–660 breaths per minute, whereas those used during HFOV (with its even smaller tidal volumes) range from 480–900 breaths per minute.

HFJV is used in tandem with a conventional mechanical ventilator, which also provides PEEP and can be used to deliver sigh breaths to help recruit lung volume and avoid atelectasis. It has been used primarily as a rescue therapy and for management of pulmonary interstitial emphysema and other thoracic air leaks. One study, conducted by Keszler et al.[22] in 1997, demonstrated a reduction in the incidence of CLD and a lower need for home oxygen therapy when HFJV was used as a primary strategy.

HFOV has a wider evidence base, although the results are no more compelling that this form of treatment can reduce CLD. The trial of Gerstmann et al.[23] showed better survival without an increase in CLD for babies treated with HFOV compared to conventional IMV. Two German studies failed to show a reduction in CLD. Rettwitz-Volk et al.[24] found no differences in any of the pulmonary outcome parameters, and Thome et al.[25] found a shorter time to extubation but no differences in the incidence of intraventricular haemorrhage, CLD, or death. The study of Moriette et al.[26] demonstrated a reduced surfactant requirement but no decrease in CLD. Two trials published in 2002 had conflicting results. The study of Courtney et al.[27] showed a modest decrease in CLD in babies weighing 601–1200 g, but the control arm of the trial used SIMV rather than A/C. The UKOS trial of Johnson et al.[28] found no change in the incidence of CLD in babies of 23–28 weeks' gestation when HFOV was compared to IMV. Although different strategies were utilised in these two trials, which might account for the discrepant conclusions, HFOV cannot be recommended as a primary strategy for RDS based on the evidence to date.[29]

CONTINUOUS MONITORING TECHNIQUES

During the era of mechanical ventilation, monitoring of the ventilated infant has been altered dramatically. Intermittent blood gas sampling and once or twice daily radiographs have given way to continuous and mostly non-invasive monitoring techniques to assess oxygenation, ventilation, and pulmonary mechanics (as well as cardiac function) on a breath-to-breath (and beat-to-beat) basis. Real-time graphic monitoring of pulmonary mechanics and waveforms allows recognition of events such as hyperinflation (Fig. 3) and gas trapping (Fig. 4) before they become clinically apparent. Monitoring has been demonstrated to be a useful adjunct in the weaning of infants from mechanical ventilation. Although there is no true evidence-base as yet, these devices and techniques can be used to optimise strategies for the individual patient, such as determining the best level of PEEP, adjusting how the gas flow is delivered (rise time), and assessing patient–ventilator synchrony.[30]

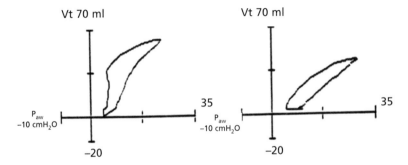

Fig. 3 Pressure–volume loops. Left: the loop demonstrates hyperinflation, with an upper inflection point on the inspiratory limb. Right: the loop has been normalised by reducing the peak inspiratory pressure (with permission from *Archives of Diseases in Childhood*).

Use of the newer modalities of ventilation, such as SIMV with PSV, mandates an understanding of real-time pulmonary graphics. However, this monitoring also enhances the ability of the clinician to choose ventilator settings which produce the best results in the individual patient.

OPTIMISING MECHANICAL VENTILATION IN THE PRETERM INFANT

Choosing the proper strategy based upon the basic principles of mechanical ventilation should optimise pulmonary gas exchange and begin to reduce lung injury. Reduction of the 'mechanical' components of VILI – barotrauma, volutrauma, atelectotrauma, and rheotrauma – can be achieved by ventilating the lung near functional residual capacity. This occurs at the mid-point of the inflationary limb of the pressure–volume loop (Fig. 5), where compliance is maximum, and the theoretical zones of lung injury can be averted. The use of higher pressures leads to both baro- and volutrauma, with increased FRC, decreased compliance, and lung overexpansion. The use of pressures below the 'safe zone' may result in atelectotrauma, with decreased FRC, lower compliance, and alveolar collapse.

Careful attention must be paid to airway and circuit flow. Flow is defined as the time rate of volume delivery. Excessive flow in the ventilator circuit can cause a greater delivery of gas volume over the same inspiratory time,

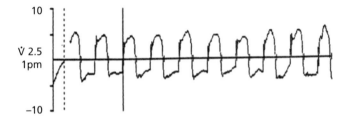

Fig. 4 Flow waveform indicative of gas trapping. On each waveform the decelerating expiratory flow never returns to baseline (zero flow state) before initiation of the next breath. Thus, more gas is entering the lung than exiting (with permission from *Archives of Diseases in Childhood*).

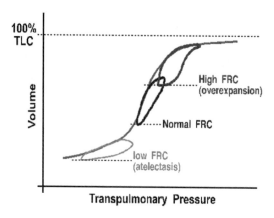

Fig. 5 Pressure–volume relationship. The best compliance is seen at the steepest slope of the curve, where ventilation occurs at normal functional residual capacity (with permission from *Archives of Diseases in Childhood*).

contributing to overdistension and an increased elastic load. Gas trapping and inadvertent PEEP may result if flow is too high or if there is inadequate expiratory time for the lung to empty completely. Conversely, if flow is set too low, gas volumes may be too small and air hunger may arise, leading to tachypnoea and, subsequently, an increased work of breathing.

Monitoring of tidal volume delivery, irrespective of whether the target variable is volume or pressure, has become much more important in recent years now that we have the ability to measure, finally, volumes at the proximal airway. Delivering a physiological tidal volume during conventional ventilation seems prudent.

CONCLUSIONS

Clinical investigation has not yet demonstrated how to avoid lung injury completely in preterm infants requiring mechanical ventilation. The reality is that CLD may be inevitable in infants delivered at a time when the lung is still in the saccular or canalicular phase of development. Nevertheless, clinicians must try to avoid contributing further damage during this time.

The ideal mode or modality of ventilation should provide and maintain adequate and consistent tidal volume delivery and minute ventilation at low airway pressures. It must be able to respond quickly to rapid or unpredictable changes in patient demand or pulmonary mechanics. It should provide the lowest possible work of breathing for the baby.

The ideal ventilator is one which satisfactorily achieves the goals of mechanical ventilation. It should provide a variety of modes and modalities that can effectively ventilate even the most challenging pulmonary diseases. It must have monitoring capabilities to assess, adequately, patient and ventilator interaction and performance. It must also have alarm safety-features and alarms that enable use of lung protective strategies. Finally, it should be managed by an experienced clinician who continues to ask the right questions and seek the right answers.

Key points for clinical practice

- Although mechanical ventilation saves lives of very preterm babies, it also causes complications such as ventilator-induced lung injury and chronic lung disease.

- Chronic lung disease is multifactorial and is cascaded through a number of factors such as immaturity of lung development itself, which in turn makes these immature lungs more susceptible to damage by ventilation, oxygen and other noxious agents such as inflammation and infection.

- Ventilator-induced lung injury is also multifactorial. Understanding of these pathophysiological processes has led to the introduction of a number of newer techniques of mechanical ventilation in newborns. These are based on a good physiological rationale but, being new, require further scientific evidence.

- There is growing interest in application of non-invasive forms of artificial respiratory support such as continuous positive airway pressure, but caution is required, especially in its use in very preterm babies as a substitute for mechanical ventilation during the early stages of respiratory distress syndrome. There is still no convincing evidence of its efficacy and safety in this population.

- On the other hand, judicious use of non-invasive respiratory support after extubation prevents re-intubation and reduces pulmonary morbidity in many patients.

- Strategic ventilation aimed to counterbalance the underlying pathophysiology is likely to reduce chronic lung disease but unlikely to eliminate it completely, as factors other than ventilator-induced lung injury are also involved and they require individual attention.

References

1. Northway WH, Rosan RC, Porter DY: Pulmonary disease following respirator therapy of hyaline membrane disease. Bronchopulmonary dysplasia. *N Engl J Med* 1967; **276**: 357–368.
2. Philip AGS. Oxygen plus pressure plus time: the etiology of bronchopulmonary dysplasia. *Pediatrics* 1975; **55**: 44–50.
3. Jobe AH. The new BPD: an arrest of lung development. *Pediatr Res* 1999; **46**: 641–643.
4. Walsh MC, Yao O, Gettner P *et al*. Impact of a physiologic definition on bronchopulmonary dysplasia rates. *Pediatrics* 2004; **114**: 3505–3511
5. Attar MA, Donn SM. Mechanism of ventilator-induced lung injury in premature infants. *Semin Neonatol* 2002; **7**: 353–360.
6. Dreyfuss D, Saumon G. Ventilator-induced lung injury: lessons from experimental studies. *Am J Respir Crit Care Med* 1998; **157**: 294–323.
7. Crowley P. Antenatal corticosteroid therapy: a meta analysis of the randomized trials 1972–1994. *Am J Obstet Gynecol* 1995; **173**: 322–325.
8. Soll RF, Morley CJ. Prophylactic versus selective use of surfactant in preventing morbidity and mortality in preterm infants. Cochrane Database System Rev 2001, Issue 2. CD000510.

9. Donn SM, Sinha SK. Invasive and non invasive neonatal mechanical ventilation. *Respir Care* 2003; **48**: 426–441.
10. Wung JT, Koons AH, Driscoll Jr JM, James LS. Changing incidence of bronchopulmonary dysplasia. *J Pediatr* 1979; **95**: 845–847.
11. Morley CJ, Davis PG, Doyle LW, Brion L, Hascoet JM, Carlin J, for the trial collaborators. A randomized controlled trial of nasal CPAP or intubation and ventilation for very preterm infants at birth: The COIN trial. *J Paediatr Child Health* 2007; **43**: A64.
12. Davis PG, Henderson-Smart DJ. Nasal continuous positive airway pressure immediately after extubation for preventing morbidity in preterm infants. Cochrane Library. Issue 1. Oxford: Update Software, 1999.
13. Kraybill EN, Runyun DK, Bose CL, Khan JH. Risk factors for chronic lung disease in infants with birth weights of 751 to 1000 grams. *J Pediatr* 1989; **115**: 115–120.
14. Mariani G, Cifuentes J, Carlo WA. Randomized trial of permissive hypercapnia in preterm infants. *Pediatrics* 1999; **104**: 1082–1088.
15. Carlo WA, Stark AR, Bauer C *et al*. Effects of minimal ventilation in a multicenter randomized controlled trial of ventilator support and early corticosteroid therapy in extremely low birthweight infants. *Pediatrics* 1999; **104**: 738–739.
16. Greenough A. Update on patient-triggered ventilation. *Clin Perinatol* 2001; **28**: 533–546.
17. Donn SM, Sinha SK. Newer modes of mechanical ventilation for the neonate. *Curr Opin Pediatr* 2001; **13**: 99–103.
18. Greenough A, Milner AD, Dimitriou G. Synchronized mechanical ventilation for respiratory support in newborn infants. Cochrane Database System Rev 2004, Issue 3. Art. No.: CD000456.
19. McCallion N, Davis PG, Morley CJ. Volume-targeted versus pressure-limited ventilation in the neonate. Cochrane Database System Rev 2005, Issue 3. Art. No.: CD003666.
20. Singh J, Sinha SK, Donn SM *et al*. A randomized controlled trial of volume control ventilation. *Pediatr Res* 2005; **57**: 1546A.
21. Schulze A, Gerhardt T, Musante G *et al*. Proportional assist ventilation in low birth weight infants with acute respiratory disease: a comparison to assist/control and conventional mechanical ventilation. *J Pediatr* 1999; **135**: 339–344.
22. Keszler M, Modanlou HD, Brudno DS *et al*. Multi-center controlled clinical trial of high-frequency jet ventilation in preterm infants with uncomplicated respiratory distress syndrome. *Pediatrics* 1997; **100**: 593–599.
23. Gerstman DR, Minton SD, Stodard RA *et al*. The Provo multicenter early high frequency oscillatory high frequency trial: Improved pulmonary and clinical outcome in respiratory distress syndrome. *Pediatrics* 1996; **98**: 1044–1057.
24. Rettwitz-Volk W, Veldman A, Roth B *et al*. A prospective, randomized, multicenter trial of high-frequency oscillatory ventilation compared with conventional ventilation in preterm infants with respiratory distress syndrome receiving surfactant. *J Pediatr* 1998; **132**: 249–254.
25. Thome U, Kossel H, Lipowsky G *et al*. Randomized comparison of high-frequency ventilation with high-rate intermittent positive pressure ventilation in preterm infants with respiratory failure. *J Pediatr* 1999; **135**: 39–46.
26. Moriette G, Paris-Llado J, Walti H *et al*. Prospective randomized multicenter comparison of high-frequency oscillatory ventilation and conventional ventilation in preterm infants with respiratory distress syndrome. *Pediatrics* 2001; **107**: 363–372.
27. Courtney SE, Durand DJ, Asselin JM *et al*. High-frequency oscillatory ventilation versus conventional mechanical ventilation for very-low-birth-weight infants. *N Engl J Med* 2002; **347**: 643–652.
28. Johnson AH, Peacock JL, Greenough A *et al*. High-frequency oscillatory ventilation for the prevention of chronic lung disease of prematurity. *N Engl J Med* 2002; **347**: 633–642.
29. Stark AR. High-frequency oscillatory ventilation to prevent bronchopulmonary dysplasia – are we there yet? *N Engl J Med* 2002; **347**: 682–684.
30. Bhutani VK. Clinical applications of pulmonary function and graphics. *Semin Neonatol* 2002; **7**: 391–399.

Kevin E. Brown

14

Parvovirus B19 infection in the fetus and child

Human parvovirus B19 (B19V) was first identified in 1975 (in a sample coded B19, hence the name), in a serum sample giving anomalous reactions in a newly developed assay for hepatitis B.[1] The virus had a small (~22 nm) non-enveloped virion, and antibody could be detected in a large number of adults indicating that infection was common in humans. It is now known that B19V is the aetiological agent of erythema infectiosum (fifth disease) and transient aplastic crisis, and a major cause of hydrops fetalis. Currently, there is no licensed vaccine to prevent B19V, but a recombinant vaccine is in development.

VIRAL CLASSIFICATION AND BIOLOGY

Members of the virus family *Parvoviridae*, are small (20–25 nm) non-enveloped viruses, with icosahedral structures, and a linear single-stranded DNA genome of about 5000 nucleotides.[2] The viruses encode no polymerase and, therefore, are dependent on either rapidly dividing host cells or helper viruses for viral replication. Members of the family infect a wide variety of animals, birds and insects, and at least four different types of parvovirus infect humans – adeno-associated viruses (AAVs), parvovirus B19 (B19V), the recently described Parv4/5 virus, and human bocavirus. To date, only B19V has definitively been shown to be a human pathogen.

B19V is classified as a member of the Erythrovirus genus, a group of mammalian viruses that are highly erythrotropic, with efficient viral replication occurring mainly in red-cell precursors. The B19V genome encodes one non-structural protein which is required for viral replication and mediates cytotoxicity, and two capsid proteins, VP1 and VP2, formed by alternative splicing. The major capsid protein VP2 makes up 95% of the viral capsid and

Kevin E. Brown MD MRCP FRCPath
Consultant Medical Virologist, Immunisation and Diagnosis, Virus Reference Department, Centre for Infections, Health Protection Agency, 61 Colindale Avenue, London NW9 5EQ, UK
E-mail: kevin.brown@hpa.org.uk

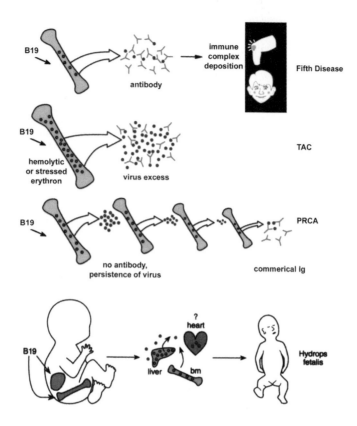

Fig. 1 Pathogenesis of B19V infection. Modified from Figure 76-7 in *Clinical Hematology*[39] © 2006 US Government

will self-assemble to form virus-like particles *in vitro*. The VP1 protein contains an additional 227 amino acids at the amino terminal of VP2; this VP1-unique sequence encodes a phospholipase motif, and is the major target for neutralising antibodies. Based on viral sequence, B19V can be divided into three distinct genotypes (genotypes 1–3), but only a single B19V antigenic type has been described. Genotypes 2 and 3 are relatively infrequently detected in Europe and the US, although genotype 3 does appear to be more common in west Africa. Animals cannot be infected with B19V, but a primate erythrovirus, simian parvovirus, has been discovered and infection with simian parvovirus mimics B19 infection in humans, including the development of hydrops in the infected fetus.

PATHOPHYSIOLOGY

The erythroid specificity of B19V tropism is, in part, due to the tissue distribution of the major receptor for parvovirus B19, the blood group P antigen.[3] Rare individuals without the blood group P antigen (blood group p phenotype) are naturally resistant to B19V infection.[4] P antigen, also known as globoside, is found in the erythrocyte precursors in the bone marrow, and in a variety of other cells and tissues including mature and immature

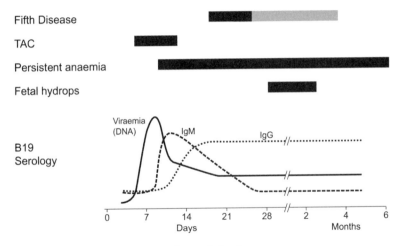

Fig. 2 Schematic of the time course of B19V infection.

megakaryocytes, endothelial cells, placental tissues, fetal myocardium and fetal liver. In addition, some of the clinical consequences of parvovirus infection, including the rash and arthropathy of fifth disease, are immune-mediated (Fig. 1).

Following respiratory acquisition, the virus targets bone marrow and induces a lytic infection of red-cell precursors. Infection of the erythroid progenitors results in high-titre viraemia, with $> 10^{12}$ virus particles/ml (or 10^{12} IU/ml B19V DNA) detectable in the blood at the height of viraemia (Fig. 2), and the virus-induced cytotoxicity results in an arrest of red-cell production and the appearance in the bone marrow of giant pronormoblasts, large cells (25–32 μm in diameter), with cytoplasmic vacuolisation, immature chromatin and large eosinophilic nuclear inclusion bodies (Fig. 3B).[40]

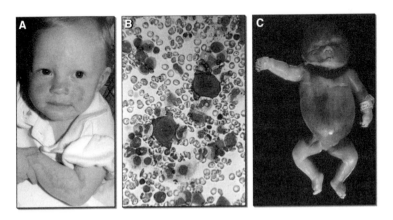

Fig. 3 Clinical manifestations of parvovirus B19 infection. (A) Typical rash of fifth disease. (B) Giant pronormoblasts seen in the bone marrow and peripheral blood of patients with transient aplastic crisis or B19V-induced chronic anaemia. (C) Hydrops fetalis following maternal B19 infection. First published: Young NS, Brown KE. Parvovirus B19. *N Engl J Med* 2004; **350**: 586–597. Copyright © 2004 Massachusetts Medical Society. All rights reserved.

In immunocompetent individuals, this viraemia and interruption of erythropoiesis is transient and resolves as the immunoglobulin (Ig) M and IgG antibody response is mounted (Fig. 2). In individuals with normal red-cell turnover, this results in only a minimal reduction in haemoglobin levels; however, in individuals with increased erythropoiesis, and especially in patients with sickle cell disease or haemolytic anaemias, the abrupt cessation of red cell production can induce a transient aplastic crisis and severe anaemia. In individuals who cannot mount an effective immune response, including the fetus following infection in pregnancy, the absence of neutralising antibody response results in a continuation of the erythroid progenitor infection, red-cell production is compromised and patients develop pure red-cell aplasia or chronic anaemia. Infection can be abrogated by administration of neutralising antibody in the form of intravenous immunoglobulin treatment. In fetal infection, the severe anaemia is confounded with infection of the fetal cardiomyocytes, leading to myocarditis and cardiac failure.

The second, or immune-mediated, phase of illness begins as the antibody response develops. Typical manifestations of this phase of the illness are the rash of fifth disease, arthralgia, and arthritis. Symptoms usually resolve in 1–2 weeks, although joint symptoms may persist for several months. In immunocompetent hosts, there is usually no clinical evidence of residual infection, although B19 DNA can be detected by polymerase chain reaction (PCR) in blood and tissues for months to years after acute infection.

IgM antibody may be detected in serum samples for 2–3 months after infection (Fig. 2), and is used as a marker of recent infection. In contrast, B19-specific IgG persists for life. In immunocompetent individuals, the early antibody response is to the major capsid protein VP2; as the immune response matures, reactivity to the minor capsid protein, VP1, dominates. Sera from patients with chronic B19 infection typically contain antibody to VP2 but not to VP1.[5]

Although the importance of the humoral arm of the immune response is shown by recovery from infection with the appearance of circulating, specific anti-virus antibody and treatment of persistent infection in immunodeficient patients with intravenous immunoglobulin, the role of the cellular immune response in containing B19V infection is less clear. CD4 and in particular CD8 responses to B19 proteins and peptides can be demonstrated,[6] and the persistent CD8 response may be crucial in controlling the low levels of B19 DNA that can be detected in tissues following acute infection.

EPIDEMIOLOGY

B19V exclusively infects humans. Infection is endemic in virtually all parts of the world with, in temperate countries at least, most infections occurring in the spring/early summer, with mini-epidemics at regular intervals several years apart. Transmission is predominantly via the respiratory route, probably by droplet spread, and is highest at the time of viraemia before the onset of rash or arthralgia.

B19 infection is a common illness of childhood; by the age of 15 years, approximately 60% of children have detectable IgG,[7] rising to > 75% of those aged 45 years or more. In pregnant women there is an estimated annual seroconversion rate of ~1%. Infections within homes and schools are common.

Secondary infection rates approach 50% in household contacts,[8] but are lower for adults in schools or other institutions.

Due to the high levels of B19V viraemia that can occur prior to symptomatic infection, detection of B19V is common in blood and blood-products. Thus, transmission can occur as a result of transfusion, most commonly of pooled components[9] especially factor VIII and IX concentrate. B19V is resistant to solvent or detergent inactivation and relatively resistant to heat treatment. To reduce the risk of transmission, plasma pools are currently screened by quantitative DNA assays and high-titre pools discarded.

CLINICAL MANIFESTATIONS IN CHILDREN

Disease manifestations of infection with B19V vary widely with the immunological and haematological status of the host (Table 1), although most infection is asymptomatic and goes unrecognised. In normal, immunocompetent children, B19V infection commonly presents as erythema infectiosum (also known as fifth disease), which can be associated with a transient polyarthropathy. In children with underlying haemolytic disorders, B19V is the primary cause of transient aplastic crisis; in immunocompromised children, persistent B19 viraemia manifests as pure red-cell aplasia and chronic anaemia.

ERYTHEMA INFECTIOSUM

Most people with B19-specific antibody have no recollection of any specific symptoms, but erythema infectiosum is the major manifestation of B19

Table 1 Presentations of B19V infection

Frequency of association	Disease	Comments
Common	Erythema infectiosum (fifth disease)	Healthy children
	Polyarthropathy syndrome	Healthy adults (especially women)
	Transient aplastic crisis	Patients with increased erythropoiesis
	Persistent anaemia/pure red-cell aplasia	Immunodeficient/ immunocompetent patients
	Hydrops fetalis/fetal death	
Unusual/ possible association	Myocarditis	
	Hepatitis	
	Neurological disease	Meningitis/encephalitis/ neuropathy
	Papular-purpuric glove and sock syndrome	
	Vasculitis	
	Arthritides	Juvenile rheumatoid arthritis, juvenile idiopathic arthritis
	Haematological disease	Thrombocytopenia, neutropenia, haemophagocytic syndrome
	Glomerulonephritis	

infection. Erythema infectiosum was well characterised clinically even before the discovery of B19V, and was probably first described by Robert Willan in 1799.[10] The disease was rediscovered in Germany when, in 1899, Sticker gave it the name erythema infectiosum. Six years later, Cheinisse classified it as the 'fifth rash disease' of the six classical exanthema of childhood.

Clinical symptoms begin with a non-specific prodromal illness, which often goes unrecognised; there may be symptoms of fever, coryza, headache, and mild gastrointestinal distress, including nausea and diarrhoea. Then, 2–5 days later, the classic slapped cheek rash appears, a fiery red eruption on the cheek accompanied by relative circumoral pallor (Fig. 3A). There may be a second stage rash within a few days, an erythematous maculopapular exanthemum on the trunk and limbs; as this eruption fades, it produces a typical lacy appearance. There is great variation in the dermatological symptoms. The classic slapped cheek is much commoner in children than adults. The second stage eruption may vary from a very faint, barely perceptible, erythema to a florid exanthema, and the rash may be transient or recurrent for weeks. Pruritus, especially on the soles of the feet, can be the dominant symptom. The rash is particularly difficult to see on a dark skin, and fifth disease may go unrecognised in these patients.

Although the characteristic rash of papular-purpuric glove and sock syndrome has been associated with B19V infection in adults, the syndrome is unusual in children, and the juvenile variant is less often associated with B19V infection.[11]

TRANSIENT ARTHROPATHY/ARTHRITIS

Although in children B19V infection is usually mild, of short duration, and of limited consequence, occasionally, but more commonly in adults, there may be an associated transient arthropathy. In adults, the arthralgia is usually symmetrical, with mainly the small joints of hands and feet involved; it generally lasts for 1–3 weeks, although may persist or recur for months. In the absence of a history of rash, the symptoms may be mistaken for acute rheumatoid arthritis, especially as B19V infection can be associated with transient rheumatoid factor and other auto-antibody production.[12] Fewer studies have been performed on arthralgia in children but, in one study of children presenting with arthropathy, > 20% had evidence of recent B19V infection (B19 IgM detected).[13] Those with detectable B19 IgM were more likely to develop chronic arthritis and to be diagnosed as having juvenile rheumatoid arthritis. Other studies have shown similar increases in B19V seropositivity (IgM and/or IgG) suggesting that B19V infection may be a trigger for the development of juvenile rheumatoid arthritis and/or juvenile idiopathic arthritis.

TRANSIENT APLASTIC CRISIS

Transient aplastic crisis, the abrupt cessation of erythropoiesis characterised by reticulocytopenia, absent erythroid precursors in the bone marrow and precipitous worsening of anaemia, was first used to describe the abrupt onset of severe anaemia with absent reticulocytes in patients with hereditary spherocytosis, and was the first clinical illness associated with B19V infection.[14] In contrast to haemolytic crises, transient aplastic crisis occurs as a single episode in the patient's life.

Although originally identified in patients with sickle cell disease, transient aplastic crisis due to B19V has now been described in a wide range of patients with underlying haemolytic disorders, including hereditary spherocytosis, thalassaemia, red-cell enzymopathies such as pyruvate kinase deficiency and autoimmune haemolytic anaemias.[15] Transient aplastic crisis can also occur under conditions of erythroid 'stress', such as haemorrhage, iron-deficiency anaemia and following kidney or bone marrow transplantation. Rarely, acute anaemia has been described in the haematologically normal person.

Patients present with symptoms typical of sudden anaemia, including lethargy, poor concentration, dyspnoea and even confusion due to the resultant hypoxia. Although the infection is ultimately self-limiting, congestive heart failure and severe bone marrow necrosis may develop and the illness can be fatal. Aplastic crisis can be the first presentation of an underlying haemolytic disease, especially in children.

Community-acquired transient aplastic crisis is almost always due to B19V[16] and, in patients with haemolytic disease, B19V infection should be the presumptive diagnosis in children over that age of 2 years with sudden onset of anaemia with reticulocytopenia. In contrast to patients with fifth disease, transient aplastic crisis patients are often viraemic at the time of presentation with concentrations of virus as high as 10^{14} genome copies/ml, and the diagnosis is readily made by detection of B19V DNA in the serum. Bone marrow appearance shows a reduction or absence of erythroid precursors, and the presence of giant pronormoblasts (Fig. 3B). As the immune response develops, B19V DNA levels fall in serum, and B19-specific IgM becomes detectable. In immunocompetent individuals, immunity is life-long following B19V infection.

Transient erythroblastopenia of childhood, the temporary failure of red-cell production in haematologically normal children, does not appear to be associated with B19V infection,[17] although a viral infection has been implicated in its aetiology. Transient erythroblastopenia of childhood generally occurs in children less than 2 years old, in contrast to B19V infection which generally affects older children. Sporadic cases of transient erythroblastopenia of childhood with thrombocytopenia have been described with evidence of recent B19V infection, whereas 'classical' transient erythroblastopenia of childhood is associated with normal or high platelet counts and/or neutropenia.

Thrombocytopenia and neutropenia

Transient aplastic crisis and B19V infection in haematologically normal patients are often associated with changes in other blood lineages, varying degrees of neutropenia and thrombocytopenia. Some cases of idiopathic thrombocytopenia purpura and Henoch-Schoenlein purpura have been reported to follow B19V infection. Transient pancytopenia after parvovirus infection is rare.

CHRONIC ANAEMIA

Persistent B19V infection resulting in pure red-cell aplasia has been reported in a wide variety of immunosuppressed patients, ranging from patients with congenital immunodeficiency, acquired immunodeficiency (AIDS), lympho-proliferative disorders and transplant patients.[18] The stereotypical presentation is with persistent anaemia rather than immune-mediated symptoms of rash or arthropathy. Patients have absent or low levels of B19V-specific antibody and persistent or recurrent B19V viraemia as detected by high-titre B19V DNA in the serum. Generally, only erythropoiesis is affected; rarely, other haematological lineages are also involved, although B19V does not cause aplastic anaemia. As in transient aplastic crisis, bone marrow examination generally reveals a reduction of erythroid precursors and the presence of scattered giant pronormoblasts. Temporary cessation of maintenance chemotherapy may lead to resolution of the anaemia.[19] Alternatively, or if this not practical, administration of immunoglobulin can be beneficial[20] and may allow temporary, or even complete, resolution of infection.

Haemophagocytosis

Virus-associated haemophagocytic syndrome is characterised by histiocytic hyperplasia, marked haemophagocytosis and cytopenia, in association with a systemic viral illness. B19V infection has been detected in cases of haemophagocytosis syndrome in both children and adults.[21] The majority of patients were previously healthy, but four patients were immunosuppressed. Further studies are required to determine if parvovirus B19V is a major cause of virus-associated haemophagocytic syndrome as well as the rate of virus-associated haemophagocytic syndrome in otherwise uncomplicated parvovirus B19V infection.

UNUSUAL PRESENTATIONS

A large number of symptoms and disease have been associated with B19V infection (Table 1). However, many of these presentations are based on case reports or the identification of B19V DNA in tissues by PCR. Increasing evidence indicates that B19V DNA can persist in tissues for years following acute infection,[22] and the interpretation of detecting low levels of B19V DNA by PCR should be treated with caution.

Neurological symptoms

A number of case reports have associated fifth disease infection with neurological symptoms including meningitis encephalitis,[23–27] with detection of B19V DNA in cerebrospinal fluid. In all these cases, there have been no long-term neurological sequelae.

Other neurological symptoms that have been related to B19V infection include brachial plexus and peripheral neuropathy. In one study, 50% of patients with classical fifth disease (confirmed serologically) experienced neurological symptoms (tingling and numbness in the fingers or toes).[28] In most of these patients, neurological examination was normal apart from decreased sensation to light touch; one patient developed more significant disease with progressive weakness of one arm. The mechanism for the neurological symptoms is unknown, but the earlier appearance of the rash suggests that the neuropathy may be immune-mediated.

Myocarditis and hepatitis

The role of B19V infection in myocarditis and cardiomyopathy is controversial. Myocarditis associated with acute B19V infection has been reported; although it is clearly unusual, the incidence is not known. In the fetus, there is good evidence for cardiac involvement in the pathogenesis of hydrops fetalis. More recently, several investigators have reported the detection of B19V DNA in cardiac tissue of patients with myocarditis and dilated myocardiopathy and suggested a more general aetiological role for B19V. However, the significance of these low levels of B19V DNA, especially in the absence of detectable viral proteins or replicating DNA, is unclear.

Similar concerns have been raised for the role of B19V in hepatic disease. Transient elevation of transaminases in B19V infection is common, but the development of frank hepatitis is unusual. The detection of B19V DNA in liver tissue is not unusual.

B19V INFECTION AND THE FETUS

HYDROPS FETALIS AND FETAL DEATH

The link between the development of B19V infection in pregnancy was first identified in 1984;[29] since then, there have been a large number of case reports of miscarriage or hydrops fetalis (Fig. 3C) secondary to maternal B19V infection during pregnancy. The clinical features have been similar: in cases where pathological studies were undertaken, the fetuses showed evidence of ascites, cardiomegaly and pericardial effusions. In the liver there were signs of a leukoerythroblastic reaction with large pale cells with eosinophilic inclusion bodies and peripheral condensation or margination of the nuclear chromatin. Human parvovirus B19 infection was confirmed by detection of B19V DNA, proteins or virions (by electron microscopy) in fetal tissues.

An adverse fetal outcome is not typical following maternal B19V infection, and the timing of maternal infection is also crucial, with the greatest risk to the fetus following infection during weeks 11–20.[30] Transplacental transmission of B19V infection has been estimated at about 33%, and discordant infection in twin pregnancies has been recorded. Transplacental transmission can occur even in the absence of maternal symptoms and there may be significant delay between maternal infection and development of hydrops, with intervals in the range 2–17 weeks. In a prospective British study of over 400 women with serologically confirmed B19V during pregnancy, the excess rate of fetal loss was confined to the first 20 weeks of pregnancy and averaged only 9%, with a risk of hydrops fetalis of 2.9% following maternal infection between weeks 9–20.[31] No abnormalities were found at birth in the surviving infants, even when there was evidence of intra-uterine infection by the presence of B19 IgM in the umbilical cord blood. Similar results were obtained in a study of over 1000 women in Germany, with serologically confirmed B19V infection.[32] In the UK group, there were no long-term sequelae of B19V infection in the 129 children followed for over 7 years, although three children were reported to have developmental delay. A similar observation of developmental delay was seen in a Dutch study of the outcome of intra-uterine blood transfusion for treatment of B19V-induced hydrops.[33]

B19V probably causes 10–15% of all cases of non-immune hydrops. Non-immune hydrops fetalis is rare (1 in 3000 births); in approximately 50% of cases, the aetiology is unknown.[34] In a study of 55 cases of non-immune hydrops, the majority were due to cardiovascular or chromosomal abnormalities, but B19V infection was diagnosed in 14% of the cases.[35]

CONGENITAL INFECTION

No systematic studies have shown evidence for congenital abnormalities following B19V infection, although there are a few case reports of congenital malformation associated with B19V infection, including ocular abnormalities, structural abnormalities, and fetal liver calcifications. Although normally there are no long-term haematological sequelae from intra-uterine B19V infection, rare infants born with chronic anaemia following a history of maternal B19V exposure and intra-uterine hydrops have been described. Similarly, B19V DNA has been detected in some cases of Diamond-Blackfan anaemia,[36] and the role of *in utero* B19V infection inducing constitutional bone marrow failure such as Diamond-Blackfan anaemia is still under investigation.

DIAGNOSIS

Diagnosis of rash, or infection in immunocompetent individuals, is generally based on detection of B19 IgM antibodies (Table 2). IgM can be detected at the time of rash in fifth disease and by the third day of transient aplastic crisis in patients with haematological disorders. IgM antibodies remain detectable for 2–3 months after infection, and then become negative, even in patients with persisting symptoms of arthralgia/arthritis. IgG antibodies are detectable by the seventh day of illness and remain detectable thereafter for life. Even in children, the seroprevalence of B19 IgG is so high that B19 IgG antibody detection is often not helpful for diagnosing acute infection.

Table 2 Diagnosis of B19V infection

Disease	IgM	IgG	PCR	Quantitative PCR
Fifth disease	Positive	Positive	Positive	Often > 10^4 genome equivalents/ml
Transient aplastic crisis			Positive	Often > 10^{12} genome equivalents/ml, but rapidly decreases
Persistent anaemia/ pure red-cell aplasia	Negative/ weak positive	Negative/ weak positive	Positive	Often > 10^{12} genome equivalents/ml, but should be > 10^6 in the absence of treatment
Hydrops fetalis (fetus)			Positive amniotic fluid/tissue/ blood	
Hydrops fetalis (mother)	Negative or positive	Positive	Not diagnostic	Not diagnostic

Even though the bone marrow in patients with transient aplastic crisis and chronic anaemia due to B19V infection has characteristic appearance, confirmation of the diagnosis by detection of B19V should be undertaken. The virus cannot be readily grown in tissue culture and detection of B19V DNA should be used for the diagnosis of chronic anaemia or early transient aplastic crisis. However, as B19V DNA can be detectable by PCR for many months and even years after infection even in healthy individuals, quantitative PCR should be used. In acute infection at the height of viraemia, $> 10^{12}$ B19V DNA genome equivalents/ml (or IU/ml) of serum can be detected, but titres fall rapidly within 2 days (Fig. 2). Patients with aplastic crisis or chronic anaemia due to B19V generally have $> 10^5$ B19V DNA genome equivalents/ml of serum. Response to treatment and relapse can be monitored by changes in the titre of B19V DNA, and rise and fall, respectively, of the reticulocyte count.

Although detection of B19V IgM can be used to confirm B19V infection in pregnancy, due to the time interval between maternal infection and fetal symptoms the B19 IgM assay may have reverted to negative at the time of investigation. In these cases, if the B19 IgG test indicates previous infection, the 'booking sample' can be investigated for evidence of earlier infection (B19 IgM) or for IgG seroconversion.[30] Even after confirmed B19V infection during pregnancy, fetal infection only occurs in about one-third of cases. However, once maternal infection has been confirmed, the pregnancy should be monitored for development of fetal anaemia and/or development of hydrops by ultrasound and measurement of middle cerebral artery peak systolic velocities. Confirmation of the diagnosis can be made by testing fetal blood and/or tissues for B19V DNA.

TREATMENT AND PREVENTION

TREATMENT

Treatment of B19V symptoms is dependent on the stage of the infection. No antiviral drugs are available for treatment of B19V infection, and treatment is either symptomatic or dependent on administration of antibody to block infection.

Erythema infectiosum and polyarthropathy syndrome
Treatment is symptomatic only and there is no evidence that administration of immunoglobulin is beneficial.

Transient aplastic crisis
Crises precipitated by parvovirus B19V infection often necessitate symptomatic treatment with blood transfusions. Patients with aplastic crisis are viraemic and should be considered infectious at the time of clinical presentation. The viraemia is transient and usually resolving at the time of diagnosis; immunoglobulin is usually of little benefit.

Pure red-cell aplasia/chronic anaemia
In patients on chemotherapy, temporary cessation of chemotherapy may result in an immune response to parvovirus B19V and resolution of infection. If

unsuccessful or not applicable, commercial immune globulin preparations (Gammagard, Sandoglobulin) from healthy blood donors can cure or ameliorate persistent B19V infection in immunosuppressed patients. Generally, the dose used is 400 mg/kg/day for 5–10 days. As for patients with transient aplastic crisis, individuals should be considered infectious. Patients should be monitored for response to treatment (drop in B19V DNA titre and increase in reticulocyte count), and may require more than one course of therapy.

Fetal hydrops

Although spontaneous resolution of fetal hydrops has been reported, there is a significantly greater chance of fetal survival following intra-uterine blood transfusion.[37] Depending how well the fetus tolerates the procedure, the transfusion may be given in one or two boluses, and the pregnancy should be followed by regular scans to ensure resolution of the hydrops.[30]

PREVENTION

Although, currently, no vaccine is approved for B19V, prospects for a vaccine are good. The presence of VP1 protein in the immunogen appears critical for the production of neutralising antibodies and recombinant capsids with supranormal VP1 content are even more efficient in inducing neutralising activity. A recombinant vaccine based on VP1-enhanced viral-like particles expressed in insect cells is under development and results of phase 1 trials were promising.[38]

Although phase 2 trials of one B19V vaccine preparation are planned, the targets for such a vaccine remain to be determined. Should only patients at high risk of severe or life-threatening disease, such as sickle cell patients, be protected? Or, in view of the wide variety of disease manifestations affecting all strata of the population, should a universal vaccine policy be pursued?

Key points for clinical practice

- B19V is a common infection in childhood and, by age 15 years, 60% of children have antibody to B19V.

- B19V infection causes a biphasic illness, and the symptomatic presentation of B19V infection is dependent of the host's immune and haematological status.

- Following acute infection, low-titre B19V DNA persists in tissues and serum for months or years with no known clinical significance. The detection of this low-level B19V DNA should not be used to diagnose B19V-associated disease.

- B19V is the cause of erythema infectiosum (fifth disease) in healthy children.

- Diagnosis of erythema infectiosum is by detection of B19 IgM.

Key points for clinical practice *(continued)*

- In children with haemolytic disease, or other causes of increased erythropoiesis, B19V infection causes transient aplastic crisis.

- Diagnosis of B19V-induced transient aplastic crisis is by detection of high-titre B19 DNA in serum.

- In immunosuppressed children, B19V infection can cause chronic anaemia or pure red cell aplasia.

- Diagnosis of chronic anaemia due to B19V infection is by detection of high-titre B19 DNA in serum or bone marrow. Patients can be treated with intravenous immunoglobulin.

- B19V infection before the 20th week of pregnancy is associated with fetal loss or hydrops fetalis.

- Fetal infection may respond to intra-uterine blood transfusion.

- A vaccine for B19V is in development.

References

1. Cossart YE, Field AM, Cant B, Widdows D. Parvovirus-like particles in human sera. *Lancet* 1975; **i**: 72–73.
2. Tattersall P, Bergoin M, Bloom ME *et al.* Parvoviridae. In: Fauquet CM, Mayo MA, Maniloff J, Desselberger U, Ball LA. (eds) *Virus Taxonomy: Classification and Nomenclature of Viruses: Eighth Report of the International Committee on Taxonomy of Viruses.* New York: Elsevier Academic Press, 2005; 353–369.
3. Brown KE, Anderson SM, Young NS. Erythrocyte P antigen: cellular receptor for B19 parvovirus. *Science* 1993; **262**: 114–117.
4. Brown KE, Hibbs JR, Gallinella G *et al.* Resistance to parvovirus B19 infection due to lack of virus receptor (erythrocyte P antigen). *N Engl J Med* 1994; **330**: 1192–1196.
5. Kurtzman GJ, Cohen BJ, Field AM, Oseas R, Blaese RM, Young NS. Immune response to B19 parvovirus and an antibody defect in persistent viral infection. *J Clin Invest* 1989; **84**: 1114–1123.
6. Norbeck O, Isa A, Pohlmann C *et al.* Sustained CD8+ T-cell responses induced after acute parvovirus B19 infection in humans. *J Virol* 2005; **79**: 12117–12121.
7. Vyse AJ, Andrews NJ, Hesketh LM, Pebody R. The burden of parvovirus B19 infection in women of childbearing age in England and Wales. *Epidemiol Infect* 2007; **e-pub**: 1–9.
8. Chorba T, Coccia P, Holman RC *et al.* The role of parvovirus B19 in aplastic crisis and erythema infectiosum (fifth disease). *J Infect Dis* 1986; **154**: 383–393.
9. Azzi A, Morfini M, Mannucci PM. The transfusion-associated transmission of parvovirus B19. *Transfus Med Rev* 1999; **13**: 194–204.
10. van Elsacker-Niele AM, Anderson MJ. First picture of erythema infectiosum? [Letter]. *Lancet* 1987; **i**: 229.
11. Hsieh MY, Huang PH. The juvenile variant of papular-purpuric gloves and socks syndrome and its association with viral infections. *Br J Dermatol* 2004; **151**: 201–206.
12. Luzzi GA, Kurtz JB, Chapel H. Human parvovirus arthropathy and rheumatoid factor [Letter]. *Lancet* 1985; **i**: 1218.
13. Oguz F, Akdeniz C, Unuvar E, Kucukbasmaci O, Sidal M. Parvovirus B19 in the acute arthropathies and juvenile rheumatoid arthritis. *J Paediatr Child Health* 2002; **38**: 358–362.
14. Serjeant GR, Topley JM, Mason K *et al.* Outbreak of aplastic crisis in sickle cell anaemia associated with parvovirus-like agent. *Lancet* 1981; **ii**: 595–597.

15. Young N. Hematologic and hematopoietic consequences of B19 parvovirus infection. *Semin Hematol* 1988; **25**: 159–172.

16. Anderson MJ, Davis LR, Hodgson J *et al*. Occurrence of infection with a parvovirus-like agent in children with sickle cell anaemia during a two-year period. *J Clin Pathol* 1982; **35**: 744–749.

17. Rogers BB, Rogers ZR, Timmons CF. Polymerase chain reaction amplification of archival material for parvovirus B19 in children with transient erythroblastopenia of childhood. *Pediatr Pathol Lab Med* 1996; **16**: 471–478.

18. Frickhofen N, Young NS. Persistent parvovirus B19 infections in humans. *Microb Pathog* 1989; **7**: 319–327.

19. Smith MA, Shah NR, Lobel JS, Cera PJ, Gary GW, Anderson LJ. Severe anemia caused by human parvovirus in a leukemia patient on maintenance chemotherapy. *Clin Pediatr (Phil)* 1988; **27**: 383–386.

20. Kurtzman GJ, Cohen B, Meyers P, Amunullah A, Young NS. Persistent B19 parvovirus infection as a cause of severe chronic anaemia in children with acute lymphocytic leukaemia. *Lancet* 1988; **ii**: 1159–1162.

21. Shirono K, Tsuda H. Parvovirus B19-associated haemophagocytic syndrome in healthy adults. *Br J Haematol* 1995; **89**: 923–926.

22. Soderlund-Venermo M, Hokynar K, Nieminen J, Rautakorpi H, Hedman K. Persistence of human parvovirus B19 in human tissues. *Pathol Biol (Paris)* 2002; **50**: 307–316.

23. Watanabe T, Satoh M, Oda Y. Human parvovirus B19 encephalopathy [Letter]. *Arch Dis Child* 1994; **70**: 71.

24. Cassinotti P, Schultze D, Schlageter P, Chevili S, Siegl G. Persistent human parvovirus B19 infection following an acute infection with meningitis in an immunocompetent patient. *Eur J Clin Microbiol Infect Dis* 1993; **12**: 701–704.

25. Okumura A, Ichikawa T. Aseptic meningitis caused by human parvovirus B19. *Arch Dis Child* 1993; **68**: 784–785.

26. Suzuki N, Terada S, Inoue M. Neonatal meningitis with human parvovirus B19 infection [Letter]. *Arch Dis Child* 1995; **73**: F196–F197.

27. Koduri PR, Naides SJ. Aseptic meningitis caused by parvovirus B19. *Clin Infect Dis* 1995; **21**: 1053.

28. Faden H, Gary Jr GW, Korman M. Numbness and tingling of fingers associated with parvovirus B19 infection [Letter]. *J Infect Dis* 1990; **161**: 354–355.

29. Brown T, Anand A, Ritchie LD, Clewley JP, Reid TM. Intrauterine parvovirus infection associated with hydrops fetalis [Letter]. *Lancet* 1984; **ii**: 1033-1034.

30. Cohen BJ, Kumar S. Parvovirus B19 infection and pregnancy. *Fetal Matern Med Rev* 2005; **16**: 123–150.

31. Miller E, Fairley CK, Cohen BJ, Seng C. Immediate and long term outcome of human parvovirus B19 infection in pregnancy. *Br J Obstet Gynaecol* 1998; **105**: 174–178.

32. Enders M, Weidner A, Zoellner I, Searle K, Enders G. Fetal morbidity and mortality after acute human parvovirus B19 infection in pregnancy: prospective evaluation of 1018 cases. *Prenat Diagn* 2004; **24**: 513–518.

33. Nagel HT, De Haan TR, Vandenbussche FP, Oepkes D, Walther FJ. Long-term outcome after fetal transfusion for hydrops associated with parvovirus B19 infection. *Obstet Gynecol* 2007; **109**: 42–47.

34. Warsof SL, Nicolaides KH, Rodeck C. Immune and non-immune hydrops. *Clin Obstet Gynecol* 1986; **29**: 533–542.

35. Ismail KM, Martin WL, Ghosh S, Whittle MJ, Kilby MD. Etiology and outcome of hydrops fetalis. *J Matern Fetal Med* 2001; **10**: 175–181.

36. Heegaard ED, Hasle H, Clausen N, Hornsleth A, Kerndrup GB. Parvovirus B19 infection and Diamond-Blackfan anaemia. *Acta Paediatr* 1996; **85**: 299–302.

37. Fairley CK, Smoleniec JS, Caul OE, Miller E. Observational study of effect of intrauterine transfusions on outcome of fetal hydrops after parvovirus B19 infection. *Lancet* 1995; **346**: 1335–1337.

38. Ballou WR, Reed JL, Noble W, Young NS, Koenig S. Safety and immunogenicity of a recombinant parvovirus B19 vaccine formulated with MF59C.1. *J Infect Dis* 2003; **187**: 675–678.

39. Brown KE, Young NS. Parvovirus B19. In: Young NS, Gerson SL, High KA. (eds) *Clinical Hematology*. Philadelphia, PA: Mosby Elsevier, 2006; 981–991.

40. Young NS, Brown KE. Parvovirus B19. *N Engl J Med* 2004; **350**: 586–597.

Esther Crawley

15

Chronic fatigue syndrome or myalgic encephalopathy

Chronic fatigue syndrome or myalgic encephalopathy (CFS/ME) is surprisingly common with prevalence figures of between 0.19 and 1% from population studies in both the US and the UK.[1–3] Life-time prevalence (up to 30 years old) of self-reported CFS/ME, uncorroborated by a physician, of 0.8% has been reported from the 1970 British Birth Cohort.[4] Life-time prevalence (aged 8–17 years) of disabling fatigue of 3 months and 6 months of 2.34% and 1.29% has been reported from a longitudinal cohort of twins.[5]

CFS/ME in children causes significant suffering. Over 50% of children who get CFS/ME are bed-bound at some stage.[6] It is probably the largest cause of long-term authorised school absence in the UK.[7]

WHAT CAUSES CFS/ME?

GENES

CFS/ME is heritable. Twin studies in adults have shown consistently higher concordance rates in monozygotic twins compared to dizygotic twins for CFS/ME (for example, MZ = 0.55; DZ = 0.19) with heritability increasing with increasingly stringent case definition.[8] This is consistent with studies of fatigue in children in the UK where carers of 670 twin pairs were questioned about disabling fatigue of more than a week and more than a month. In both cases, the concordance was higher in monozygotic twins compared to dizygotic twins (0.81 versus 0.59 for one week; 0.75 versus 0.47 for one month).[9,10] Candidate genes of interest are those with potential biological explanations for symptoms. This includes the hypothalamic-pituitary-adrenal axis, tryptophan and serotonin pathway, sympathetic system and pro-inflammatory cytokines.

Esther Crawley BA BM BCH FRCPCH PhD
Senior Clinical Lecturer, Bristol University, and Consultant Paediatrician and Clinical Lead of the Bath/Bristol Paediatric CFS/ME Service, Royal National Hospital for Rheumatic Disease, Upper Borough Walls, Bath BA1 1RL, UK. E-mail: esther.crawley@bristol.ac.uk

INFECTION

As with many complex illnesses, gene–environmental interaction may be the best model for this illness. In children and young people, an environmental trigger, such as a viral infection, appears to be relatively common. One of the best studied environmental triggers is Epstein-Barr virus (EBV) infection.[11] Other infections can also trigger CFS/ME and there is some evidence that the risk for developing CFS/ME is related to the severity of the infection.[12]

MOOD

Between 25–75% of young people with CFS/ME have an increased risk of suffering from low mood, somatisation or anxiety.[1,13–15] However, none of these studies has been able to show the direction of causality, in other words whether the mood is primary or secondary to suffering from a severe chronic disabling condition. The only longitudinal study, to date,[4] showed that childhood or adolescent psychological distress was not associated with the risk of life-time self-reported or physician-diagnosed CFS/ME.

WHO GETS CFS/ME?

CFS/ME is indiscriminate in whom it affects. There is no social class gradient, no gender preference and all ethnic groups are affected.[1–3] There is some evidence that it is less common in children of primary school age, but few studies have been done in this age group.[16]

HOW DOES CFS/ME PRESENT?

The Royal College of Paediatrics and Child Health (RCPCH) describes CFS/ME as 'disabling fatigue without another medical or psychological cause'. However, it lists a range of common symptoms associated with CFS/ME (Table 1).[17] The US Centers for Disease Control (CDC) definition only applies to adults but the symptom list can be helpful in guiding paediatricians

Table 1 RCPCH definition and symptoms

RCPCH description for CFS/ME
Generalised fatigue persisting after routine tests and investigations have failed to identify an obvious underlying 'cause'. In CFS/ME, the fatigue is likely to be associated with other classical symptoms and is often exacerbated by effort (both mental and physical)

Other classical symptoms
Severe malaise, headaches, sleep disturbances, concentration difficulties, memory impairment, depressed mood, myalgia/muscle pain at rest and on exercise, nausea, sore throat, tender lymph nodes, abdominal pain and arthralgia/joint pain

Symptoms reported less often
Feeling too hot or cold, dizziness, cough, eye pain/increased sensitivity to light (photophobia), vision or hearing disturbances (hyperacusis), weight loss or gain, muscle weakness, lack of energy for usual activities and diarrhoea

Table 2 Requirements to fulfil the 1994 Centers for Disease Control definition for CFS/ME

(1) *The presence of fatigue for a minimum of 6 months*

(2) *The fatigue must be*
- Clinically evaluated
- Unexplained
- Persistent or relapsing
- New or definite onset (not life-long)
- Not the result of on-going exertion
- Not substantially relieved by rest
- Results in substantial reduction in previous levels of occupational, educational, social or personal activities

(3) *Four or more of the following symptoms*
- Substantial impairment in short-term memory or concentration
- Sore throat
- Tender cervical or axillary lymph nodes
- Muscle pain
- Multiple joint pain without joint swelling or redness
- Headaches of a new type, pattern or severity
- Unrefreshing sleep
- Postexertional malaise lasting more than 24 h

towards a diagnosis (Table 2). The CDC definition requires disabling fatigue that lasts 6 months. This is thought to be too long for children. The RCPCH report suggested fatigue duration of 3 months.[17] This has been echoed in the Chief Medical Officer report.[18] Good practice is described in the UK National Service Framework for Children exemplar for CFS/ME[19] and the RCPCH guidelines with the suggestion that CFS/ME is thought about early, investigations started and treatment offered even if a formal diagnosis is not given until the child has had fatigue for 3 months.

SCREENING TESTS

All children presenting with possible CFS/ME must have a full history and examination. In addition, as CFS/ME is a diagnosis of exclusion, screening tests must be done in all children even those who present with typical symptoms of CFS/ME. The screening tests recommended are listed in Table 3. Additional tests should be done, if necessary, according to the history and examination. Viral tests are not recommended apart from testing for EBV if there is a good history of possible EBV infection associated with the start of the illness, as there is some evidence that prognosis may be better in this group of patients.[20]

MANAGEMENT

When the diagnosis of CFS/ME has been made, the child or young person should be offered a rehabilitation programme which aims to enable the child or young person to fulfil their goals. The management of CFS/ME includes specific management strategies for symptoms such as the sleep disturbance,

225

Table 3 Recommended screening tests for CFS/ME and diagnosis excluded

Full blood count	Anaemia and leukaemia
ESR or viscosity and C-reactive protein	Inflammatory conditions and auto-immune disorders
Ferritin	Iron deficiency
Urea and electrolytes, creatinine	Renal impairment or endocrine abnormality
Random glucose	Diabetes mellitus
Liver function tests	Hepatitis
Creatine kinase	Muscle disease
Thyroid function	Hypothyroidism
Coeliac screen	Coeliac disease
Urine test for protein, glucose and blood	Renal disease, diabetes mellitus, urinary tract infection

pain and nausea as well as general management for the CFS/ME; both are discussed separately below. It is important to involve the child and family in discussions over the different options and review the programme regularly so that the management plan can be adapted and improved in consultation with the child and family.

SPECIFIC MANAGEMENT STRATEGIES

Children and young people with CFS/ME will have a variety of symptoms that may be part of their CFS/ME. It is important that a full history and examination is carried out for each symptom and that other co-morbid disorders are excluded. For example, just because headache is a common symptom in CFS/ME, it is important that children with headache are examined and, if necessary, investigated in the same way as a child without CFS/ME. Many symptoms will get better as the CFS/ME improves. The areas that are probably worth special mention, however, are sleep disturbance, pain, nausea and hypersensitivity.

Sleep problems

One of the symptoms described as part of the CDC definition for CFS/ME is unrefreshing sleep (see Table 2). Adult studies have demonstrated prolonged sleep latency, low sleep efficiency index and a low percentage of slow-wave sleep.[21]

Many children present with difficulty getting off to sleep and difficulty waking. This is then exacerbated by excessive sleeping during the day, which is known to reduce restorative sleep further at night. This can, in some cases, lead to day–night reversal or a shift in the timing of sleep. Some of these abnormalities could be explained by abnormalities in tryptophan metabolism or changes in the diurnal rhythm of the hypothalamic-pituitary-adrenal axis.[22]

Table 4 Suggestions to improve sleep quality

	ACTION
Make sure you only sleep in your bedroom	If possible, do not watch TV or do computer work in bedroom or close to your bed
	If you need to rest during the day, try and rest on a day bed which is different to your night bed and, if possible, in a different room
Have a sleep routine	Have a routine before going to bed, *e.g.* bath, warm drink which will cue your brain that it is now time to get ready to sleep
Try not to stimulate yourself just before bed	Try to reduce physical or mental stimulation (TV or reading for some people) just before bedtime
Avoid day–night reversal	Watch our for day–night reversal. Be consistent about the time you wake up and go to sleep
	Try and expose your brain to as much sunlight during the day as feasible. Some young people have tried light boxes in the winter
Do not sleep too much during the day and correct day–night reversal	Long sleeps decrease sleep quality so keep hours of sleep at night only slightly more then age-appropriate levels. Work this out from peers
	If day–night reversal is a problem, start getting up a few minutes earlier each day to reverse this (maximum 60 min/week)
Limit day time sleeps	Try to rest not sleep during the day
	If you have to sleep keep it to less than 40 min before 3 pm

Before deciding on the appropriate management for sleep problems, a good sleep history must be taken and the clinician needs to exclude other causes for abnormal sleep such as obstructive sleep apnoea. It is important to explain to the child or young person and their family why they feel so tired in the morning and why they find it hard to get to sleep at night.

Getting back to a good sleep pattern involves the following steps (see Table 4 for further details).

1. Ensure the young person has good sleep hygiene and a good routine for going to bed.

2. Reduce and, if possible, stop day-time sleeps as this reduces the quality of the night-time sleep. If the child has to sleep, then help them limit this to less than 30 min before 3 pm.

3. Support the child or young person to wake up earlier each morning. You will need to explain that, initially, they will feel worse as they will have less sleep and for a while it will continue to be of poor quality; however, after a few weeks, the relative sleep deprivation will mean that sleep quality improves and they will feel better in the morning.

There is no good evidence on the rate of change for morning wake-up time. We normally recommend that children and young people get up 30–60 min earlier every few days until they are getting up regularly at a reasonable time in the morning. Some children will need to go slower than this.

Pain

Many children with CFS/ME will experience pain and this may be abdominal pain, headaches or severe muscle and joint pain. If no other cause for the pain can be discovered, a neuropathic or chronic pain type problem will need to be considered. This type of pain typically does not respond to pain killers which children describe as 'just taking the edge off'. It is important to explain what the pain is. The pain pathway model can be a useful way of explaining how a child or young person can experience such high levels of pain without doctors finding an underlying reason. This model is analogous to phantom-limb pain. The explanation is that although there was an original reason for the pain, the reason went away (amputation in the case of phantom-limb pain) but the pain continues. This is supported by studies in adults using functional MRI (reviewed by Borsook and Becerra[23]).

The general management of this type of pain is essentially the same as the general management of CFS/ME with the additional explanation of what the pain is, how unhelpful it is and with some suggestions on how to deal with it. Additional approaches to try might be a referral to the pain clinic where some children benefit from intervention procedures for pain, such as nerve blocks or the trial of additional medication for neuropathic pain. It may also be worth trying low-dose amitriptyline 30 min before bed, which can be stared at 5 mg and increaseduntil it is effectiveup to a maximumof 20 or 25 mg. Amitriptyline has the additional advantage of helping some children get off to sleep and possibly improving the quality of sleep.

Nausea

Many children experience significant nausea which can be very hard to deal with. If other causes for the nausea are excluded, and it is thought to be part of the CFS/ME, then it is worth looking carefully at the child or young person's diet. Sometimes, small, regular, simple meals of complex carbohydrate seem to help. There is currently no evidence that exclusion diets are useful, although many families will want to try them. If an exclusion diet is adopted, this should be undertaken with the supervision of a dietitian. There is no evidence that medication helps. Once again, the symptoms tend to resolve when the CFS/ME gets better.

Hypersensitivity to touch, light or noise

Many children describe hypersensitivity to touch, light or noise at some stage in their illness. These symptoms are almost universal for children and young people who are severely affected (see below) but even children who are mild-to-moderately affected can experience problems at some point in their illness. As with the other symptoms, it is important to take a full history and examine the young person or child. If it is felt that the symptoms are part of the CFS/ME, then a desensitisation programme can be discussed as a treatment option. Desensitisation follows the same principles as described below for noise and light – finding a baseline level and then gradually increasing exposure. This is often very important for noise before re-integration to school is attempted, otherwise the noise levels experienced in school will be too painful for the child or young person. For touch, a desensitisation programme can involve first the child and then perhaps a carer massaging the affected area. Sometimes, light touch can be more exquisitely painful then firm touch so the child and young person will have to experiment. The principle is regular (hourly perhaps) touch to the affected area. In some cases, actually touching the affected area is too difficult and so massaging from outside in may be helpful.

ACTIVITY MANAGEMENT AND COGNITIVE BEHAVIOURAL THERAPY

There is good evidence for activity management, graded exercise and cognitive behavioural therapy in the management of adults with mild-to-moderate CFS/ME. There is some evidence for these treatment strategies for children including one randomised, controlled trial which demonstrated improved outcome for children with cognitive behavioural therapy versus waiting list and one open trial which demonstrated improved outcome for children using graded activity and family work versus supportive care alone.[4,24,26]

There are several methods described for managing activities and energy and many overlap. Three commonly used approaches which are very similar (although the descriptions vary) are activity management, energy management or pacing. The RCPCH guidelines[17] have a more detailed description but a brief, useful and pragmatic approach is described here.

As with all rehabilitation methods, it is very important to find out, and work with, the goals set by the child or young person. Some children will just want to get back to school but others will want to get fit, or see their friends more. For children who are severely affected (see below), the goals may be very limited, such as sitting out of bed for a few minutes every day.

The stages of activity management are to recognise the boom–bust pattern of activity, find a baseline and then increase activity slowly.

Recognise the boom–bust pattern

Most children and young people will use a boom–bust strategy for managing their CFS/ME. This means that they will make a decision on what they will do depending on how they feel. On a good day, they might go to school or if they are severely affected get out of bed. On a bad day, they have an increase in symptoms and, therefore, reduce their activity. This means they may miss school or, for those who are severely affected, stay in bed. Some children set up their weeks so that they can 'boom' during the week and 'bust' at the weekend. The bust is not just an increase in tiredness but an increase in all the other symptoms associated with the child or young person's illness. The child or young person will often look more ill. It is often called payback as it is a result of the increased activity previously. It may by delayed by several hours or a day or two. It is often very difficult for the young person and their family to see that the increase in symptoms are not just occurring by chance but are secondary to over-doing it on a good day.

When trying to understand what a child or young person does every day, it is important to remember that activity is not just physical but can be cognitive and emotional as well. It is worth going through the various activities of the

Table 5 Examples of different types of activity

High-energy activity	**Physical**: exercise, PE, walking. If the young person is severely affected then brushing hair, sitting up or eating may all be high energy
	Cognitive: school, school work, computer and computer games. Often reading and games such as Suduko. Watching TV that the young person is engaged in
	Emotional: worries or arguments
Low-energy activity	Watching TV that the young person is not particularly engaged in (background noise), reading easy books or magazines, repetitive easy tasks such as beading can be low energy unless the young person is severely affected
Rest	Not doing anything physical or cognitive. Relaxation exercises, deep breathing, guided imagery, progressive relaxation or listening to music

child, and discussing with them whether they are high- or low-energy activity (see Table 5 for examples of activity). They are then in a good position to start to monitor their activity and find their baseline.

Find the baseline

This is tricky and children and their families may need quite a lot of support whilst they try and find the baseline. The baseline is the level of activity they can do on a good day and a bad day. It is often around half of what they can do on a good day. On a good day, they should feel like they want to do more and on a bad day they should feel they can just about manage it. So if the young person was managing some full days at school and on some days was not able to go in to school at all, their baseline would normally be half-days at school. If on a good day they were managing an hour of home tuition and two hours on the computer but were unable to manage anything on a bad day, their baseline is probably about 30 min of 'tricky' work during the home tuition and maybe 30 min of 'low-energy work' and an hour on the computer. However, they then need to do that every day including an equivalent amount of activity at the weekend (see Fig. 1 for an example).

Increase activity

Once a young person has successfully found their baseline, they can then increase this but by no more than about 10–15% a week. This means that if the child or young person is doing four hours at school one week, the next week they add in 25–35 extra minutes of activity. If the young person is doing a 10-min walk one week, the following week it will be 11 min. The increase should be especially focused and driven by their own goals. It often helps to work out what they will need to achieve their goal and work towards this slowly. For example, if they have identified getting back to school as a goal, then they may need to work on getting fitter and being able to increase their time concentrating on academic work as well as getting used to noisy environments. The child and young person can continue to increase the activity as long as they are not getting payback and as long as they do not have a setback.

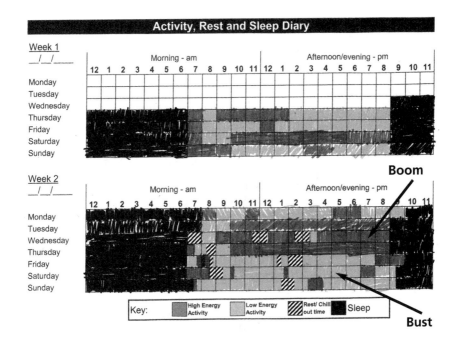

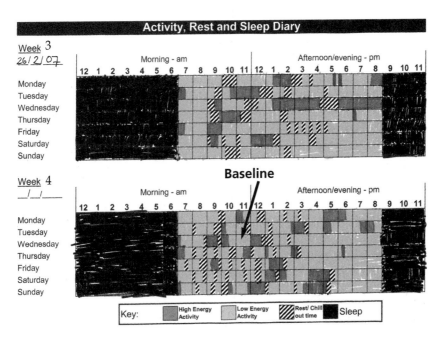

Fig. 1 Example of activity charts filled in by an 11-year-old boy over a 4-week period. These are the charts that we use. In the first week after the assessment on the Wednesday, he had high activity on the Thursday and Saturday, and collapsed (bust) on the Friday, Sunday and Monday. He then did more high-energy work on the Tuesday, Wednesday and Thursday before having a really bad day on the Friday. His mother realised what was going on and tried to find a baseline of activity for him which was sustainable. She managed to achieve this by the fourth week. Note the regular small amounts of activity and regular rests. By this week, he was feeling much better with a decrease in symptoms and no 'bad' days. We then started to increase activity gradually by 10–15% a week.

Graded exercise therapy

Graded exercise therapy is a structured and supervised programme of exercise agreed between the therapist and the child or young person and their family. It follows the same principles as described above of finding a baseline and then increasing activity but concentrates on physical activity rather than on physical, cognitive and emotional uses of energy. The fact that graded exercise therapy is supervised is an important element of the programme. Telling a child or young person to 'just do more exercise' is unlikely to be helpful.

Cognitive behavioural therapy

Cognitive behavioural therapy has two elements. The cognitive element which identifies and modifies thoughts, beliefs and assumptions which may change the patients understanding of the illness and the behavioural element which aims to introduce, gradually and consistently, a change in behaviour. As with all the treatment options, treatment needs to be tailored to the needs of the child or young person.

There is currently no evidence to predict which children need and are likely to benefit from cognitive behavioural therapy. The potential advantages and disadvantages should be discussed with the child and their family. Children with increased anxiety or low mood or those who are particularly stuck may be the most to benefit.

Rest

All the above approaches incorporate regular rests during the day. Rest is when the child or young person does not perform either physical or cognitive activity. It is usually better to rest in a room which is not the bedroom. Watching TV is not resting but a low-energy activity. Children and young people can learn techniques to help them rest such as deep breathing, guided imagery or progressive relaxation.

Setbacks

Setbacks are an increase in symptoms which last longer than the normal payback. They are sometimes caused by the child or young person getting another illness such as the 'flu but sometimes it is difficult to see why they have happened. Setbacks are a normal part of CFS/ME and it is sensible to warn children and young people so they do not become too despondent when they happen. When a child or young person goes through a setback, it is a good idea to have a think about why it may have happened to try and avoid it happening in the future. Then reset the baseline, review other areas such as sleep and symptom control and start again.

EDUCATION

Working closely with teachers and home tutors in the management of a child or young person is an important part of the rehabilitation programme. Teachers may need to understand that although a child looks well on one day, that he is could be unwell the next day. Home tutors who go into the home daily can be an invaluable support to the child and family if they understand about CFS/ME. Keeping Education Welfare Officers in the picture means they can be supportive and helpful to families. Many children will need extra time in examinations and a quiet room. Some young people will need to delay GCSEs or A-levels and will need tremendous support and advocacy as they negotiate a change at this time in their lives.

DIET

There is no good evidence that elimination diets help children or young people with CFS/ME but, as mentioned above, many children and young people will try eliminating various foods from their diet in an attempt to control symptoms. Some standard dietary suggestions are: have a well balanced diet; avoid too much sugary food during the day; if they are feeling very nauseated then try 5 or 6 small meals a day; include iron and vitamin C in the diet as low iron levels can make you feel tired. If a child or young person needs further advice, referral to a dietitian can be helpful.

MANAGEMENT OF CHILDREN AND YOUNG PEOPLE WHO ARE SEVERELY AFFECTED

The prevalence of children and young people who are severely affected is not known; however, one study suggested that over 50% of children had been house-bound at some stage.[6]

It is important to remember that the randomised, controlled trials described in this chapter recruited children and young people who could attend outpatient appointments and, therefore, excluded the severely affected. However, many of the principles described above appear to be helpful but they need to be offered with care, in consultation with the child and family, and the management plan needs to be reviewed frequently.

Activity management can be very difficult in children who are severely affected as activities that health professionals assume are low-energy activity may be exhausting for the children or young person. For example, the child may get significant payback after getting out of bed for 30 min on a good day and be unable to get out of bed the following day. In addition, activities such as watching TV or reading may become high-energy activities. Taking very careful history and detailed activity plans usually show where the problems lie and, in consultation with the child and family, it is usually possible to find a baseline and enable the child to increase activity very slowly towards their goals.

It is important that the child or young person has access to a multi-disciplinary team while they are severely affected. An assessment by an occupational therapist is usually very helpful to make sure that the child is as mobile as possible. A physiotherapist can help with an extremely gentle stretching or passive exercise programme and a paediatrician in collaboration with the general practitioner can help with symptom control. Social care can play an important role in helping with disability benefits and also adaptations to the house. The management of children who are severely affected can be complex and difficult. If a child is not making anticipated progress then getting a second opinion from a specialist in paediatric CFS/ME may be helpful.

PROGNOSIS AND OUTCOME

The prognosis for children and young people with CFS/ME who access a service is good, with over 90% of children getting much or completely better.[25] It is much better than in adults and this is an important point to tell families where there is also a parent involved as some children believe they may never get better.

Key points for clinical practice

- CFS/ME is surprisingly common and can affect children from any ethnic group and any socio-economic class. CFS/ME can occur in primary school aged children although it appears to be less common.

- There is good evidence that CFS/ME is genetically heritable; therefore, it is not surprising, indeed it should be expected, that it runs in families.

- Before making a diagnosis of CFS/ME, it is important to exclude other illnesses which may present with fatigue. This means that screening investigations need to be carried out on all children.

- When a diagnosis is made, the child or young person and their family should be able to access an appropriate treatment programme for their needs. This is likely to include a combination of symptom-specific and CFS/ME management strategies.

- Children and young people with CFS/ME should be offered activity management, energy management, pacing, cognitive behavioural therapy or components of all these to create an individual programme for rehabilitation. These may be delivered by one clinician or by a multidisciplinary team.

- It is important to review children and young people and their families fairly frequently, especially in the early days when they are finding their baseline and increasing activity.

- Children or young people who are severely affected should be assessed and offered an appropriate management package of care at home. If necessary, a second opinion from a specialist in CFS/ME may be helpful, particularly with diagnosis.

- The prognosis for CFS/ME in children and young people is good if they are able to access a service.

References

1. Chalder T, Goodman R, Wessely S, Hotopf M, Meltzer H. Epidemiology of chronic fatigue syndrome and self reported myalgic encephalomyelitis in 5–15 year olds: cross sectional study. *BMJ* 2003; **327**: 654–655.
2. Jordan KM, Ayers PM, Jahn SC *et al*. Prevalence of fatigue and chronic fatigue syndrome-like illness in children and adolescents. *J Chronic Fatigue Syndrome* 2000; **6**: 3–21.
3. Jones JF, Nisenbaum R, Solomon L, Reyes M, Reeves WC. Chronic fatigue syndrome and other fatiguing illnesses in adolescents: a population-based study. *J Adolesc Health* 2004; **35**: 34–40.

4. Viner R, Hotopf M. Childhood predictors of self reported chronic fatigue syndrome/myalgic encephalomyelitis in adults: national birth cohort study. *BMJ* 2004; **329**: 941.

5. Farmer A, Fowler T, Scourfield J, Thapar A. Prevalence of chronic disabling fatigue in children and adolescents. *Br J Psychiatry* 2004; **184**: 477–481.

6. Rangel L, Garralda ME, Levin M, Roberts H. The course of severe chronic fatigue syndrome in childhood. *J R Soc Med* 2000; **93**: 129–134.

7. Dowsett EG, Colby J. Long-term sickness absence due to ME/CFS in UK schools: an epidemiological study with medical and educational implications. *J Chronic Fatigue Syndrome* 1997; **3**: 29–42.

8. Buchwald D, Herrell R, Ashton S *et al*. A twin study of chronic fatigue. *Psychosom Med* 2001; **63**: 936–943.

9. Farmer A, Scourfield J, Martin N, Cardno A, McGuffin P. Is disabling fatigue in childhood influenced by genes? *Psychol Med* 1999; **29**: 279–282.

10. Fowler TA, Rice F, Thapar A, Farmer A. Relationship between disabling fatigue and depression in children: genetic study. *Br J Psychiatry* 2006; **189**: 247–253.

11. White PD, Thomas JM, Sullivan PF, Buchwald D. The nosology of sub-acute and chronic fatigue syndromes that follow infectious mononucleosis. *Psychol Med* 2004; **34**: 499–507.

12. Hickie I, Davenport T, Wakefield D *et al*. Post-infective and chronic fatigue syndromes precipitated by viral and non-viral pathogens: prospective cohort study. *BMJ* 2006; **333**: 575.

13. Carter BD, Kronenberger WG, Edwards JF, Michalczyk L, Marshall GS. Differential diagnosis of chronic fatigue in children: behavioral and emotional dimensions. *J Dev Behav Pediatr* 1996; **17**: 16–21.

14. Garralda ME, Rangel L. Annotation: Chronic Fatigue Syndrome in children and adolescents. *J Child Psychol Psychiatry* 2002; **43**: 169–176.

15. Van MH, Geenen R, Kuis W, Heijnen CJ, Sinnema G. Psychological adjustment of adolescent girls with chronic fatigue syndrome. *Pediatrics* 2001; **107**: e35.

16. Chalder T, Goodman R, Wessely S, Hotopf M, Meltzer H. Epidemiology of chronic fatigue syndrome and self reported myalgic encephalomyelitis in 5–15 year olds: cross sectional study. *BMJ* 2003; **327**: 654–655.

17. Chalder T, Goodman R, Wessely S, Hotopf M, Meltzer H. Epidemiology of chronic fatigue syndrome and self reported myalgic encephalomyelitis in 5–15 year olds: cross sectional study. *BMJ* 2003; **327**: 654–655.

18. Lloyd AR, Hickie I, Boughton CR, Spencer O, Wakefield D. Prevalence of chronic fatigue syndrome in an Australian population. *Med J Aust* 1990; **153**: 522–528.

19. Royal College of Paediatrics and Child Health. *Evidence Based Guideline for the Management of CFS/ME (Chronic Fatigue Syndrome/Myalgic Encephalopathy) in Children and Young People*. London: RCPCH, 2004.

20. CFS/ME Working Group. *A report to the chief medical officer of an independent working group*. London: CFS/ME Working Group, 2002.

21. *Chronic fatigue syndrome/myalgic encephalopathy (CFS/ME). Change for children – every child matters*. London: Gateway ref: 3779, 2004.

22. Carter BD, Edwards JF, Kronenberger WG, Michalczyk L, Marshall GS. Case control study of chronic fatigue in pediatric patients. *Pediatrics* 1995; **95**: 179–186.

23. Van Hoof E, De Becker P, Lapp C, Cluydts R, De Meirleir K. Defining the occurrence and influence of alpha-delta sleep in chronic fatigue syndrome. *Am J Med Sci* 2007; **333**: 78–84.

24. Di GA, Hudson M, Jerjes W, Cleare AJ. 24-Hour pituitary and adrenal hormone profiles in chronic fatigue syndrome. *Psychosom Med* 2005; **67**: 433–440.

25. Borsook D, Becerra LR. Breaking down the barriers: fMRI applications in pain, analgesia and analgesics. *Mol Pain* 2006; **2**: 30.

26. Viner R, Gregorowski A, Wine C, Bladen M, Fisher D, Miller M, *et al*. Outpatient rehabilitative treatment of chronic fatigue syndrome (CFS/ME). Arch Dis Child 2004; **89**: 615–619.

27. Joyce J, Hotopf M, Wessely S. The prognosis of chronic fatigue and chronic fatigue syndrome: a systematic review. *Quart J Med* 1997; **90**: 223–233.

28. Chalder T, Tong J, Deary V. Family cognitive behaviour for chronic fatigue syndrome: an uncontrolled study. Arch Dis Child 2002; 86: 95–97

Delane Shingadia

16

Diagnosis of tuberculosis

The natural history of tuberculosis (TB) has traditionally been divided into 'infection' and 'disease'. Initial exposure to an infectious individual (primarily sputum smear positive pulmonary disease) results in tuberculosis infection characterised by tuberculin skin test (TST) conversion. Subsequent development of disease is characterised by the development of signs and symptoms and/or radiological changes. While differentiation between 'infection' and 'disease' may be difficult, especially in children, the management of the two will be significantly different.

CLINICAL SPECTRUM OF DISEASE IN CHILDREN

Following initial exposure to an infectious individual, inhalation of an aerosolised particle containing tubercle bacilli results in infection in the lung. The initial encounter with the bacilli results in a series of immunological events, particularly a cell-mediated immune response, resulting in the formation of a sub-pleural granuloma (called the Gohn focus) with accompanying regional mediastinal lymphadenitis (called the primary or Gohn complex). In most children, the primary complex resolves spontaneously with

Box 1	Abbreviations used	
	TB	tuberculosis
	TST	tuberculin skin test
	MT	miliary tuberculosis
	LTBI	latent tuberculosis infection
	PPD	purified protein derivative (tuberculin)
	BCG	bacille Calmetté-Guerin vaccine
	PCR	polymerase chain reaction

Delane Shingadia MB ChB DCH DTM&H MPH MRCP FRCPCH
Consultant in Infectious Diseases, Department of Infectious Diseases, Great Ormond Street Hospital
for Children, Great Ormond Street, London WC1N 3JH, UK. E-mail: shingd@gosh.nhs.uk

residual calcification or scarring at the site of the Gohn focus. However, in some children, particularly infants, the primary complex may result in progressive and persistent lymphadenopathy, which may compress surrounding structures such as the bronchi.[1] Inability to control infection within the primary parenchymal infiltrate results in the development of a caseating lesion, known as progressive primary tuberculosis. Invasion and rupture into surrounding structures, such as pleural or pericardial spaces, will result in disease at those sites. Erosion of caseating lesions into intrathoracic vessels can result in haematogenous dissemination within the lung and also extrathoracic anatomical sites. The most common manifestation of this is miliary tuberculosis (MT), which involves the lungs, as well as liver and spleen. MT usually occurs as an early complication of primary infection and usually affects infants and young children. In the majority of children, initial infection is successfully controlled and the primary complex resolves without the development of any symptoms. Persistence of bacilli within the lung (called latent TB infection or LTBI) and subsequent re-activation at a later stage occurs in 3–5% of individuals following infection (called post-primary tuberculosis). Older children and adults will develop re-activation pulmonary disease which typically follows infection acquired after 7 years of age and commonly occurs at the time of puberty.[2] Post-primary TB is characterised by extensive pulmonary infiltration and cavitation, especially of the upper lobe of the lung, and are usually found on chest X-ray. Compared with progressive primary disease, post-primary disease is characterised by large numbers of bacilli within the pulmonary cavities, resulting in higher yields on microbiological testing of samples (see below).

Progressive primary tuberculosis with haematogenous dissemination and subsequent spread to extrathoracic sites results in extrapulmonary tuberculosis. Extrapulmonary disease is more common in children than adults, occurring in approximately 25% of infants and young children < 4 years of age.[3] Superficial lymphadenitis is the most common form of extrapulmonary TB in children, typically involving the supraclavicular, anterior cervical, tonsillar and submandibular nodes. Without treatment, cold abscess and chronic sinus formation may occur. Central nervous system disease, especially TB meningitis, is the most serious complication of tuberculosis in children and occurs in about 4% of children with tuberculosis.[4] The overall mortality has been reported to be 13%, with approximately half of survivors developing permanent neurological sequelae.[5] Tuberculomas of the central nervous system infection may occur and are usually characterised by solitary brain lesions, sometimes occurring after commencement of antituberculous treatment. Musculoskeletal disease primarily involves weight-bearing bones and joints, particularly the vertebrae (called Pott's disease).[6] Other, less common extrapulmonary manifestations of TB include gastrointestinal or renal disease. Renal disease is particularly rare in children mainly because the long incubation following haematogenous dissemination will mean that disease will often not develop until adulthood.

DIAGNOSIS

MICROSCOPY AND CULTURE

'In the diagnosis of pulmonary tuberculosis examination, and constantly repeated examination, of the sputum must be carried out'; so said Riviere in his text *The Early Diagnosis of Tubercle* published in 1921.[7] Microscopic examination of clinical samples for identification of tubercle bacilli using acid-fast staining techniques, such as the Ziehl-Neelsen stain, has been a standard tool for the diagnosis of TB. Acid-fast smears of sputum have become the cornerstone of TB diagnosis in many countries and, in some settings, the only test used to diagnose TB. Microscopic examination can detect 60–70% of culture positive samples with a lower limit of detection of 5×10^3 organisms/ml. Detection is increased by collection of multiple samples and concentration of samples (cumulative proportion positive for three smears for concentrated specimens were 74%, 83% and 91% and for direct smears were 57%, 76% and 81%).[8] Detection will depend on numbers of bacilli in the sample and, therefore, also the type of disease (*i.e.* progressive primary disease versus post-primary disease). Newer, fluorochrome stains, such as the auramine and rhodamine, appear to have higher detection when compared with the Ziehl-Neelsen stain.[9] These tests are generally easy to perform, cheap and give rapid results. However, young children and infants may be unable to produce sputum and, when they do, microscopic examination is often negative because they have progressive primary disease. As an alternative to obtaining sputum, early morning gastric aspirate samples are often collected by aspiration of overnight gastric contents via a nasogastric tube. This takes advantage of the fact that infants and young children will often swallow respiratory secretions which are pooled in the stomach overnight and which can be collected prior to ingestion of food in the morning. The yield from microscopy of gastric aspirate samples in children with proven pulmonary TB is less than 20%, compared with 75% in adults.[10] In a study of Haitian children, the sensitivity, specificity and positive predictive value of fluorescence microscopy of gastric washings compared with culture were 58%, 95% and 81%, respectively.[11]

The rates of detection on microscopy from other extrapulmonary samples, such as cerebrospinal fluid, are even lower mainly because of the paucibacillary nature of disease at these sites.

Culture of gastric aspirates has provided a more useful method of diagnosis in children with suspected pulmonary tuberculosis. Three consecutive morning gastric aspirates yield *Mycobacterium tuberculosis* in 30–50% of cases and may be as high as 70% in infants.[12] The culture yield from other body fluids or tissues from children with extrapulmonary tuberculosis is usually less than 50% due to lower numbers of mycobacteria in these sites of disease.[13] A recent study from South Africa has shown that bacteriological yields in children with intrathoracic disease manifestations other than uncomplicated lymph node disease were as high as 77% compared with those with uncomplicated lymph node disease alone where yield was only 35%.[14]

The role of bronchoscopy in the diagnosis of pulmonary TB remains controversial. Cultures from broncho-alveolar lavage fluid in children with suspected pulmonary TB has a low yield and does not significantly aid bacteriological confirmation.[15] Comparison of culture yields from a single bronchoscopic sample were lower than for three gastric aspirates.[16] Bronchoscopy may, however, play a useful role in the diagnosis of certain forms of TB such as endobronchial tuberculosis or bronchial obstruction, especially if transbronchial biopsy is performed.[17] Bronchoscopy may also be useful in excluding other causative agents such as opportunistic infections particularly in immunocompromised children and children with HIV were the radiological findings might be similar.

Sputum induction with nebulised, hypertonic (5%) saline has recently been used to obtain sputum from young infants and children in resource-limited settings. In this study, a single induced sputum sample had equivalent yield to that from three consecutive early morning gastric aspirates.[18] The microbiological yield from sputum induction did not differ between HIV-infected and HIV-uninfected children with pulmonary TB and all sputum induction procedures were well tolerated with only minor side-effects including increased coughing, epistaxis, vomiting, or wheezing.[19] However, there are concerns regarding the infection control aspects of this procedure particularly with respect to other immunocompromised patients and transmission of resistant TB. It is, therefore, advisable that sputum induction be performed with appropriate infection control procedures (*e.g.* negative-pressure cubicles), and by appropriately trained and protected staff.

The string test is a novel approach that has recently been evaluated in adults for its ability to retrieve *M. tuberculosis* from the upper gastrointestinal tract. This test was developed for the diagnosis of enteric parasites, such as *Giardia lamblia*. In a study of HIV-positive adults in Peru, the string test was shown to be safe and effective for retrieval of useful clinical specimens for diagnosis of pulmonary tuberculosis, and was at least as sensitive as sputum induction.[20] A recent study showed that the string test is well-tolerated in children as young as 4 years; however, there are no published data on bacteriological yield in children compared with other sample collection methods.[21] Further studies are needed to evaluate the utility of this test, particularly in young children where sputum samples may be difficult to obtain.

Laboratory cultivation of *M. tuberculosis* using solid growth media, such as Lowenstein-Jensen media, was one of the great advances in mycobacteriology during the 20th century. In microscopy positive samples, cultures make take from 2–4 weeks to become positive whereas in microscopy negative samples this may take from 4–8 weeks. More recently, rapid culture methods have been developed, with the potential advantages of more rapid growth and increased culture yields than with solid media.[22]

TUBERCULIN SKIN TEST

Tuberculin was developed in the early part of the 20th century, as a treatment for TB, but subsequently as a test of sensitivity to mycobacterial infection. In essence, tuberculin contains tuberculoproteins and is available in solubilised form as purified protein derivative (PPD). The tuberculin skin test (TST) relies on an individual's delayed-type hypersensitivity reaction to these tuberculoproteins following infection, past or present. A positive TST reaction is, therefore, regarded as a hallmark of primary infection with *M. tuberculosis*. In most children, tuberculin reactivity becomes apparent within 3–6 weeks after initial infection but, occasionally, can take up to 3 months. Tuberculin reactivity due to *M. tuberculosis* infection usually remains positive for the life-time of the individual, even after treatment.[23]

The Mantoux test is the standard TST currently in use and uses 5–10 tuberculin units of PPD. The Mantoux test is the standard method used in

Table 1 Summary of interpretation of positive tuberculin skin test results for Mantoux test in children[24]

NICE guidelines (UK)
> 6 mm (no BCG)
> 15 mm (BCG)

WHO
> 10 mm (no BCG)
> 15 mm (BCG)

American Academy of Pediatrics (USA)

> 5 mm and one or more of the following

- Children in close contact with known or suspected contagious case of tuberculosis disease, *i.e.* households with active or previously active cases if treatment cannot be verified as adequate before exposure, treatment was initiated after the child's contact or re-activation of latent tuberculosis infection is suspected

- Children suspected to have tuberculosis disease, *i.e.* chest radiograph consistent with active or previously active tuberculosis; or clinical evidence of tuberculosis disease

- Children receiving immunosuppressive therapy or with immuno suppressive conditions including HIV infection

> 10 mm and one or more of the following:

- Children at increased risk of disseminated disease, *i.e.* younger than 4 years of age or other medical condition, including Hodgkin's disease, lymphoma, diabetes mellitus, chronic renal failure or malnutrition

- Children with increased exposure to tuberculosis disease, *i.e.* born or whose parents were born in high-prevalence regions of the world; or are frequently exposed to adults who are HIV-infected, homeless, users of illicit drugs, residents of nursing homes, incarcerated or institutionalised, and migrant farm workers

> 15 mm
- Children 4 years of age or older without any risk factors

---

many countries for detecting infection by *M. tuberculosis*. This test involves the intradermal injection of PPD solution into the most superficial layer of the skin of the forearm, which raises an immediate wheal. The reaction is measured as millimetres of induration (not erythema) after 48–72 h. Sometimes, with strongly positive Mantoux tests, there may be marked induration, blister formation and ulceration at the site of intradermal injection. Percutaneous, multipuncture devices, such as the Heaf test and Tine test, are no longer in common use. Interpretation of TST results differs around the world and is summarised in Table 1.[24]

TST suffers from both poor sensitivity (false-negative results) and specificity (false-positive results). The TST has the lowest sensitivity in younger children. Up to 10% of otherwise normal children with culture-proven tuberculosis do not react to tuberculin initially.[13] Most of these children will become reactive during treatment, suggesting that tuberculosis disease may itself contribute to immunosuppression. False-negative TST may also occur in children with severe tuberculosis disease, those with debilitating or immunosuppressive illnesses, malnutrition, or other severe infections. The rate of false-negative TST in children with tuberculosis who are infected with HIV, is unknown, but it is certainly higher than 10% and is dependent on the degree of immunosuppression, particularly the CD4 count.

False-positive TST results may also occur. Bacillus Calmette–Guérin (BCG) is a vaccine derived from an attenuated strain of *Mycobacterium bovis* and, because of antigenic similarities with *M. tuberculosis*, may transiently cause a reactive TST. However, most children who received BCG as infants will have a non-reactive TST at 5 years of age.[25] A recent meta-analysis suggests that the effect of BCG on TST measurements was less after 15 years, and induration greater than 15 mm was more likely to be due to tuberculosis infection than BCG.[26] Among older children or adolescents who receive BCG, most develop a reactive TST initially; however, by 10–15 years post-vaccination, the majority will have lost tuberculin reactivity.[27] Recent studies have shown that BCG vaccination had little impact on the interpretation of TST in children being tested as part of a contact investigation.[28] Another reason for false-positive TST is that of infection or exposure to non-tuberculous mycobacteria (also called environmental mycobacteria). This phenomenon may arise through antigenic cross-reactivity with tuberculin.[29] Skin reactivity can also be boosted, probably through antigenic stimulation, by serial testing with TST in many children and adults who received BCG.[30]

SEROLOGICAL DETECTION

Serological assays for detecting TB antibodies have so far been disappointing. No serological assay is sufficiently accurate to replace conventional tests and, so far, serological assays have found little place in the routine diagnosis of children with tuberculosis. ELISA has been used to detect antibodies to a host of *M. tuberculosis* antigens including protein-purified derivative, killed *M. tuberculosis*, and antigen A60.[31–33] A recent study to evaluate the efficacy of ELISA serological tests (IgG antibodies against specific glycolipid antigen and ESAT-6 antigen of *M. tuberculosis*) compared with bacteriological tests (Ziehl-Neelsen stain, solid media culture and polymerase chain reaction [PCR]) in children with pulmonary, central nervous system, lymph node, and gastrointestinal tuberculosis showed higher sensitivity and comparable specificity except in pulmonary disease.[34] It has been suggested that ELISA tests have a promising future in the diagnosis of childhood tuberculosis; however, at present, these methods have had a limited role in routine use in the diagnosis of tuberculosis in children and further studies are needed.

Serological tests for tuberculosis have focused on detection of mycobacterial antigens, therefore, like skin tests, can be confounded by cross-reactivity with non-pathogenic mycobacteria or previous immunisation with BCG. Recent advances in proteonomic fingerprinting have proposed diagnostic tests based on the distinctive configurations of serum circulating proteins which may be characteristic of individual disease states such as tuberculosis. In serum samples from adults with active tuberculosis collected in Uganda, The Gambia and the UK, proteonomic profiles provided diagnostic accuracy of 94% (sensitivity 93.5%, specificity 94.9%) and was unaffected by HIV status.[35] The investigators proposed that these tests could be adapted to field use by incorporation of defined biomarkers into dipstick-type formats. Further studies are needed in large-scale, longitudinal studies of tuberculosis and other difficult diagnostic categories, such as sputum-negative TB, extrapulmonary TB and paediatric TB.

RADIOLOGY

Chest radiology has been an important tool in the diagnosis of pulmonary tuberculosis. Radiological changes will depend on the type and stage of disease. Primary complex and progressive primary disease (most often seen in household contacts of smear-positive adults) will result in intrathoracic lymphadenopathy (hilar or mediastinal; Fig. 1). Following resolution and containment of the primary complex, a subpleural area of fibrosis or calcification may be visible on chest radiography. Endobronchial disease may occur with progressive primary disease and is characterised by multiple, small, acinar shadows in the lower lobes indicating bronchogenic spread . Other radiological features of progressive primary disease include segmental hyperinflation, atelectasis, alveolar consolidation, pleural effusion/empyema and, rarely, a focal mass. Miliary tuberculosis following haematogenous dissemination is characterised by fine bilateral reticular shadowing, described as a 'snowstorm' appearance (Fig. 2). Cavitary disease is relatively rare in young children but is more common in adolescents (Fig. 3), who may develop adult-type post-primary disease and are hence more likely to be infectious.[36] Re-activation disease characteristically shows upper lobe infiltrates and/or cavitation on chest radiograph.

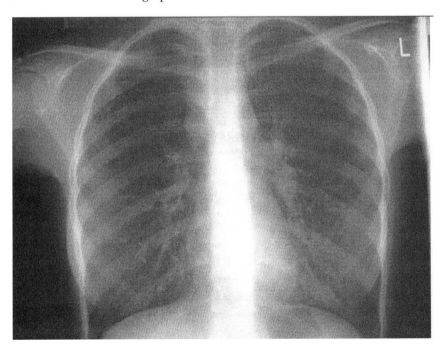

Fig. 1 Chest radiograph showing intrathoracic hilar lymphadenopathy.

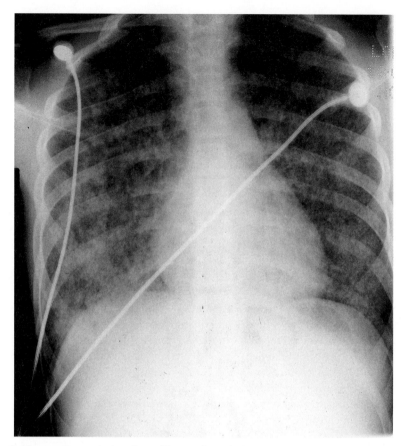

Fig. 2 Chest radiograph showing military tuberculosis or 'snow storm' appearance.

Newer radiological investigations, such as computed tomography (CT) and high-resolution CT has been useful in demonstrating early pulmonary disease such as cavitation often in the absence of any abnormality on chest radiography (Fig. 4). CT is also better than chest radiography in demonstrating bronchial involvement such as bronchial compression and bronchiectasis. CT may also be useful in detecting intrathoracic hilar lymphadenopathy including in those with normal chest x-rays.[37–39] There is, however, interobserver variability in the detection of mediastinal and hilar lymph nodes on CT in children with suspected pulmonary tuberculosis and diagnostic accuracy might be improved by refining radiological criteria for lymphadenopathy.[40]

CT has also been used for evaluation of pericardial effusions which, when associated with mediastinal lymphadenoapthy and a positive TST, are strongly suggestive of tuberculous disease.[41] Central nervous system disease, such as tuberculous meningitis or tuberculoma, may also be identified on CT. TB meningitis is characterised by basilar meningeal enhancement (Fig. 5).

Magnetic resonance imaging (MRI) has been found to be useful for musculoskeletal and soft tissue tuberculosis, particularly involving bones and joints.[42] Figure 6 shows a Pott's fracture of the spine, which was identified on MRI.

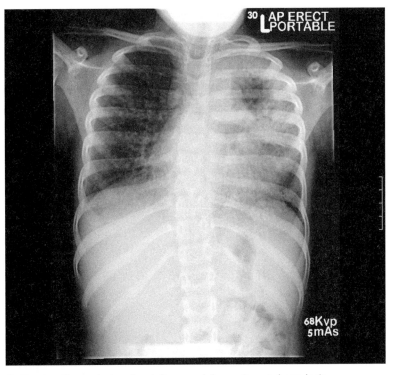

Fig. 3 Chest radiograph showing left upper lobe cavitary tuberculosis.

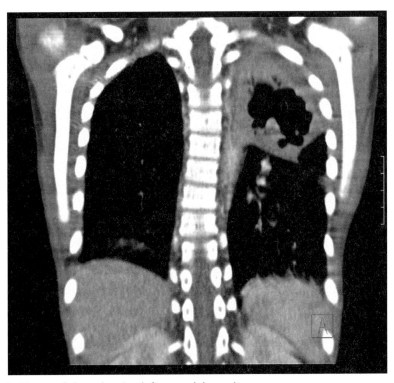

Fig. 4 CT scan of chest showing left upper lobe cavity.

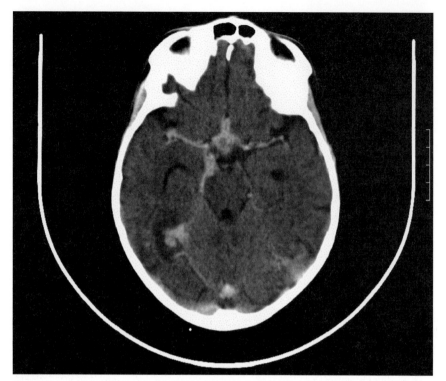

Fig. 5 Head CT scan showing basilar enhancement consistent with TB meningitis.

DIAGNOSTIC APPROACHES IN CHILDHOOD TUBERCULOSIS

The diagnosis of tuberculosis in children is based mainly on a combination of history of contact with an adult infectious case, clinical signs and symptoms, and investigations mentioned above, particularly chest radiograph and tuberculin skin testing. However, symptoms may often be non-specific with over half of children being asymptomatic with early disease.[36] A positive history of contact with a case of tuberculosis, especially if the source case was a parent or other member of the household who was also bacteriologically positive, has been strongly associated with disease in a child.[43] These epidemiological, clinical, and diagnostic parameters have been used to devise simple, cheap, and reliable tests to enable accurate diagnosis of tuberculosis in children especially in low-income countries. Several diagnostic approaches exist and most are grouped, broadly, into four families based on point-scoring systems, diagnostic classifications, diagnostic algorithms, or combinations of these.[44] An example of a diagnostic approach is that recommended by the World Health Organization (WHO) which relies on stratified categories of suspected, probable, and confirmed tuberculosis.[45] Most of these diagnostic approaches have not been standardised, making comparison difficult, and few have been properly validated.[44] Some diagnostic approaches have been modified for populations where HIV is prevalent; however, only one diagnostic approach has been specifically designed to diagnose tuberculosis in such a population.[46] In a high HIV-prevalent population, clinical scoring

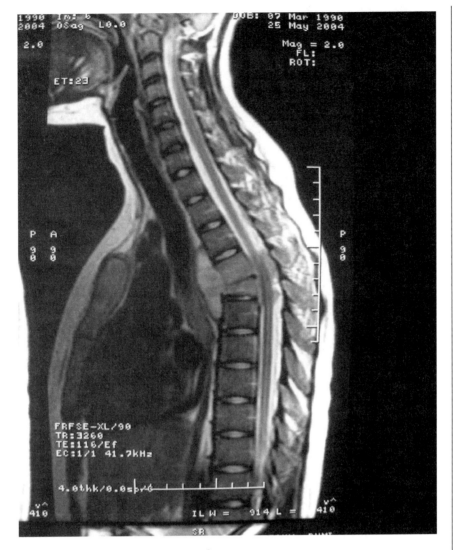

Fig. 6 MRI scan of spine showing Pott's fracture.

systems have been found to have low specificity (25%) resulting in over-diagnosis of tuberculosis.[47] A recent, prospective, community-based study from South Africa has suggested that combining symptoms of a persistent non-remitting cough of more than 2 weeks' duration, documented failure to thrive (in the preceding 3 months) and fatigue provided reasonable diagnostic accuracy in HIV-uninfected children (sensitivity, 82.3%; specificity, 90.2%; positive predictive value, 82.3%).[48] However, this symptom-based approach offered little diagnostic value in HIV-infected children diagnosed with pulmonary tuberculosis. Further studies are, therefore, needed to develop standardised diagnostic approaches that are relevant to developing countries with limited resources with a high burden of tuberculosis, malnutrition, and HIV/AIDS.

MOLECULAR DIAGNOSTICS

Due to the slow growth of most pathogenic mycobacteria, even with automated liquid culture methods, investigations have been developed for microbial detection directly from clinical specimens. Nucleic acid amplification tests have been developed and rely on amplification of small amounts of bacterial nucleic acid using techniques such as PCR. PCR has been used successfully in identifying many infectious agents, allowing early diagnosis and initiation of therapy. Although the specificity of a well-developed PCR can be high, the sensitivity is significantly less than that of the use of culture. The sensitivity of a good quality PCR would be expected to be 90–100% and 60–70% on smear-positive and smear-negative culture-positive respiratory samples, respectively.[49–51] However, there are several problems with applying this technique to routine clinical care, including variations in methodology, high cost, and high risk of contamination resulting in false positives. A recent systematic review of nucleic acid amplification tests showed that accuracy was higher when applied to respiratory samples as opposed to other body fluids. While specificity of nucleic acid amplification tests was high, sensitivity was poor to rule out disease, especially in smear-negative (paucibacillary) disease where clinical diagnosis is equivocal and where the clinical need is greatest.[52]

Several studies in children have found the PCR test on clinical samples to have a sensitivity of 40–60% compared with clinical diagnosis(53–56). This compares favourably to standard cultures, which have a sensitivity of 30–40%. The specificity of PCR ranges from 80–96% but is dependent on the type of assay used. Furthermore, up to 39% of children with no radiographical or clinical evidence of tuberculous disease also had positive PCR results.[57] With the limitations that exist, the results of PCR alone are insufficient to diagnose tuberculosis in children. PCR detection in other body fluids or tissues, such as cerebrospinal fluid, appears to have been even less successful.

In view of the problems highlighted above, PCR methods have a limited role in the diagnosis of tuberculosis in children; however, they may be useful where the diagnosis is not easily established using standard clinical, microbiological, and epidemiological methods. PCR may also have a future role in the diagnosis of tuberculosis in immunocompromised children, or those with extrapulmonary tuberculosis.

Molecular methods have also been used for species confirmation, detection of rifampicin resistance and for molecular typing as part of epidemiological investigation. Species confirmation will allow differentiation between *M. tuberculosis* complex organisms (*M. tuberculosis, M. bovis* and *Mycobacterium africanum*) and environmental mycobacteria. Species identification may sometimes be possible directly from the specimen but these tests are most effective when applied to samples in which mycobacteria have been detected microscopically. They may also be important in confirming tuberculosis before a large contact-tracing exercises is conducted. Molecular probes looking for mutations of the *rpoB* gene may be useful particularly as a marker of multidrug resistant tuberculosis. Molecular typing of *M. tuberculosis* strains, using techniques such as restriction fragment length polymorphism, may be a useful epidemiological tool to identify potential links between patients and impact on diagnosis and transmission of tuberculosis in a community.[58]

IMMUNODIAGNOSIS

The TST suffers from poor specificity due to cross-reactivity with BCG immunisation and non-tuberculous mycobacteria. Furthermore, false negatives may occur in individuals with altered immunity such as HIV infection, immunodeficiency or immunosuppression, advanced tuberculosis and malnutrition. New diagnostic tests have been the developed based on *in vitro* T-cell based interferon-γ (IFN-γ) assays. These tests measure IFN-γ production by sensitised T cells exposed to specific tuberculosis antigens. Initial assays used PPD as the stimulating antigen; however, assays have now been developed utilising antigens more specific to *M. tuberculosis,* such as the early secretory antigenic target-6 (ESAT-6) antigen and culture filtrate protein 10 (CFP-10). These antigens are present in *M tuberculosis* complex but absent from all strains of *M. bovis* BCG (lost during attenuation process), and most non-tuberculous mycobacteria. Two commercial IFN-γ assays, the QuantiFERON-TB Gold assay (Cellestis Limited, Carnegie, Victoria, Australia), and the T SPOT-TB assay (Oxford Immunotec, Oxford, UK) are currently available. Both tests measure IFN-γ release from T cells following stimulation with ESAT-6 and CFP-10. The enzyme-linked immunospot (ELISPOT) assay, commercially available as the T-SPOT TB test, requires separation of peripheral blood mononuclear cells and incubation with stimulating antigens.[59] When interferon is produced by individual cells, it binds to specific antibody on the base of the ELISPOT wells, producing spots each representing a single cell producing interferon. The QuantiFERON-TB GOLD is a whole blood assay where heparinised whole blood is incubated with stimulating agents. Following incubation, interferon is measured in the supernatant using a sandwich ELISA The QuantiFERON-TB Gold test has been approved by the US Food and Drug Administration (FDA) for diagnosis of TB infection and disease. The T SPOT-TB test is currently approved for use in Europe and is awaiting FDA approval. In the US, the Centers for Disease Control and Prevention has published guidelines for use of the QuantiFERON-TB test which will be used in all circumstances in which the TST is currently used, including contact investigations, evaluation of immigrants and serial testing of healthcare workers. The guidelines do acknowledge that there are few data regarding the performance of this test in children, particularly less than 5 years of age. In the UK, the National Institute for Health and Clinical Excellence (NICE) guidelines recommend an increased role of IFN-γ tests in diagnosing latent infection, particularly following a positive TST in previously BCG-vaccinated individuals. The guidelines do not differentiate between the two available tests but do acknowledge that further studies are needed for these tests, particularly in population groups including children.[60]

In a large study in the UK, school children were tested by ELISPOT following a school tuberculosis outbreak. The ELISPOT assay showed improved sensitivity when compared with TST and showed better correlation with degree of exposure to an active case of tuberculosis.[61] In South Africa, Liebeschuetz *et al.*[62] assessed the usefulness of the ELISPOT assay in children with tuberculosis, including some with HIV co-infection. In children with tuberculosis, sensitivity of ELISPOT was 83%, significantly higher than the 63% sensitivity of TST. Sensitivity of TST fell significantly in children younger than 3 years (51%), with HIV co-infection (36%) or with malnutrition (44%) while sensitivity of ELISPOT was unaffected in these groups.[62]

In a study of 979 Turkish children who were household contacts of adults with sputum-smear positive tuberculosis, previous BCG vaccination was more likely to be associated with a positive TST but negative ELISPOT assay. Risk factors associated with positive TST and ELISPOT included number of TB cases in the household, being a first-degree relative of a TB case and increasing age. Interestingly, BCG-vaccinated children had a lower odds ration (0.60) for tuberculosis infection compared with non-vaccinated children suggesting some protection from BCG against TB infection.[63] However, a study from The Gambia of children who were TB contacts showed similar rates of positive TST and ELISPOT (32.5% and 32.3%, respectively) with overall agreement between the two tests of 83%. Interestingly, previous BCG did not seem to have any impact on either of the tests. The ELISPOT assay did appear to be less sensitive in this study.[64]

Connell *et al.*[65] used the QuantiFERON assay to test 106 children with a risk of latent TB infection or TB disease. There was poor correlation between the QuantiFERON test and TST for the diagnosis of latent infection. The QuantiFERON assay appeared to have lower sensitivity than TST and also yielded inconclusive results in 17% of children due to failure of positive or negative controls.[65]

Current evidence suggests that IFN-γ assays have the potential to become useful diagnostic tools in clinical and public-health settings. Studies in different populations suggest that these tests have greater specificity (> 90%) compared to TST, although sensitivity may be equivalent or less, especially for latent infection. The accuracy and reliability of these studies in diagnosing both TB infection and TB disease in infants and children's needs to be established. Furthermore, there are limited data from specific populations, particularly children and immunosuppressed individuals. Nevertheless, new guidelines have incorporated IFN-γ testing as an alternative and/or adjunct to TST. However, the cost-effectiveness and utility of these tests, especially in certain population groups, remains unclear.

Key points for clinical practice

- Tuberculosis is the most prevalent infection in the world, with two-thirds of the global population infected.

- Children with TB are generally less infectious than adults and are almost always infected by an infectious adult.

- Most infection is asymptomatic (latent TB infection); however, children are at risk of uncontrolled, progressive, primary infection.

- Adult-type post-primary or re-activation disease is more commonly seen in older children and adolescents.

- Compared with adults, microbiological tests are less likely to be positive in children; in most cases, a diagnosis is made clinically.

Key points for clinical practice *(continued)*

- Gastric aspirates should be obtained in young children and infants who are unable to cough or produce a sputum sample.

- Tuberculin skin tests suffer from both poor sensitivity (false-negative results) and specificity (false-positive results).

- Computed tomography, especially at high-resolution, may be useful in demonstrating early pulmonary disease such as cavitation often when there is no abnormality on chest radiograph.

- Molecular diagnostic tests, such as polymerase chain reaction, may be less useful in children and in extrapulmonary disease.

- Interferon-γ assays have the potential to become useful diagnostic tools although the accuracy and reliability of these assays in infants and children needs to be established.

References

1. Daly J, Brown D, Lincoln E. Endobronchial tuberculosis in children. *Dis Chest* 1952; **22**: 380.
2. Lincoln E, Gilbert L, Morales S. Chronic pulmonary tuberculosis in individuals with known previous tuberculosis. *Dis Chest* 1960; **38**: 473.
3. Jacobs R, Starke J. Tuberculosis in children. *Med Clin North Am* 1993; **77**: 1335–1351.
4. Kumar D, Watson J, Charlett A. Tuberculosis in England and Wales in 1993: results of a national survey. *Thorax* 1997; **52**: 1060–1067.
5. Farinha N, Razali K, Holzel H, Morgan G, Novelli V. Tuberculosis of the central nervous system in children: a 20-year survey. *J Infect* 2000; **41**: 61–68.
6. Janssens J, de Haller R. Spinal tuberculosis in a developed country. *Clin Orthop* 1990; **256**: 67.
7. Riviere C. *The early diagnosis of tubercle*, 3rd edn. London: Oxford Medical, 1921.
8. Peterson E, Nakasone A, Platon-DeLeon J, Jang Y. Comparison of direct and concentrated acid-fast smears to identify specimens culture positive for *Mycobacterium* spp. *J Clin Microbiol* 1999; **11**: 3564–3568.
9. Ba F, Rieder H. A comparison of fluorescence microscopy with the Ziehl-Neelsen technique in the examination of sputum for acid-fast bacilli. *Int J Tubercul Lung Dis* 1999; **3**: 1101–1105.
10. Strumpf I, Tsang A, Syre J. Reevaluation of sputum staining for the diagnosis of pulmonary tuberculosis. *Am Rev Respir Dis* 1979; **119**: 599–602.
11. Laven G. Diagnosis of tuberculosis in children using fluorescence microscopic examination of gastric washings. *Am Rev Respir Dis* 1977; **115**: 743–749.
12. Vallejo J, Ong L, Starke J. Clinical features, diagnosis and treatment of tuberculosis in infants. *Pediatrics* 1994; **94**: 1–7.
13. Starke J, Taylor-Watts K. Tuberculosis in the pediatric population of Houston, Texas. *Pediatrics* 1989; **84**: 28–35.
14. Marais B, Hesseling A, Schaaf H, Enarson D, Beyers N. The bacteriologic yield in children with intrathoracic tuberculosis. *Clin Infect Dis* 2006; **42**: e69–e71.
15. Bibi H, Mosheyev A, Shoseyov D, Feigenbaum D, Kurzbat E, Weiller Z. Should bronchoscopy be performed in the evaluation of suspected pediatric pulmonary tuberculosis? *Chest* 2002; **122**: 1604–1608.
16. Abadco D, Steiner P. Gastric lavage is better than bronchoalveolar lavage for isolation of *Mycobacterium tuberculosis* in childhood tuberculosis. *Pediatr Infect Dis J* 1993; **11**: 735–738.
17. de Blic J, Azevedo I, Burren C, Le Bourgeois M, Lallemand D, Scheinmann P. The value of flexible bronchoscopy in childhood pulmonary tuberculosis. *Chest* 1991; **100**: 688–692.

18. Zar H, Tannenbaum E, Apolles P, Roux P, Hanslo D, Hussey G. Sputum induction for the diagnosis of pulmonary tuberculosis in infants and young children in an urban setting in South Africa. *Arch Dis Child* 2000; **82**: 305–308.

19. Zar H, Hanslo D, Apolles P, Swingler G, Hussey G. Induced sputum versus gastric lavage for microbiological confirmation if pulmonary tuberculosis in infants and young children: a prospective study. *Lancet* 2005; **365**: 130–134.

20. Vargas D, Garcia L, Gilman R *et al*. Diagnosis of sputum-scarce HIV-associated pulmonary tuberculosis in Lima, Peru. *Lancet* 2005; **365**: 150–152.

21. Chow F, Espiritu N, Gilman R *et al*. *La cuerda dulce* – a tolerability and acceptability study of a novel approach to specimen collection for diagnosis of paediatric pulmonary tuberculosis. *BMC Infect Dis* 2006; **6**: 67.

22. NHS Health Technology Assessment Programme. *The clinical and cost-effectiveness of diagnostic tests for the detection of mycobacterial infection*. London: NHS, 2004.

23. Hsu K. Tuberculin reaction in children treated with isoniazid. *Am J Dis Child* 1983; **137**: 1090–1092.

24. Shingadia D, Novelli V. Diagnosis and treatment of tuberculosis in children. *Lancet Infect Dis* 2003; **3**: 624–632.

25. Lifschitz M. The value of the tuberculin skin test as a screening test for tuberculosis among BCG-vaccinated children. *Pediatrics* 1965; **36**: 624–627.

26. Wang L, Turner M, Elwood R, Schulzer M, Fitzgerald J. A meta-analysis of the effect of Bacille Calmetté Guerin vaccination on tuberculin skin test measurements. *Thorax* 2002; **57**: 804–809.

27. Menzies R, Vissandjee B. Effect of bacille Calmetté-Guerin vaccination on tuberculin reactivity. *Am Rev Respir Dis* 1992; **141**: 621–625.

28. Almeida L, Barbieri M, Da Paixao A, Cuevas L. Use of purified protein derivative to assess the risk of infection in children in close contact with adults in a population with high Calmetté-Guerin bacillus coverage. *Pediatr Infect Dis J* 2001; **20**: 1061–1065.

29. Larsson L, Bentzon M, Lind A *et al*. Sensitivity to sensitins and tuberculin in Swedish children. Part 5: A study of school children in an inland rural area. *Tubercle Lung Dis* 1993; **74**: 371–376.

30. Sepulveda R, Burr C, Ferrer X, Sorensen R. Booster effect of tuberculin testing in healthy 6-year-old school children vaccinated with bacille Calmetté-Guerin at birth in Santiago, Chile. *Pediatr Infect Dis J* 1988; **7**: 578–582.

31. Barrera L, Miceli I, Ritacco V. Detection of circulating antibodies to purified protein derivative by enzyme-linked immunosorbent assay: its potential for the rapid diagnosis of tuberculosis. *Pediatr Infect Dis J* 1989; **8**: 763–767.

32. Hussey G, Kibel M, Dempster W. The serodiagnosis of tuberculosis in children: an evaluation of an ELISA test using IgG antibodies to *M. tuberculosis*, strain H37RV. *Ann Trop Paediatr* 1991; **11**: 113–118.

33. Delacourt C, Gobin J, Gaillard J-L, de Blic J, Veran M, Scheinmann P. Value of ELISA using antigen 60 for the diagnosis of tuberculosis in children. *Chest* 1993; **104**: 393–398.

34. Dayal R, Sirohi G, Singh M *et al*. Diagnostic value of ELISA serological tests in childhood tuberculosis. *J Trop Pediatr* 2006; **52**: 433–437.

35. Agranoff D, Fernandez-Reyes D, Papadopoulos M *et al*. Identification of diagnostic markers for tuberculosis by proteonomic fingerprinting of serum. *Lancet* 2006; **368**: 1012–1021.

36. Khan E, Starke J. Diagnosis of tuberculosis in children: increased need for better methods. *Emerg Infect Dis* 1995; **1**: 115–123.

37. Delacourt C, Mani T, Bonnerot V. Computed tomography with normal chest radiograph in tuberculosis infection. *Arch Dis Child* 1993; **69**: 430–432.

38. Uzum K, Karahan O, Dogan S, Coskun A, Topcu F. Chest radiography and thoracic computed tomography findings in children who have family members with active pulmonary tuberculosis. *Eur J Radiol* 2003; **48**: 258–262.

39. Andronikou S, Joseph E, Lucas S *et al*. CT scanning for the detection of tuberculous mediastinal and hilar lymphadenopathy in children. *Pediatr Radiol* 2004; **34**: 232–236.

40. Swingler G, Du Toit G, Andronikou S, van der Merwe L, Zar H. Diagnostic accuracy of chest radiography in detecting mediastinal lymphadenopathy in suspected pulmonary tuberculosis. *Arch Dis Child* 2005; **90**: 1153–1156.

41. Cherian G, Uthaman B, Salama A, Habashy A, Khan N, Cherian J. Tuberculous pericardial

effusion: features, tamponade and computed tomography. *Angiology* 2004; **55**: 431–440.

42. De Backer A, Mortele K, Vanhoenacker F, Parizel P. Imaging of extraspinal musculoskeletal tuberculosis. *Eur J Radiol* 2006; **57**: 119–130.

43. Fourie P, Becker P, Festenstein F *et al*. Procedures for developing a simple scoring method based on unsophisticated criteria for screening children for tuberculosis. *Int J Tubercul Lung Dis* 1998; **2**: 116–123.

44. Hesseling A, Schaaf H, Gie R, Starke J, Beyers N. A critical review of diagnostic approaches used in the diagnosis of childhood tuberculosis. *Int J Tubercul Lung Dis* 2002; **6**: 1038–1045.

45. World Health Organization. *WHO tuberculosis programme framework for effective tuberculosis control*. Geneva: WHO, 1994.

46. Kiwanuka J, Graham S, Coulter J *et al*. Diagnosis of pulmonary tuberculosis in children in an HIV-endemic area, Malawi. *Ann Trop Paediatr* 2001; **21**: 5–14.

47. Van Rheenen P. The use of the paediatric tuberculosis score chart in an HIV-endemic area. *Trop Med Int Health* 2002; **7**: 435–441.

48. Marais B, Gie RP, Hesseling AC *et al*. A refined symptom-based approach to diagnose pulmonary tuberculosis in children. *Pediatrics* 2006; **118**: 1350–1359.

49. Eisenach K, Sifford M, Cane M, Bates J, Crawford J. Detection of *Mycobacterium tuberculosis* in sputum samples using a polymerase chain reaction. *Am Rev Respir Dis* 1991; **144**: 1160–1163.

50. Noordhoek A, Kolk A, Bjune G. Sensitivity and specificity of polymerase chain reaction for detection of *Mycobacterium tuberculosis*: a blind comparison study among seven laboratories. *J Clin Microbiol* 1994; **32**: 277–284.

51. Watterson S, Drobniewski F. Modern laboratory diagnosis of mycobacterial infections. *J Clin Pathol* 2000; **53**: 727–732.

52. Dinnes J, Deeks J, Kunst H *et al*. A systematic review of rapid diagnostic tests for the detection of tuberculosis infection. *Health Technol Assess* 2007; **11**: 3.

53. Starke J, Ong L, Eisenach K. detection of *M. tuberculosis* in gastric aspirate samples from children using polymerase chain reaction. *Am Rev Respir Dis* 1993; **147**: A801.

54. Smith K, Starke J, Eisenach K, Ong L, Denby M. Detection of *Mycobacterium tuberculosis* in clinical specimens from children using a polymerase chain reaction. *Pediatrics* 1996; **97**: 155–160.

55. Gomez-Pastrana D, Torronteras R, Caro P *et al*. Diagnosis of tuberculosis in children using a polymerase chain reaction. *Pediatr Pulmonol* 1999; **28**: 344–351.

56. Fauville-Dufaux M, Waelbroeck A, Mol P *et al*. Contribution of the polymerase chain reaction to the diagnosis of tuberculous infection in children. *Eur J Pediatr* 1996; **155**: 106–111.

57. Delacourt C, Poveda J-D, Churean C. Use of polymerase chain reaction for improved diagnosis of tuberculosis in children. *J Pediatr* 1995; **126**: 703–709.

58. Ruddy M, Davies A, Yates M, Yates S. Outbreak of isoniazid resistant tuberculosis in north London. *Thorax* 2004; **59**: 279–285.

59. Lalvani A, Nagvenkar P, Udwadia Z *et al*. Enumeration of T cells specific for RD1-encoded antigens suggest a high prevalence of latent *Mycobacterium tuberculosis* infection in healthy urban Indians. *J Infect Dis* 2001; **183**: 469–477.

60. National Institute for Health and Clinical Excellence. *Tuberculosis: clinical diagnosis and management of tuberculosis, and measures for its prevention and control*. London: NICE, 2006.

61. Ewer K, Deeks J, Alvarez L. Comparison of T-cell-based assay with tuberculin skin test for diagnosis of *Mycobacterium tuberculosis* infection in a school tuberculosis outbreak. *Lancet* 2003; **361**: 1168–1173.

62. Liebeschuetz S, Bamber S, Ewer K, Deeks J, Pathan A, Lalvani A. Diagnosis of tuberculosis in South African children with a T-cell-based assay: a prospective cohort study. *Lancet* 2004; **364**: 2196–2203.

63. Soysal A, Millington K, Bakir M *et al*. Effect of BCG vaccination on risk of *Mycobacterium tuberculosis* infection in children with household tuberculosis contact: a prospective community-based study. *Lancet* 2005; **366**: 1443–1451.

64. Hill C, Brookes R, Adetifa I *et al*. Comparison of enzyme-linked immunospot assay and tuberculin skin test in healthy children exposed to *Mycobacterium tuberculosis*. *Pediatrics* 2006; **117**: 1542–1548.

65. Connel T, Curtis N, Ranganathan S, Buttery J. Performance of a whole blood interferon gamma assay for detecting latent infection with *Mycobacterium tuberculosis* in children. *Thorax* 2006; **61**: 616–620.

Index

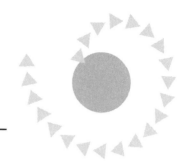